Genodermatoses

A Clinical Guide to Genetic Skin Disorders

Genodermatoses

A Clinical Guide to Genetic Skin Disorders

Second Edition

Joel L. Spitz, M.D.

Department of Dermatology

*Columbia University College of Physicians
and Surgeons
New York Presbyterian Hospital
New York, New York*

Illustrations by Vaune J. Hatch
Deep River, Connecticut

LIPPINCOTT WILLIAMS & WILKINS
A **Wolters Kluwer** Company

Philadelphia • Baltimore • New York • London
Buenos Aires • Hong Kong • Sydney • Tokyo

Acquisitions Editor: Danette Somers
Developmental Editor: Joanne Bersin
Marketing Manager: Kathy Neely
Project Manager: Bridgett Dougherty
Senior Manufacturing Manager: Ben Rivera
Production Services: Maryland Composition Inc
Printer: QuebecorWorld Kingsport

The publisher is not responsible (as a matter of product liability, negligence or otherwise) for an injury resulting from any material contained herein. This publication contains information relating to general principles of medical care which should not be constructed as specific instruction for individual patients. Manufacturer's product information should be reviewed for current information, including contraindications, dosages, and precautions.

Printed in the United States of America

Library of Congress Cataloging-in-Publication Data

Genodermatoses : a full-color guide to genetic skin disorders / [edited by] Joel L. Spitz ; illustrations by Vaune J. Hatch.—2nd ed.
    p. ; cm.
  Includes bibliographical references and index.
  ISBN 0-7817-4088-6
1. Skin—Diseases—Genetic aspects. I. Spitz, Joel L.
  [DNLM: 1. Skin Diseases—genetics—Handbooks. WR 39 G335 2005]
RL793.G46 2005
616.5′042—dc22

2004022073

The publishers have made every effort to trace copyright holders for borrowed material. If they have inadvertently overlooked any, they will be pleased to make the necessary arrangements at the first opportunity.

To purchase additional copies of this book, call our customer service department at **(800) 638-3030** or fax orders to **(301) 824-7390**. For other book services, including chapter reprints and large quantity sales, ask for the Special Sales department.

For all other calls originating outside of the United States, please call **(301) 714-2324**.

Visit Lippincott Williams & Wilkins on the Internet: **http://www.lww.com**. Lippincott Williams & Wilkins customer service representatives are available from 8:30 am to 6:30 pm, EST, Monday through Friday, for telephone access.

To Jackie, Sophia, Jonah, Ava,
Mom and Dad,
My loyal support team
—Joel L. Spitz, M.D.

To my parents and husband with love
—Vaune J. Hatch

Foreword

Academic dermatologists have recognized for many decades that a great number of dermatologic conditions have a major genetic component. While a substantial proportion of these is caused by single gene defects, a number of others represent dermatologic components of either single gene or multifactional diseases primarily affecting other organ systems. Recognition of these "genodermatoses" is not only important for accurate diagnosis but for appropriate counseling of families to take advantage of a rapidly growing number of newly available therapeutic modalities.

This book, in a highly pictorial fashion, provides current facts to allow correct diagnoses by the physician. The shorthand descriptions of the genetics and key features of the individual conditions, as well as availability of prenatal diagnosis and management, is well thought out and relates directly to the excellent illustrations. An unusual component is found in the "clinical pearls" which are quotes from experts in the field, emphasizing important points in the diagnosis and management of the diseases.

The author has clearly devoted a great deal of thought and legwork to compiling this unique collection and should be commended for making available a book that will be useful not only for dermatologists but for pediatricians, internists, and other primary care practitioners. It will allow all of these to have at hand a quick reference that will lead them in most cases to the correct diagnosis and plan of action. Of equal importance is the collection in one place of the current state of the science so as to provide a basis for the understanding of the pathophysiology of skin diseases.

Kurt Hirschhorn, M.D.
Professor of Pediatrics, Genetics, and Medicine
Chairman Emeritus, Department of Pediatrics
Mount Sinai School of Medicine
New York, New York

Preface

The idea for this book came to me one evening while I was studying for my in-service board exams as a second-year dermatology resident. I was doing my best to cram the facts into my head just as I had done through the past decade of pre-med college, medical school, and the beginning of residency. When I came upon the genodermatoses, I was inundated with more information about the patients' skin, their peculiar facies, their gait, as well as their livers, hearts, lungs, and spleens. In order to remember, I needed to synthesize the facts, to see these patients as a whole. I went to the textbooks to see full-body pictures and transform these words into a real live person. There were none. Sure, there was a snapshot of a toe, an ear, or a face; however, the complete picture was usually missing. A look at their livers or hearts was even harder to come by. For me, visual cues have always been the key to remembering. Thus, the transparent full-body drawing became the cornerstone of a new textbook on the genodermatoses. One must keep in mind that these are idealized drawings attempting to capture the most common findings in each syndrome. By no means do the illustrations attempt to depict a specific patient. Likewise, in our attempt to draw the patient's entire body, the figure must be placed at a distance to fit all the findings. In doing so, we lost a bit of detail on some cutaneous manifestations. In most cases I believe the color photographs help correct this limitation when it occurs.

The standard texts covered this subject with dense prose, sometimes impossible to get through, let alone memorize. There was an obvious need to "bulletize" information. This I've tried to accomplish.

As I thought about this subject, I began to think like a clinician. How would I work up a patient in my office? What were his/her particular needs or worries? How could I help them maintain a decent quality of life? My first instinct would be to call the expert in handling such a patient. This led to the "Clinical Pearls" section, a kind of medical textbook conference call in which the reader can eavesdrop on a telephone conversation between the expert and a clinician in practice.

Serendipitously, my desire to present the genodermatoses in a new light came about as the meteoric rise in genetic discoveries began to be chronicled on the front pages of *The New York Times*. Ten years later, the speed and breadth of continued genetic discovery has been nothing short of astonishing. A majority of the syndromes covered in the text now have a clearly defined mutation at its pathogenic core. In addition, since the first edition, progress continues towards definitive genetic diagnosis, treatment, and cure. The entire human genome has been described, preimplantation diagnosis in certain forms of EB has been accomplished, and retroviral vectors have genetically transferred DNA and temporarily "cured" diseases such as Severe Combined Immunodeficiency.

Dr. Ervin Epstein has been called upon once again to update his introduction from the first edition. While he and others zoom in on our DNA and discover the genetic mechanisms that produce these syndromes, we need to remain clinically sharp, to pick up on subtleties that may elude the unsuspecting and thus ill-prepared physician. I have never met a more astute clinician than Kurt Hirschhorn, who is Chairman Emeritus of Pediatrics at Mount Sinai Hospital in New York City and a world leader in the field of medical genetics. It is a great honor for me to have him write the foreword to this book.

Acknowledgments

Wow! It's been a real fun ride watching the incredible success of the first edition. I am really proud and honored that it was so well-received by the dermatology and primary care communities. A special thank you to all the dermatology residents and programs whom have made the book an integral part of their training curriculum.

While the first edition was written in relative "personal life" calm as a dermatology resident with one child, this edition was undertaken while being a busy practitioner, father of three with two home moves, and a teacher with responsibilities at three hospitals. Needless to say, this edition required a team effort and a few people really stand out. First and foremost, I could never have completed the project without the help of Lisa Weisfelner, my medical assistant-turned-medical student and future surgeon who worked tirelessly in researching articles, finding new photos, and gathering Clinical Pearls over a 2 year period. In addition, Barbara Crisci lent her critical skills in organizing the Clinical Pearls, photos, and Suggested Readings section of the book. My entire staff at North Shore Dermatology in Williston Park, NY, chipped in and helped whenever I needed them at various points in the making of this edition.

I thank all of my editors, including Hal Pollard, James Merritt, Danette Somers, Joanne Bersin, and Heidi Pongratz for guiding and pushing me to the finish line. I am indebted to my close friends, Herb and Dena Mauthner who graciously provided a luxurious office, good conversation, and warm cups of coffee in the midst of one of the coldest Januarys on record in New York City. To Vaune, once again I feel lucky to have you contribute your creative talents to the book.

Most of all, the making of this edition was toughest on my family. To Jackie and my children, Sophia, Jonah, and Ava, I can only say thanks for hanging in there and I'm all yours again!

Contributors

Jean L. Bolognia, M.D.
Professor of Dermatology
Yale University School of Medicine
Attending Physician, Dermatology
Yale-New Haven Hospital
New Haven, Connecticut

Vincent A. DeLeo, M.D.
Chair of Dermatology
St. Lukes Roosevelt and Beth Israel Medical Centers
New York, New York

Lawrence F. Eichenfield, M.D.
Clinical Professor of Pediatrics and Medicine
(Dermatology)
University of California San Diego School of Medicine
Chief, Pediatric and Adolescent Dermatology
Children's Hospital and Health Center
San Diego, California

DGR Evans, M.D., MRCP
Department of Medical Genetics
St. Mary's Hospital
Manchester, United Kingdom

Ilona J. Frieden, M.D.
Clinical Professor of Dermatology and Pediatrics
University of California San Francisco School of Medicine
San Francisco, California

Kurt Hirschhorn, M.D.
Professor of Pediatrics, Genetics, and Medicine
Chairman Emeritus, Department of Pediatrics
Mount Sinai School of Medicine
New York, New York

Bernice R. Krafchik, M.D.
Associate Professor
Department of Pediatrics and Medicine (Dermatology)
University of Toronto
Head, Division of Dermatology
The Hospital for Sick Children
Toronto, Ontario, Canada

Moise L. Levy, M.D.
Professor of Dermatology and Pediatrics
Baylor College of Medicine
Chief, Dermatology Service
Texas Children's Hospital
Houston, Texas

Leonard M. Milstone, M.D.
Professor of Dermatology
Yale University School of Medicine
Attending Physician, Dermatology
Yale-New Haven Hospital
New Haven, Connecticut

Seth J. Orlow, M.D.
Samuel Weinberg Professor of Pediatric Dermatology
Professor of Cell Biology and Pediatrics
Departments of Dermatology, Cell Biology, and Pediatrics
New York University Medical Center
New York, New York

Amy S. Paller, M.D.
Professor and Chair
Department of Dermatology
Professor of Pediatrics
Northwestern University Feinberg School of Medicine
Department of Dermatology
Children's Memorial Hospital
Chicago, Illinois

Gabrielle Richard, M.D.
Associate Professor
Departments of Dermatology & Cutaneous Biology
and Medicine
Division of Genetics and Preventative Medicine
Thomas Jefferson University, Jefferson Medical College
Philadelphia, Pennsylvania

William Rizzo, M.D.
Professor of Pediatrics
University of Nebraska Medical Center
Omaha, Nebraska

Richard K. Scher, M.D., FACP
Professor of Clinical Dermatology
Columbia University
Attending Physician, Dermatology
New York Presbyterian Hospital
New York, New York

Jouni Uitto, M.D., Ph.D.
Professor and Chairman
Department of Dermatology and Cutaneous Biology
Professor of Biochemistry and Molecular Pharmacology
Thomas Jefferson University, Jefferson Medical College
Director, Jefferson Institute of Molecular Medicine
Program Director, Jefferson Dermatology Residency
Training Program
Philadelphia, Pennsylvania

David A. Whiting, M.D., FRCP
Clinical Professor of Dermatology and Pediatrics
University of Texas Southwestern Medical Center
Medical Director, Baylor Hair Research
and Treatment Center
Dallas, Texas

Judith P. Willner, M.D.
Associate Professor of Human Genetics and Pediatrics
Mount Sinai School of Medicine
Director, Clinical Genetics
Department of Human Genetics
Mount Sinai Medical Center
New York, New York

Introduction

A century ago a combination of strategic insights and technical innovations combined to permit an explosion of knowledge about one important class of ancient diseases of mankind. The insight was that bacteria came from other bacteria—spontaneous generation was understood not to occur. The innovations were heat sterilizable-media and the cotton plug, which allowed media at the bottom of the test tube to equilibrate with air but which blocked the passage of bacteria. This class of diseases of course was those caused by bacterial infection, and in a few years the cause of multiple ancient scourges, e.g., tuberculosis, anthrax, plague, streptococcal and staphylococcal pyodermas, was found to be bacterial and not the wrath of the gods.

We seem today to be in the midst of a similar explosion of understanding, this time not of diseases due to bacterial infection but rather of diseases due to mutations in DNA. The strategic insights underlying this explosion have been developed over the 20th century—one gene - one protein, DNA as the carrier of heritable information, the physical configuration of DNA into a double helix. The technical innovations have come more recently—Southern analyses, the polymerase chain reaction, and more recently the reading of the entire set of blueprints for making humans—the sequencing of our entire DNA. Just as a century ago investigators tried to be first to culture new bacteria from each infectious disease, today's investigators have vied to be the first to identify the gene whose mutations cause each hereditary disease and to use that information not only to understand deranged pathophysiology but to better understand normal function.

This explosion has affected our understanding of skin diseases profoundly, and within the past $1\frac{1}{2}$ decade mutations have been described for the first time in genes underlying, e.g., multiple types of ichthyoses, epidermolysis bullosa, and xeroderma pigmentosa, and prenatal diagnoses already have been accomplished. In fact, just since the publication of the first edition of this book, the genes, whose mutations underlie an amazingly high percentage of those diseases described in this volume, have been identified. All of these diseases are rare to be sure but many are diseases that make life miserable and some cases even end the life of the afflicted. The field of molecular genetics applied to the investigation of skin diseases seems sure to grow as attention is directed to finding the gene defects not only in the remaining Mendelian hereditary skin diseases but also in the "everyday" diseases such as psoriasis, atopic dermatitis, and even severe acne. Today the way forward to identify their genetic underpinnings seems of great difficulty and highly uncertain of success but surely that was the case for the Mendelian diseases but two decades ago.

The publication of the first edition of Genodermatoses came at an especially propitious time, for general knowledge of the clinical characteristics of heritable skin diseases paradoxically has been harder to come by than was knowledge of the new molecular genetics insights. On the face of it, that might seem unlikely in an era of immediate access via the Internet to compendia such as McKusick's Mendelian Inheritance in Man. Nonetheless, simple thumbing the pages of this book reminds the reader of the pleasures and benefits to be derived from selection of data by experts and presentation of these data in a logical, organized fashion in the ultimately user friendly format—a book. The second edition expands on the strengths of the first and brings this compendium of this fast-moving field up to date.

Its perusal is a reminder not only of the immense diversity of the "experiments of Nature" that can be so instructive about normal functioning but that perusal also is a reminder that Nature unfortunately has "visited" these experiments on patients who deserve the benefit of all our collective wisdom and experience, not just to develop cures for their afflictions in the ultimate future but also to care for them and so to lighten their burden as much as possible in the here and now.

The finding of a "generic solution" to the problem of bacterial disease—penicillin—took a half century. Hope remains high that such a generic solution to the problem of disease caused by DNA abnormalities—gene therapy—will take much less time. Since the publication of the first edition of this book, significant technical advances have been made using both in vitro cell culture and powerful mouse models whose construction was based on the knowledge of the genetic flaws, and these advances do give some optimism that disorders of the skin actually might be treatable in the not too distant future by changing the DNA of the cells. Until the success of this approach, and no doubt even after, careful clinical classification and application of the best ameliorative therapies are the inescapable responsibility of all who "care" for the patient. Hence the utility and importance of this book can only increase.

Ervin Epstein, Jr.
November 2004

Contents

Chapter Five

Disorders with Malignant Potential

Clinical Pearls by Lawrence Eichenfield, M.D. (LE)

Chapter Six

Epidermolysis Bullosa

Clinical Pearls by Juoni Uitto, M.D., Ph.D. (JU)

Chapter Seven

Disorders of Porphyrin Metabolism

Clinical Pearls by Vincent DeLeo, M.D. (VD)

Chapter Eight

Disorders with Photosensitivity

***Clinical Pearls by Moise Levy, M.D. (ML),
Kurt Hirschhorn, M.D. (KH), Judith Willner, M.D.
(JW), and Leonard Milstone, M.D. (LM)***

Chapter Nine

Disorders with Immunodeficiency

Clinical Pearls by Moise Levy, M.D. (ML)

Chapter Ten

Disorders of Hair and Nails

***Clinical Pearls by David Whiting, M.D. (DW),
Bernice Krafchik, M.D. (BK), Richard Scher, M.D.
(RS), Kurt Hirschhorn, M.D. (KH), and
Judith Willner, M.D. (JW)***

Chapter Eleven

Disorders of Metabolism

***Clinical Pearls by Kurt Hirschhorn, M.D. (KH) and
Judith Willner, M.D. (JW)***

Chapter 1

Disorders of Cornification

Clinical Pearls

Leonard Milstone, M.D. (LM), William Rizzo, M.D. (WR), and Gabrielle Richard M.D. (GR)

Ichthyosis Vulgaris

Inheritance	Autosomal dominant; gene locus unknown
Prenatal Diagnosis	None
Incidence	1:250–1:2,000; M=F
Age at Presentation	Three months to 1 year of life
Pathogenesis	Retention hyperkeratosis with normal epidermal proliferation; defect in profilaggrin synthesis with subsequent decreased levels of profilaggrin in keratinocytes; most likely polygenic disease
Key Features	**Skin** Fine, whitish, adherent scale sparing flexures with increased involvement on extensor extremities; face usually spared but may involve cheeks and forehead Atopic dermatitis (>50%) Keratosis pilaris Palmoplantar markings accentuated; rarely frank keratoderma
Differential Diagnosis	Atopic dermatitis Xerosis Acquired ichthyosis X-linked ichthyosis (p. 4) Lamellar ichthyosis (p. 10)
Laboratory Data	Skin biopsy from anterior shin—absent granular layer Electron microscopy—small, poorly formed keratohyalin granules
Management	Referral to dermatologist—topical emollients
Prognosis	Improves in summer and with age; also improves in warm, moist environment

Clinical Pearls

This is a surprisingly difficult diagnosis to make with certainty—no genetic markers, no characteristic scale, and absent granular layer in only a small minority...Since the stratum corneum does not retain water well becaue of its inadequate endogenous humectant production, emollients containing urea or alpha-hydroxy acids work best.
LM

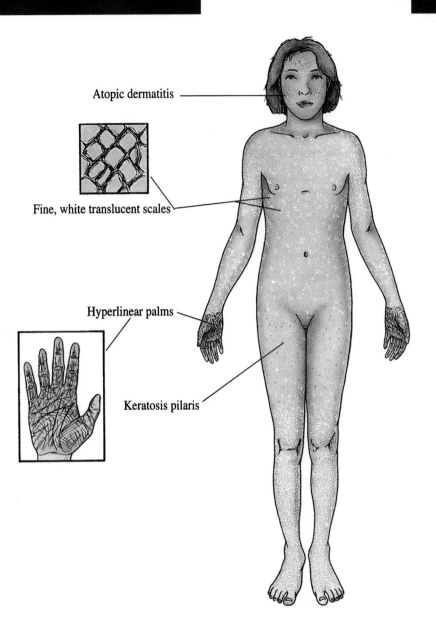

Atopic dermatitis

Fine, white translucent scales

Hyperlinear palms

Keratosis pilaris

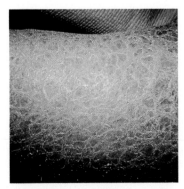

1.1. Translucent, adherent scale on extremity (1).

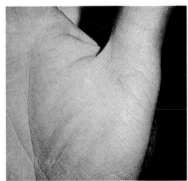

1.2. Accenuated palmar markings (1).

X-linked Ichthyosis

Synonym	Steroid sulfatase deficiency
Inheritance	X-linked recessive: steroid sulfatase gene (STS) on Xp22.32 Gene deletions most common mutation (90%); contiguous gene deletion syndrome (10%)
Prenatal Diagnosis	Amniocentesis/chorionic villus sampling (CVS)—steroid sulfatase assay, increased dehydroepiandrosterone sulfate (DHEAS) levels DNA analysis Maternal estriol (serum/urine) and dehydroepiandrosterone levels
Incidence	1:2,000–1:6,000 males
Age at Presentation	Two to 6 weeks old
Pathogenesis	Steroid sulfatase gene deletion leads to decreased steroid sulfatase activity in stratum corneum with increased cholesterol sulfate and decreased cholesterol levels; may play a role in retention hyperkeratosis Contiguous gene deletion syndrome may result in Kallmann syndrome and X-linked recessive chondrodysplasia punctata Failure of labor to begin or progress in mother carrying affected fetus because of decreased placental sulfatase and estrogen and increased fetal DHEAS

Key Features	**Skin**
	    Brown, firmly adherent scale increased on extensors, posterior neck, trunk with relative sparing of flexures; sparing of palms, soles, face
	Eyes
	    Comma-shaped corneal opacities—asymptomatic
	    (50% of adult males, some female carriers)
	Obstetrics
	    Placental sulfatase deficiency—failure of labor to begin or progress in mother carrying affected fetus
	Genitourinary
	    Cryptorchidism (20%) with possible increase in testicular cancer

Differential Diagnosis	Ichthyosis vulgaris (p. 2) Epidermolytic hyperkeratosis (p. 6) Lamellar ichthyosis (p. 10) Contiguous gene syndromes
Laboratory Data	Steroid sulfatase activity assay in scales, cultured fibroblasts, leukocytes Lipoprotein electrophoresis—increased mobility of low-density lipoproteins Serum cholesterol sulfate levels—increased
Management	Thorough physical examination by pediatrician Referral to dermatologist—topical emollients Referral to pediatric urologist if symptomatic Advise obstetrician of potential complications
Prognosis	Cutaneous involvement waxes and wanes throughout life with seasonal variation

Clinical Pearls

A significant number of these cases are caused by chromosomal deletions...Indeed, most of my recent new cases have been referred to me after prenatal fluorescent *in situ* hybridization (FISH) screening...Such cases need follow-up for contiguous gene syndromes...All should be checked for undescended testes and risk for testicular carcinoma is increased even in absence of undescended testes...Scaling can be quite variable, even for an individual...Boys with extensive cradle cap at birth can have little/no scale at 1 year of age and then develop characteristic extensor scaling at 4 to 5 years of age...Small, tightly adherent scales on flanks often give a wrinkled or pseudoatrophic appearance...Water is critical for these folks...Some with marked scale in the dry winter have little or none during humid summers...I like alphahydroxy acids for RXLI.   *LM*

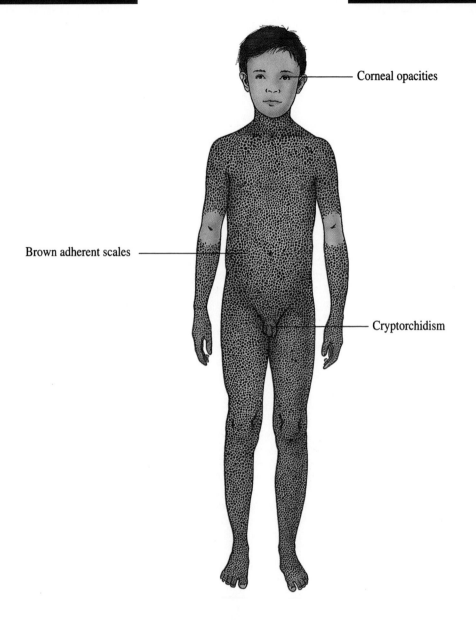

Corneal opacities

Brown adherent scales

Cryptorchidism

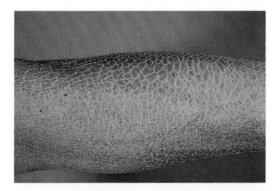

1.3. Adherent, "dirty" brown scale (2).

1.4. Schematic diagram depicting comma-shaped corneal opacities (3).

Epidermolytic Hyperkeratosis

Synonym
Bullous congenital ichthyosiform erythroderma
Bullous ichthyosis

Inheritance
Autosomal dominant; 50% spontaneous mutations; keratin K1, K10 genes on 12q, 17q respectively

Prenatal Diagnosis
Fetal skin biopsy at 20 to 22 weeks—clumped keratin filaments on electron microscopy
DNA analysis: K1 and K10 mutations if defect in family known, linkage analysis if kindred is large

Incidence
Rare—approximately 3,000 Americans afflicted; M=F

Age at Presentation
Birth

Pathogenesis
Heterogeneous gene defects in K1, K10 leads to defective keratin filaments in the upper epidermis with subsequent tonofilament clumping and bullae formation; arg res 156 of K10 is most common site for mutation with greatest severity at terminal rod regions
Extensive epidermal nevi (ichthyosis hystrix) reflect a somatic mosaicism for K1/K10 mutations; if gonadal mosaicism, then may have offspring with fullblown epidermolytic hyperkeratosis

Key Features
Skin
Newborn
Widespread bullae, erythroderma, denuded skin; secondary sepsis, electrolyte imbalance; ± focal areas of hyperkeratosis
Later Infancy to Adulthood
Localized to generalized hyperkeratosis with rare, focal bullae secondary to infection (*Staphyloccus aureus,* gram-negative bacteria); dark, warty scales with spiny ridges, increased in flexures; secondary bacterial infection with foul odor in macerated, intertriginous areas; scales shed with full-thickness stratum corneum leaving tender, denuded base; prominent palmoplantar keratoderma (in some patients); secondary nail dystrophy

Differential Diagnosis
Newborn
Epidermolysis bullosa (p. 200)
Staphylococcal scalded skin syndrome
Toxic epidermal necrolysis
Other causes of blistering
Later Infancy to Adulthood
Other ichthyoses

Laboratory Data
Skin biopsy for hematoxylin and eosin (H&E), frozen section (in newborn), and electron microscopy
Bacterial culture

Management

Newborn

Transfer to neonatal intensive care unit—monitor fluid, electrolytes, sepsis work-up; intravenous (IV) broad-spectrum antibiotics until cultures negative; gentle handling, protective isolation

Later Infancy to Adulthood

Avoid topical keratolytics, salicylic acid, corticosteroids; systemic retinoids—short course in adulthood for flares; emolliation; antistaphylococcal, gram-negative antibiotic coverage; antibacterial soaps—Betadine, Chlorhexidine, Clorox in bath

Prognosis

Widespread blistering clears after newborn period; hyperkeratotic scale usually lifelong; generalized involvement may improve to localized disease after puberty

Clinical Pearls

Although scale is the major manifestation of this disease, this is a disease of keratinocyte fragility...Friction is the cause of most blisters, and repeated shear at body folds causes accentuated scale in those locations. Blisters in the absence of friction suggest *Staphylococcus aureus*...For most of my patients Aquaphor is their favorite topical...Strong topical keratolytics remove too much stratum corneum and leave the skin surface denuded and raw...Itching is unexplained, but can be severe...Oral retinoids are very effective for many, not all...Pregnancy and skeletal toxicity are ongoing concerns of oral retinoid use...Odor is a problem, somewhat reduced by hypochlorite (0.05% or 1:100 Clorox) and salt (2–3%) baths. Watch out for contractures, especially of palms, secondary to pain and/or blisters...Early referral to F.I.R.S.T., the patient support. *LM*

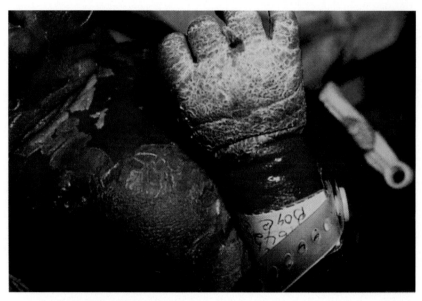

1.5. Infant with erythroderma, erosions, and hyperkeratosis (4).

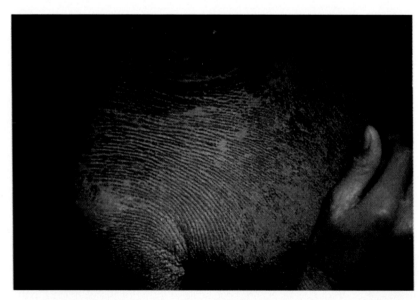

1.6. Adult with generalized hyperkeratosis. Note corrugated pattern to scale (1).

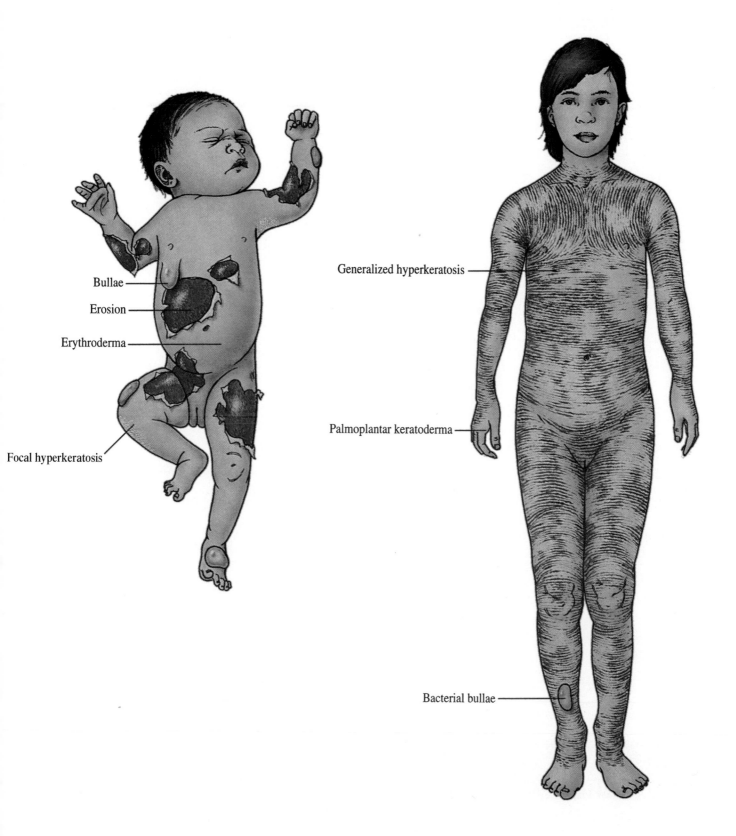

Bullae

Erosion

Erythroderma

Focal hyperkeratosis

Generalized hyperkeratosis

Palmoplantar keratoderma

Bacterial bullae

Lamellar Ichthyosis

Inheritance	Autosomal recessive; transglutaminase 1 (*TGM1*) gene on 14q11
Prenatal Diagnosis	Chorionic villus sampling (CVS)/amniocentesis: *TGM1* gene mutation or linkage analysis in families where molecular defect is known; fetal skin biopsy at 22 weeks
Incidence	Less than 1:300,000; M=F
Age at Presentation	Birth
Pathogenesis	Heterogeneous mutations in the *TGM1* gene interfere with the normal cross-linking of structural proteins in the protein and lipid envelope of the upper epidermis leading to defective cornification and desquamation

Key Features

Skin
> Newborn
>> Collodion baby with translucent membrane encasing body, ectropion, eclabium, generalized erythroderma; at risk for secondary sepsis, hypernatremic dehydration; membrane shed in first few days to weeks of life
> Child/Adult
>> Generalized large, dark, platelike scale increased in flexures; erythroderma; ectropion; palmoplantar keratoderma; decreased sweating with heat intolerance

Hair
> Scarring alopecia

Nails
> Secondary dystrophy with nail fold inflammation

Differential Diagnosis
Epidermolytic hyperkeratosis (p. 6)
X-linked ichthyosis (p. 4)
Congenital ichthyosiform erythroderma (p. 12)
Netherton syndrome (p. 24)
Trichothiodystrophy (p. 246)

Laboratory Data
Skin biopsy-*in situ* detection of transglutaminase-1 expression and activity
Light microscopic hair examination (if alopecia)
Sepsis workup (newborn)

Management

Newborn
> Transfer to neonatal intensive care unit—monitor fluids, electrolytes, and for sepsis; emolliation, high-humidity chamber

Child/Adult
> Retinoids
> Emolliation
> Counsel regarding: avoiding strenuous activity, overheating

Prognosis
Severe involvement throughout life; normal life span

Clinical Pearls

Great variability in size and thickness of scales...Ectropion results from thick scale on the eyelids...I've had success using topical retinoids to reduce ectropion...but oral retinoids work better...Most patients try oral retinoids at one time or another, but retinoids unmask the underlying erythema and some patients would rather be scaly than red...Pregnancy and skeletal toxicity are ongoing concerns with retinoids...Educate patients about heat stroke and normal activity can be pursued...One of my patients ran crosscountry in college, another played lacrosse...Early F.I.R.S.T referral can be helpful.   *LM*

Collodion baby

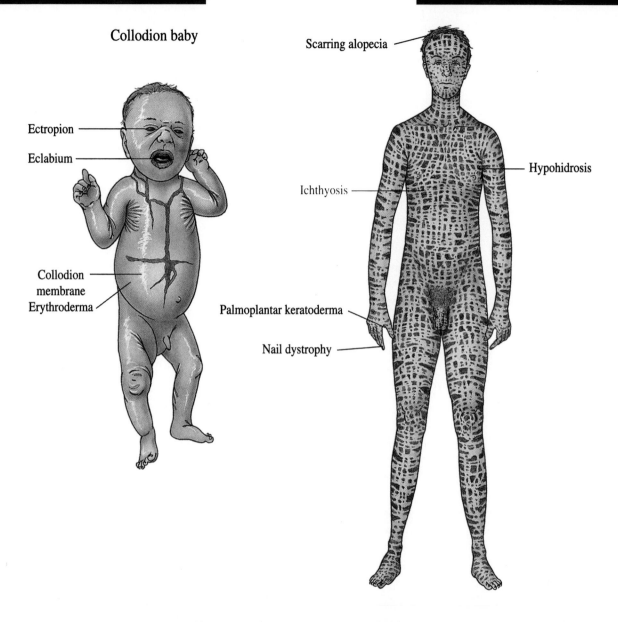

Ectropion

Eclabium

Collodion membrane
Erythroderma

Scarring alopecia

Hypohidrosis

Ichthyosis

Palmoplantar keratoderma

Nail dystrophy

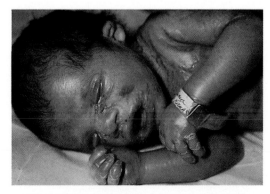

1.7. Collodion baby with ectropion, eclabium (5).

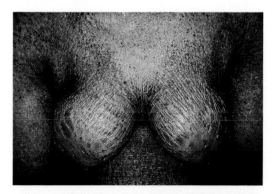

1.8. Generalized scale on trunk and extremities (1).

Congenital Ichthyosiform Erythroderma (CIE)

Synonym	Nonbullous CIE
Inheritance	Autosomal recessive; heterogeneous genetic loci
Prenatal Diagnosis	Fetal skin biopsy at 22 weeks
Incidence	1:180,000; more common than lamellar ichthyosis; M=F
Age at Presentation	Birth
Pathogenesis	*TGM1* gene mutations have been identified in some patients (much more closely identified with lamellar ichthyosis); other gene loci have been linked as well; accelerated epidermal cell turnover rate

Key Features

Skin
  Newborn
    Collodion baby (see lamellar ichthyosis, p. 10)
  After infancy
    Generalized erythroderma with fine, white scale, flexures involved; extensor legs with large, platelike, dark scale; ± palmoplantar keratoderma; hypohidrosis with heat intolerance
Hair
  Cicatricial alopecia
Eyes
  Ectropion

Differential Diagnosis
Neutral lipid storage disease (NLSD)
Lamellar ichthyosis (p. 10)
Ichthyosis vulgaris (p. 2)
Netherton syndrome (p. 24)

Laboratory Data
Complete blood count (CBC)—differentiate from NLSD with lipid vacuoles in leukocytes and monocytes in NLSD
Skin biopsy—differentiate from NLSD with lipid vacuoles in basal epidermis in NLSD

Management

Newborn
  Transfer to neonatal intensive care unit—monitor fluids, electrolytes, and for sepsis; emolliation, high-humidity chamber
Child/Adult
  Topical keratolytics, topical retinoids, emolliation
  Oral retinoids (short course)

Prognosis
Usually unremitting course but may improve at puberty

Clinical Pearls

These patients lose considerable water and energy through their skin...Children should be encouraged to eat and drink more than their unaffected sibs...I have a low threshold for recommending protein and calorie supplementation...Itching is usually mild; increased itching should prompt a search for chronic fungal infection. Most of my patients prefer emollients (Vaseline/aquaphor) to keratolytics/humectants. Early referral to the patient support group F.I.R.S.T. can be very helpful.   *LM*

Collodion Baby

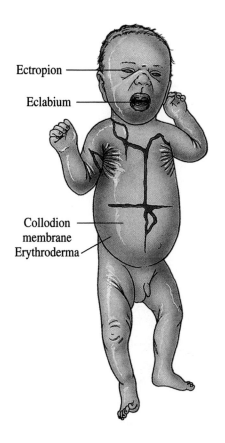

Ectropion

Eclabium

Collodion membrane
Erythroderma

Alopecia

Ectropion

Generalized white scale

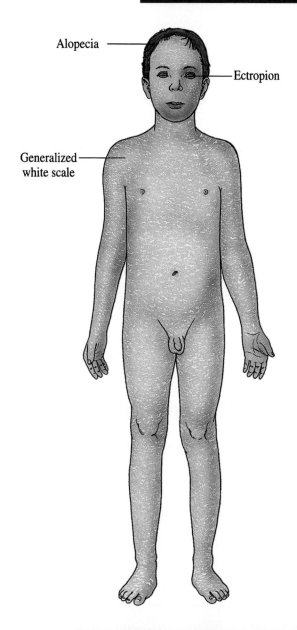

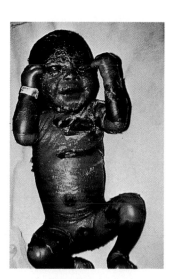

1.9. Collodion baby at 2 weeks of age (1).

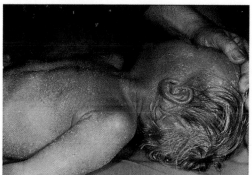

1.10. Erythroderma with fine, white scale on young boy (6).

13

Harlequin Fetus

Inheritance	Autosomal recessive most likely; genetic heterogeneity with recent description of *de novo* deletion of 18q21
Prenatal Diagnosis	Amniocentesis—abnormal morphology of amniotic fluid cells Ultrasound Fetal skin biopsy—electron microscopy with absent lamellar bodies
Incidence	Less than 1:300,000; M=F
Age at Presentation	Birth
Pathogenesis	Heterogeneous molecular and genetic causes have been described; all patients have the following in common: defective keratinization with abnormal keratinocyte biochemical and morphologic differentiation and excessive hyperkeratosis; an error in lipid metabolism with lipid accumulation in stratum corneum; absent normal lamellar granules, defective profilaggrin conversion to filaggrin and a decrease in calpain (a calcium-activated protease important in calcium-mediated signaling and normal differentiation) may play a role in phenotype; 3 subtypes have been described based on different keratin protein expression, profilaggrin presence and size and number of lamellar granules
Key Features	**Skin** Massive hyperkeratotic plates with deep fissures encasing newborn Severe ectropion, eclabium, absent/deformed ears, nose, fingers, toes; poor temperature regulation Generalized scaling with erythroderma in survivors of the neonatal period
Differential Diagnosis	Severe congenital ichthyosiform erythroderma (p. 12) Severe lamellar ichthyosis (p. 10)
Laboratory Data	Sepsis workup
Management	Transfer to neonatal intensive care unit—monitor fluids, electrolytes, and for sepsis; systemic antibiotics, humidified incubators Retinoids may help shed scale and contribute to survival; If survival beyond neonate, referral to surgeon—correction of ectropion, hand/feet deformities; referral to dermatologist—-retinoids, emolliation Referral to ophthalmologist—manage ectropion, secondary keratitis
Prognosis	If not stillborn, most die within the first few days of life as a result of sepsis or respiration and feeding complications from severe constriction of the chest and abdomen; survival has been reported with retinoid therapy

Clinical Pearls

Is not the uniformly fatal disease once thought...Support in a good pediatric intensive care unit (PICU) seems most critical for survival past postnatal period...Early intervention with oral retinoids may facilitate shedding of thick natal scale, but there are well-documented cases of survival without retinoids...Barrier is extremely poor so these kids need emollients 4–5 times a day...Call F.I.R.S.T. for names of physicians with experience. *LM*

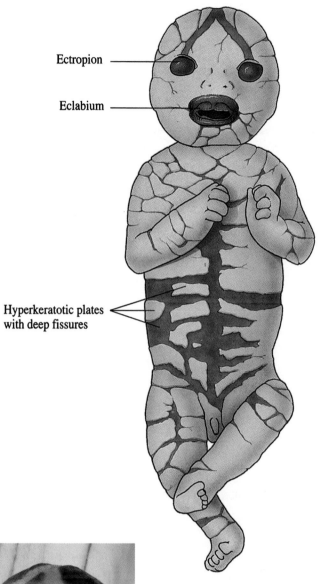

Ectropion

Eclabium

Hyperkeratotic plates
with deep fissures

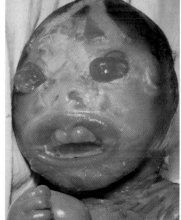

1.11. *Newborn with severe eclabium,
ectropion, deep fissures. (7)*

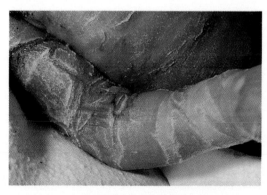

1.12. *Close-up of thick, hyperkeratotic plates. (7)*

Sjögren-Larsson Syndrome

Inheritance	Autosomal recessive; Fatty aldehyde dehydrogenase (FALDH) gene 17p11.2
Prenatal Diagnosis	CVS/amniocentesis: fatty aldehyde dehydrogenase or fatty alcohol oxidoreductase assay; DNA mutation analysis if gene defect is known Fetal skin biopsy at 23 weeks
Incidence	More than 200 cases reported, many from northern Sweden
Age at Presentation	Infancy (ichthyosis); by age 2–3 years old (central nervous system [CNS])
Pathogenesis	Over 50 mutations in the *FALDH* gene have been identified leading to a decrease in fatty-alcohol: NAD oxidoreductase (FAO) activity and subsequent defective conversion of fatty alcohol to fatty acid; this pathway is important in epidermal lipid synthesis as well as catabolism of phospholipids and sphingolipids in CNS myelin; accumulation of fatty alcohol, fatty aldehyde-modified lipids and leukotriene B4, which contributes to pruritus

Key Features

Skin
 Infancy
  Generalized ichthyosis with erythroderma, areas of fine scaling, areas of large lamellar scaling, hyperkeratosis, pruritus
 After Infancy
  Generalized darker scale without erythema accentuated in flexures, lower abdomen and back/sides of neck; spares central face

Central Nervous System
 Mental retardation, spastic di-tetraplegia with scissor gait, speech deficits, epilepsy

Eyes
 Atypical retinal pigment degeneration in macula—glistening white dots in a perimacular distribution; (many but not all cases) retinal pigmentary changes in some patients

Differential Diagnosis	Lamellar ichthyosis (p. 10) Congenital ichthyosiform erythroderma (p. 12) NLSD Multiple sulfatase deficiency
Laboratory Data	Enzyme assay in cultured fibroblasts; DNA mutation analysis if defect known
Management	Referral to dermatologist—emolliation, retinoids Referral to neurologist, ophthalmologist, orthopedist Zileuton inhibits leukotriene B4 synthesis and may help pruritus
Prognosis	Dependent on severity of CNS complications—if wheelchair-bound and severely retarded, prognosis is guarded; otherwise patients typically live well into adulthood

Clinical Pearls

Pruritis in Sjögren-Larsson syndrome (SLS) is a distinguishing feature from other clinically similar diseases and it may respond to Zileuton therapy, which reduces leukotriene B4 levels...In some patients, the ichthyosis may wax and wane every few weeks...Photophobia is a common complaint...Retinal glistening white dots, if present in a patient with suspected SLS, is a reliable diagnostic sign, but its absence does not rule out SLS...Alopecia or nail dystrophy in not seen in this disease...The neurologic symptoms of SLS are not typically progressive, though spasticity symptoms may worsen with age if the patient does not get regular physical therapy...Anecdotal reports that the ichthyosis improves with administration of a low-fat diet supplemented with medium-chain fatty acids have not been reproduceable.   *WR*

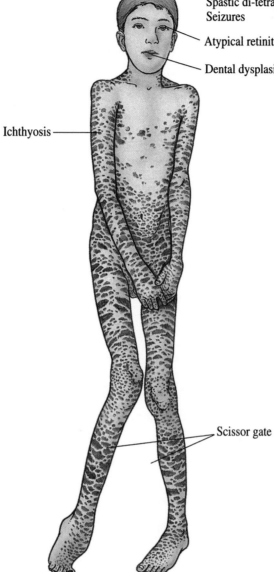

Mental retardation
Spastic di-tetraplegia
Seizures

Atypical retinitis pigmentosa

Dental dysplasia

Ichthyosis

Scissor gate

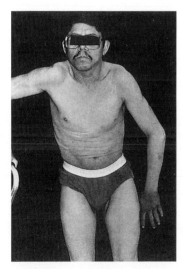

1.13. *Patients with ichthyosis, moderate spasticity and paresis (8).*

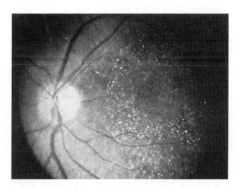

1.14. *Atypical retinitis pigmentosa with "glistening dots" patterns (9).*

Refsum Syndrome

Synonym	Phytanic acid storage disease Heredopathia atactica polyneuritiformis
Inheritance	Autosomal recessive; PAHX gene on 10p, PEX7 gene on 6q
Prenatal Diagnosis	CVS/amniocentesis: phytanic acid oxidase assay on cultured cells; DNA analysis
Incidence	Rare; approximately 100 cases reported; M=F
Age at Presentation	Neurologic symptoms start in childhood; cutaneous changes usually occur as an adult
Pathogenesis	Mutations in the *PAHX* gene create a deficiency in phytanoyl-CoA hydroxylase, a peroxisomal enzyme responsible for the catalyzation of phytanic acid; deficient enzyme leads to an accumulation of phytanic acid in serum and replacement of the normal fatty acids in epidermal lipids and other tissues throughout the body; can also be caused by mutations in the *PEX7* gene that encodes peroxin 7, a receptor important in targeting enzymes to peroxisomes; defective *PEX7* leads to a deficiency in multiple peroxisomal enzymes
Key Features	**Skin** Mild ichthyosis (i.e., ichthyosis vulgaris) usually beginning after neurologic symptomatology **Central Nervous System** Cerebellar ataxia, progressive peripheral polyneuropathy **Eyes** Retinitis pigmentosa with salt and pepper pigment, secondary night blindness **Ear-Nose-Throat** Sensorineural deafness **Cardiac** Arrhythmias with heart block, cardiac failure **Musculoskeletal** Symmetric muscular wasting, variety of skeletal anomalies
Differential Diagnosis	Peroxisomal deficiency disorders Ichthyosis vulgaris (p. 2) Vitamin B deficiency
Laboratory Data	Increased serum phytanic acid; decreased phytanic acid oxidase activity in cultured fibroblasts Skin biopsy revealing lipid-filled vacuoles in basal keratinocytes Increased cerebrospinal fluid (CSF) protein without cells
Management	Dietary restriction of phytanic acid-decrease green vegetables, dairy products and ruminant fats Plasma exchange removal of phytanic acid Referral to neurologist, ophthalmologist, cardiologist, dermatologist, otolaryngologist, and physiatrist
Prognosis	If diet and exchange instituted early on, progression of disease can be halted; if untreated, symptomatology is progressive with remissions and exacerbations culminating in premature sudden death from cardiac arrythmias (heart block) or respiratory failure (medullary depression)

Clinical Pearls

Signs and symptoms are very dependent on diet; therefore onset and severity are very variable...Neurologists usually make the diagnosis...Ichthyosis is usually mild and responsive to diet...These low vegetable/animal fat diets are tough to follow.
LM

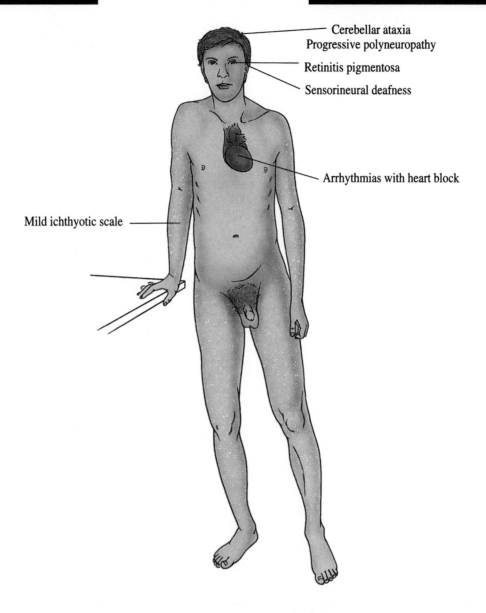

Cerebellar ataxia
Progressive polyneuropathy

Retinitis pigmentosa

Sensorineural deafness

Arrhythmias with heart block

Mild ichthyotic scale

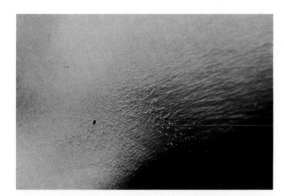

1.15. *Fine, white scales in flexures (2).*

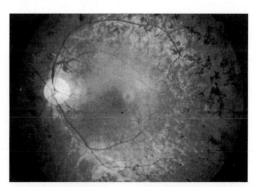

1.16. *Retinitis pigmentosa with typical "salt-and-pepper" pattern (10).*

Conradi-Hünermann Syndrome

Synonym	X-linked dominant chondrodysplasia punctata; Conradi-Hunermann-Happle syndrome
Inheritance	X-linked dominant; Emopamil-binding protein (*EBP*) gene on Xp11
Prenatal Diagnosis	Ultrasound evaluation of long bones
Incidence	Rare; usually lethal in males; reports of surviving males both with/without 47, XXY
Age at Presentation	Birth
Pathogenesis	Mutation in the *EBP* gene or 3β-hydroxysteroid-Δ^8-Δ^7-isomerase leads to a defect in cholesterol biosynthesis and can explain skeletal phenotype
Key Features	**Skin** Ichthyosiform erythroderma in Blaschko's lines in infancy; resolves with follicular atrophoderma and/or hyperpigmentation **Hair** Coarse, patchy alopecia **Eyes** Asymmetric focal cataracts **Musculoskeletal** Stippled epiphyses (punctate calcifications), asymmetric limb shortening, short stature, scoliosis **Cranofacial** Frontal bossing, macrocephaly, flat nasal root, asymmetric **Central Nervous System** Mental retardation (rare)
Differential Diagnosis	Autosomal recessive rhizomelic chondrodysplasia punctata X-linked recessive chondrodysplasia punctata with steroid sulfatase deficiency CHILD syndrome Incontinentia pigmenti
Laboratory Data	Bone films Neonatal skin biopsy—may reveal calcium in the epidermis with von Kossa's stain Peroxisomal function in cultured fibroblasts
Management	Referral to orthopedist, dermatologist, ophthalmologist Examine first-degree relatives
Prognosis	Ichthyosis and stippled epiphyses resolve after infancy; orthopedic complications predominate with normal life span

Clinical Pearls

If an erythrodermic baby has hyperkeratosis in a linear or whorled pattern, look for epiphyseal stippling on x-ray...By several years of age, the epiphyseal stippling is usually gone and the erythema more limited...Severity of skin and skeletal disease varies greatly between individual adults, and there are no good early predictors yet...Follicular atrophoderma seems to be a nearly constant finding in adults.   *LM*

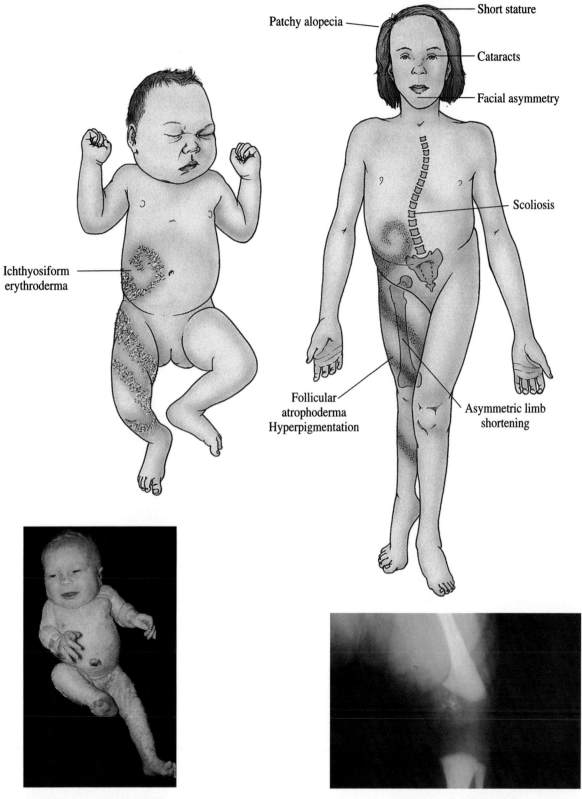

Short stature

Patchy alopecia

Cataracts

Facial asymmetry

Ichthyosiform erythroderma

Scoliosis

Follicular atrophoderma
Hyperpigmentation

Asymmetric limb shortening

1.17. *Infant with ichthyosiform erythroderma in Blaschko's lines (11).*

1.18. *Stippled epiphyses (12).*

CHILD Syndrome

Synonym
Congenital **h**emidysplasia with **i**chthyosiform erythroderma and **l**imb **d**efects **(CHILD)**
Unilateral congenital ichthyosiform erythroderma

Inheritance
X-linked dominant; *NSDHL* gene on Xq28

Prenatal Diagnosis
Ultrasound detection of limb/organ defects

Incidence
Rare; lethal in males

Age at Presentation
Birth to 1 month old

Pathogenesis
Mutations in the *NSDHL* gene encoding for 3β-hydroxysteroid dehydrogenase are most common; *EBP* gene defect (i.e. Conradi's) has been described; both enzymes involved in cholesterol biosynthesis

Key Features

Skin
Unilateral ichthyosiform erythroderma with sharp midline cutoff involving trunk and limbs; ± linear or segmental involvement on contralateral side; lesions tend to improve with age but may persist in skin folds (ptychotropism)
Hair
Ipsilateral alopecia
Nails
Severe dystrophy
Musculoskeletal
Hypoplasia to agenesis of limbs ipsilateral to ichthyosis; other ipsilateral bones may be involved; ± stippled epiphyses
Internal Organs
Hypoplasia to agenesis of organs below ichthyosis–variety of organs reported including CNS, cardiovascular, renal, and genitourinary involvement

Differential Diagnosis
Conradi-Hünermann syndrome
Inflammatory linear verrucous epidermal nevus

Laboratory Data
Computed tomography/magnetic resonance imaging (CT/MRI) scan of ipsilateral side

Management
Referral to dermatologist—topical therapy
Referral to orthopedist
Referral to organ-specific subspecialist

Prognosis
Dependent on which organs are affected—can range from normal life span to incompatible with life

Clinical Pearls

Experienced clinicians made a connection long ago between the constellation of findings in CHILD and Conradi-Hünermann, so it was satisfying to learn that their gene defects share a common biochemical pathway...In CHILD syndrome, the skin lesions can look like inflammatory linear epidermal nevi...Excision can be curative for individuals with relatively narrow, nevoid bands.   *LM*

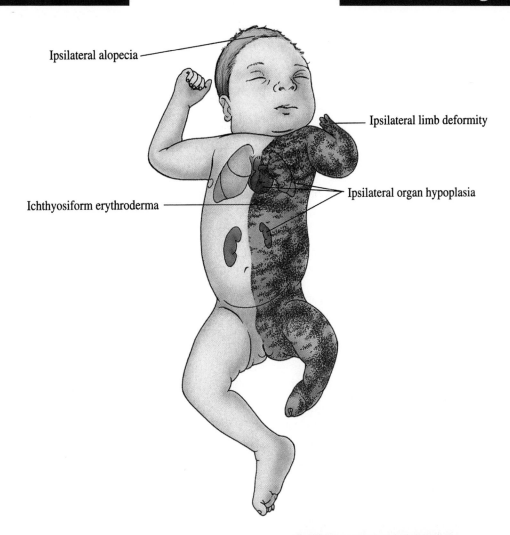

Ipsilateral alopecia

Ipsilateral limb deformity

Ipsilateral organ hypoplasia

Ichthyosiform erythroderma

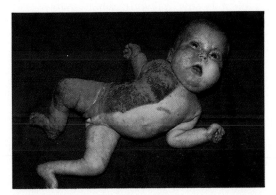

1.19. *Unilateral ichthyosiform erythroderma with ipsilateral limb hypoplasia (13).*

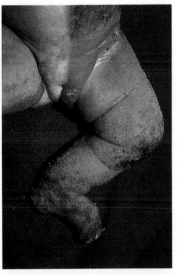

1.20. *Close-up of thick hyperkeratosis of the left foot and leg (13).*

23

Netherton Syndrome

Synonym	Ichthyosis linearis circumflexa (ILC)
Inheritance	Autosomal recessive; *SPINK5* gene on 5q32
Prenatal Diagnosis	DNA mutation analysis if defect known in family
Incidence	Rare with a few dozen case reports; M=F; observed M:F=1:2
Age at Presentation	Birth to first few months of life
Pathogenesis	Mutations in *SPINK5* gene encoding LEKT1, a serine protease inhibitor that may be important in downregulating inflammatory pathways; LEKT1 also associated with atopy

Key Features

Skin
> **Birth–Few Months**
> > Generalized erythema and scaling with secondary hypernatremia, failure to thrive
>
> **Later in Infancy**
> > Migratory erythematous, polycyclic, serpiginous plaques with double-edged scale along the margins (ILC)
> > > Atopic dermatitis with flexural lichenification and pruritus
> > > Seborrheic-like scale and erythema on face, scalp, eyebrows

Hair
> Trichorrhexis invaginata (ball-and-socket configuration; bamboo hair)—most characteristic; may also have pili torti or trichorrhexis nodosa; eyebrow hair may be most common site
> Short, sparse

Immunology
> Anaphylactic reactions to foods

Differential Diagnosis	Congenital ichthyosiform erythroderma (p. 12) Seborrheic dermatitis Dermatophytosis
Laboratory Data	Light microscope—examination of hair shaft Increased serum immunoglobulin E (IgE) KOH
Management	Monitor in infancy for hypernatremia, and failure to thrive Referral to dermatologist—topical therapy, retinoids; avoid keratolytics (can worsen condition) and tacrolimus ointment (increased absorption from compromised skin barrier with increased risk of toxicities) Referral to allergist—radioallergosorbent assay test (RAST)
Prognosis	May have partial remissions and may improve at puberty; normal life span

Clinical Pearls

These folks have extremely poor barrier function, so they lose lots of water and calories and absorb anything we put on their skin...Characteristic bamboo shafts may not be seen in all hairs and may not appear until second year of life...Lateral eyebrows are a good place to look...Characteristic scales of ILC may be fleeting and are never generalized...Most patients look mostly like CIE...Many develop vegetating intertriginous plaques of unknown etiology, though some may have HPV...These patients usually have adverse reactions to topical keratolytics and oral retinoids...Topical calcineurin inhibitors may be helpful for itch and erythema, but absorption to very high serum levels limits use...Early referral to the patient support group F.I.R.S.T. can be very helpful. *LM*

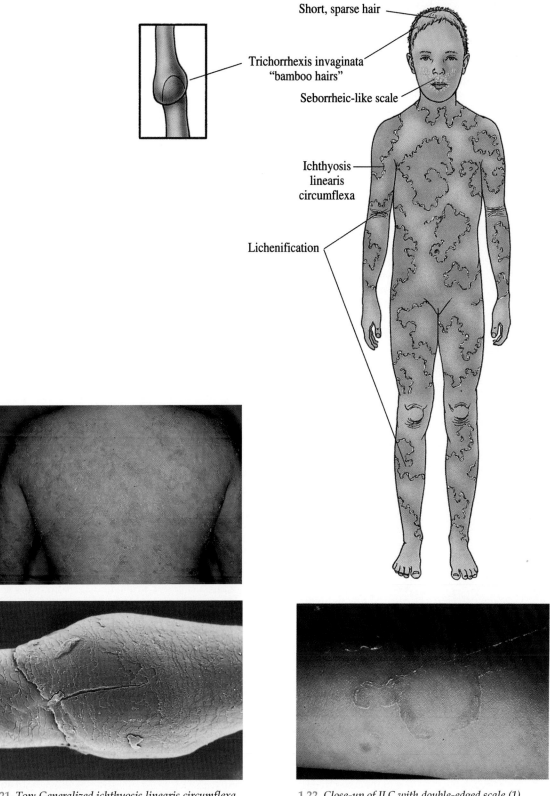

Short, sparse hair

Trichorrhexis invaginata
"bamboo hairs"

Seborrheic-like scale

Ichthyosis
linearis
circumflexa

Lichenification

1.21. *Top: Generalized ichthyosis linearis circumflexa (ILC) in an adult (1). Bottom: Scanning electron micrograph revealing trichorrhexis invaginata in a different patient (13a).*

1.22. *Close-up of ILC with double-edged scale (1).*

Erythrokeratoderma Variabilis

Synonym	Mendes da Costa syndrome
Inheritance	Autosomal dominant; *GJB3* gene on 1p35
Prenatal Diagnosis	DNA analysis for GJB3 or GJB4 mutations if defect in family known
Incidence	Rare, more than 200 case reports; majority from northern and middle European ancestry; M=F
Age at Presentation	Birth to 1 year old; may develop later in life
Pathogenesis	Mutations in *GJB3, GJB4* genes encoding for connexin 31, 30.3 respectively; connexins are membrane components in gap junction channels and are responsible for intercellular communication and signaling; defects in these channels impair epidermal differentiation and the skin's response to external stimuli

Key Features	**Skin**
	    Well-demarcated, geographic patches of erythema with changing shape and position day to day; increased on face, buttocks, extensor extremities; cold, wind, heat, emotional upset may induce lesions
	    Fixed focal hyperkeratotic plaques; may be generalized with palms and soles involved

Differential Diagnosis	Conditions associated with figurate erythema Symmetrical progressive erythrokeratoderma Psoriasis Parapsoriasis
Laborartory Data	None
Management	Referral to dermatologist—symptomatic erythematous patches-mask with makeup and camouflage; mild sedative antihistamines in case of pruritus and burning; avoid skin irritation and triggering factors Hyperkeratotic plaques—topical retinoic acid, salicylic acid, lactic acid, and other alpha-hydroxy acids in petrolatum Acitretin or isotretinoin (relative low doses) Examine first-degree relatives
Prognosis	Worsens until puberty and then enters a stable, chronic course; normal life span with general health unaffected

Clinical Pearls

Erythrokeratoderma variabilis (EKV) usually responds exceptionally well to systemic retinoid therapy; complete clearing of hyperkeratosis and significant moderation of the erythema has been reported...Systemic retinoid treatment should be considered carefully because long-term therapy is required to achieve continuing results...The minimal effective dose for persons with EKV is usually low...Erythematous patches are more conspicuous during childhood and may be completely absent in adults...Erythematous patches with pronounced, circinate or gyrate borders appear to be associated with *GJB4* mutations...Despite the finding that *GJB3* (Cx31) mutations may also cause sensorineural hearing loss and peripheral neuropathy, EKV is not associated with any of these disorders...Approximately 35% of patients report burning sensations that precede or accompany erythematous lesions. *GR*

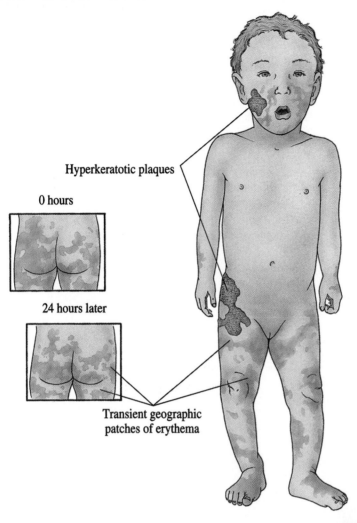

Hyperkeratotic plaques

0 hours

24 hours later

Transient geographic
patches of erythema

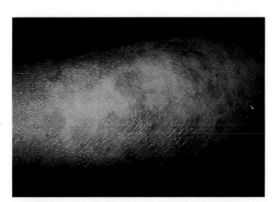

1.23. *Fixed hyperkeratotic plaques with geographic erythematous patches (5).*

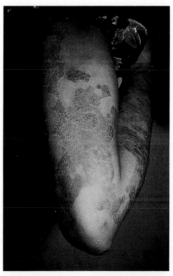

1.24. *Well-demarcated dark, hyperkeratotic plaques with patches of erythema (5).*

KID Syndrome

Synonym	**K**eratitis-**i**chthyosis-**d**eafness syndrome
Inheritance	Autosomal dominant and recessive transmission reported; *GJB2* gene on 13q11–12
Prenatal Diagnosis	Mutation analysis if defect known
Incidence	Approximately 30 cases reported; M=F
Age at Presentation	Birth
Pathogenesis	Mutations in *GJB2*, the gene encoding for connexin 26, a gap junction protein responsible for intercellular communications in the epidermis and cochlea, produces phenotype

Key Features	**Skin**
	    Generalized mild hyperkeratosis with follicular plugging
	    Erythematous, keratotic plaques on face, extremities > trunk
	    Palmoplantar keratoderma with stippled surface
	    Recurrent bacterial and fungal infections
	    Squamous cell carcinoma of skin, tongue not rare
	Hair
	    Alopecia in scalp, eyelashes, eyebrows
	Nails
	    Dystrophic
	Ear-Nose-Throat
	    Nonprogressive sensorineural deafness
	Eyes
	    Progressive bilateral vascularized keratitis—secondary blindness may occur

Differential Diagnosis	Keratosis follicularis spinulosa decalvans
Laboratory Data	Audiologic testing Skin cultures
Management	Referral to dermatologist—antibiotics, systemic antifungals, topical emollients, keratolytics; oral retinoids may exacerbate corneal neovascularization Referral to ophthalmologist—topical cyclosporine has helped keratitis Referral to otolaryngologist
Prognosis	Dependent on degree of hearing loss and blindness, may have severe sensory handicap; otherwise normal life span

Clinical Pearls

Many of these individuals seem to have increased susceptibility to fungal (especially candida) infection and there have been several reports of squamous cell carcinomas in patients with KID (unusual in other ichthyoses)...Therefore, I have a low threshold for repeated use of antifungals and biopsy of unusual looking keratotic papules...Early reports suggest that topical calcineurin inhibitors may be valuable for erosive keratitis and that cochlear implants may improve hearing. *LM*

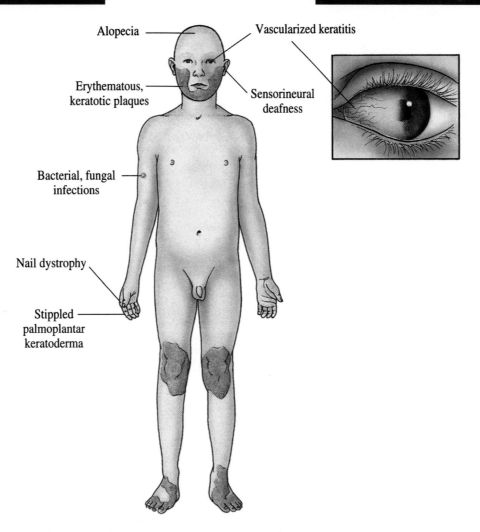

Alopecia

Vascularized keratitis

Erythematous, keratotic plaques

Sensorineural deafness

Bacterial, fungal infections

Nail dystrophy

Stippled palmoplantar keratoderma

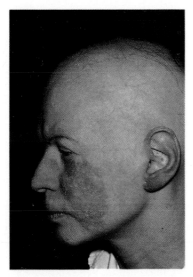

1.25. Sharply demarcated erythematous plaques on malar face, nose (14).

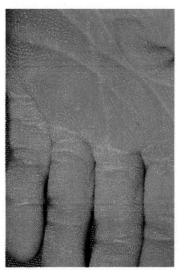

1.26. Stippled palmoplantar keratoderma (14).

Diffuse Palmoplantar Keratoderma (PPK)

Synonym	Vörner PPK or Epidermolytic PPK Unna-Thost PPK or Nonepidermolytic PPK
Inheritance	Autosomal dominant; Vörner: Keratin genes 9 (most common) and 1 (17q21 and 12q13 respectively) Unna-Thost: keratin 1 gene
Prenatal Diagnosis	DNA linkage analysis or mutation detection
Incidence	Most common inherited PPK (most patients with Vörner histopathology); 1:200 in northern Sweden; 1:40,000 in Northern Ireland; M=F
Age at Presentation	Shortly after birth to 1 year old
Pathogenesis	Mutations in keratin genes 9 and 1 disrupt keratin filament assembly within palmoplantar skin
Key Features	**Skin** Diffuse bilateral, symmetric hyperkeratosis of palms and soles with white-yellow hue; well-demarcated with erythematous border; no transgrediens (extension to dorsum); secondary painful fissuring, dermatophytosis Hyperhidrosis ± bromhidrosis; may have keratotic lesions of the doral surface of hands, feet, knees, elbows and volar wrists in Unna-Thost variant; abnormal gait secondary to pain
Differential Diagnosis	Other forms of PPK
Laboratory Data	Skin biopsy: Unna variant—orthokeratosis Vörner variant—epidermolytic hyperkeratosis
Management	Referral to dermatologist—topical emollients, keratolytics, oral retinoids, topical and oral antifungals, bath PUVA (oral administration of psoralen and exposure to long-wavelength ultraviolet light) has helped one reported patient Referral to podiatrist—customized in-soles, mechanical debridement
Prognosis	Persists throughout life; normal life span

Clinical Pearls

The clinical feature that Unna, Thost, and Vörner were emphasizing in their patients a century ago was a waxy keratoderma limited to the palms and soles, without transgrediens. Vörner's patient turns out to have had epidermolytic histology and so did Thost's. At least one family with Unna-type nonepidermolytic PPK has a mutation in keratin 1. Other causes for NEPPK are sure to be found. We should probably move away from using the eponyms for keratodermas, until they are genetically as well as clinically defined. Treatment is very difficult because most patients are not motivated to keep it up...I like saltwater soaks (3% NaC1 for 30 minutes) followed by 40% urea under occlusion overnight to quickly reduce hyperkeratosis and fissures...Paring with a sharp knife is acceptable, but avoid rubbing and scraping in this disease of keratinocyte fragility.   *LM*

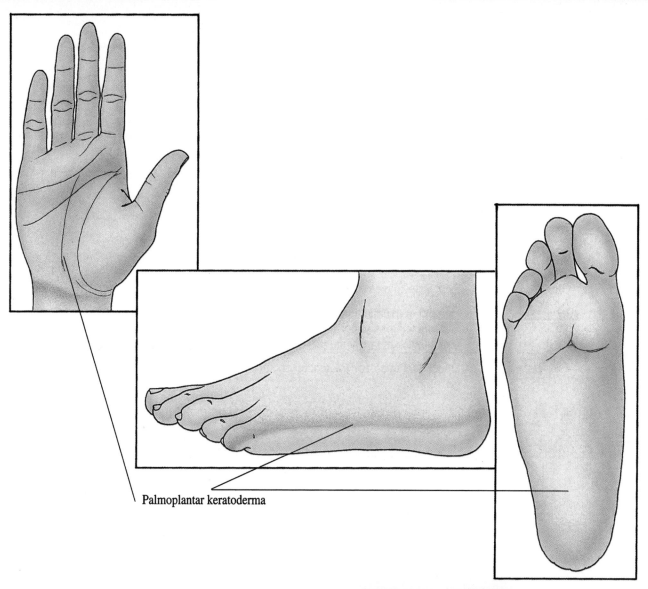

Palmoplantar keratoderma

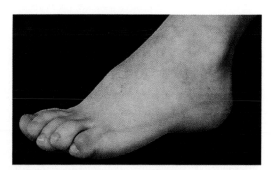

1.27. Well-demarcated plantar hyperkeratosis with yellow hue and erythematous border (15).

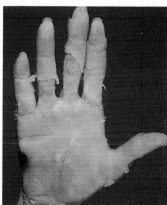

1.28. Desquamating palmar hyper-keratosis (16).

Howel-Evans Syndrome

Inheritance	Autosomal dominant; tylosis and oesophageal cancer (*TOC*) gene locus on 17q25
Prenatal Diagnosis	DNA linkage analysis in large kindred
Incidence	Rare; described in a few kindreds in United Kingdom, United States, and Germany; M=F
Age at Presentation	Second decade to adulthood (keratoderma); after third decade (esophageal carcinoma)
Pathogenesis	Mutation within the *TOC* gene locus on 17q distal to keratin 1 gene cluster plays a role in this condition as well as sporadic esophageal carcinomas; envolplakin is not the gene defect within the *TOC* locus

Key Features	**Skin**
	   Focal, weight-bearing, symmetric, non-transgrediens palmoplantar keratoderma
	Gastrointestinal
	   Esophageal carcinoma
	Mouth
	   Oral leukoplakia in one kindred

Differential Diagnosis	PPK with esophageal carcinoma (acquired)
Laboratory Data	Endoscopy if palmoplantar keratoderma present with family history
Management	Referral to gastroenterologist—periodic endoscopic evaluation, oral cavity examination Referral to dermatologist—topical therapy, oral retinoids Examination of family members
Prognosis	Dependent upon early detection of carcinoma

Clinical Pearls

The follicular and leukoplakic changes in this family have stimulated a reclassification of this as a focal palmoplantar ectodermal defect. Feet are affected more than hands, and the hyperkeratosis is not truly diffuse, occurring mainly over points of pressure. Unfortunately, there are still no genetic or clinical clues (other than a family history) of risk for cancer in someone with acquired keratoderma. Soaking in salt water followed by urea creams reduces hyperkeratosis; prolonged bedrest reportedly leads to great improvement. *LM*

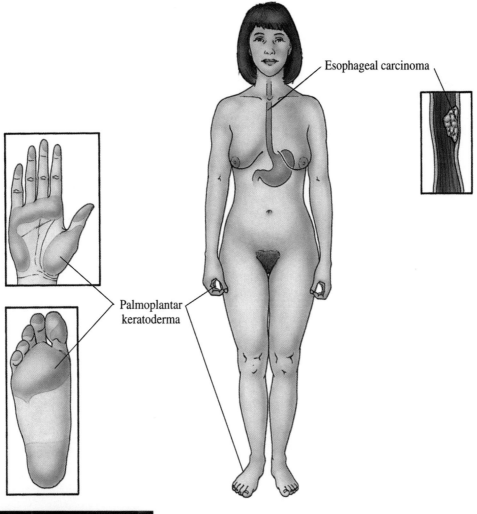

Esophageal carcinoma

Palmoplantar keratoderma

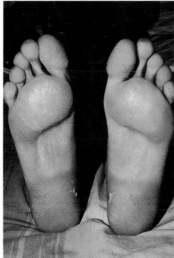

1.29. *Thick plantar keratoderma on weight-bearing surface (17).*

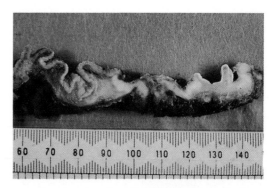

1.30. *Cross-section of esophagus revealing carcinoma in a patient with Howel-Evans syndrome (17).*

Vohwinkel Syndrome

Synonym
PPK mutilans
Keratoderma hereditaria mutilans

Inheritance
Autosomal dominant: classic form with deafness: *GJB2* gene on 13q11–12
Loricrin-variant: loricrin gene on the epidermal differentiation complex (EDC) on 1q21

Prenatal Diagnosis
DNA analysis if gene defect known

Incidence
Rare; M=F

Age at Presentation
Infancy to early childhood; pseuodainhum/autoamputation later childhood-adulthood

Pathogenesis

Classic variant with deafness caused by a *GJB2* gene mutation encoding connexin 26, a gap junction protein
A mutation in the loricrin gene, a protein important in the formation of the cornified cell envelope produces the phenotype associated with ichthyosis and not deafness

Key Features
Skin
Diffuse honeycombed PPK
Digital constriction bands with autoamputation (pseudo-ainhum)-increased on the fifth digit
Starfish-shaped keratotic plaques on dorsum of hands, feet, elbows, and knees; linear keratoses of elbows and knees; mild, generalized ichthyosis with flexural accentuation in loricrin-variant
Hair
Scarring alopecia
Ear-Nose-Throat
High-frequency, nonprogressive hearing loss (classic variant)

Differential Diagnosis
Other forms of PPK

Laboratory Data
Hand/foot films

Management
Referral to dermatologist—topical therapy, oral retinoids
Referral to hand surgeon—surgical release of constriction bands
Hearing testing

Prognosis
Normal life span with potential for loss of digits and persistent keratoderma

Clinical Pearls

Here is a good example of how genetics will help us clean up our syndromes. Vohwinkle's patient probably had a connexin mutation and clinically had honeycomb keratoderma, starfish keratoses, pseudoainhum, hearing defect, but no ichthyosis. The Vohwinkle variant described by Camisa had a loricrin mutation and clinically had no hearing defect but did have mild, generalized ichthyosis. Clearly, these are different diseases, not the same disease on a different background. I have had several cases of keratoderma with pseudoainhum respond well to oral retinoid vond avoided surgery or autoamputation. *LM*

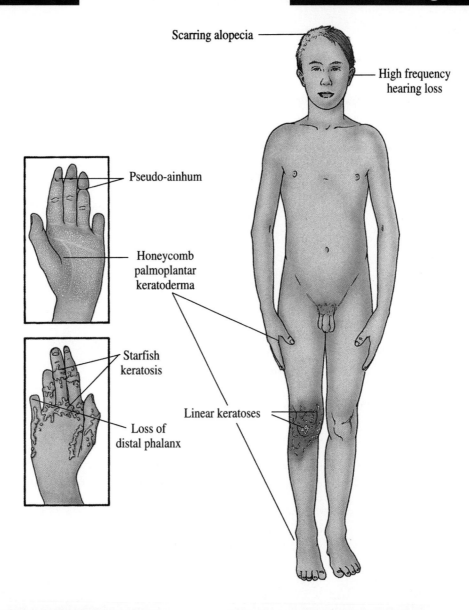

Scarring alopecia

High frequency hearing loss

Pseudo-ainhum

Honeycomb palmoplantar keratoderma

Starfish keratosis

Loss of distal phalanx

Linear keratoses

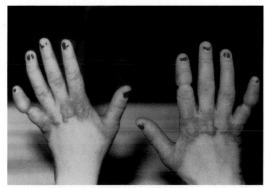

1.31. Pseudo-ainhum with keratotic plaques on the dorsum of both hands (18).

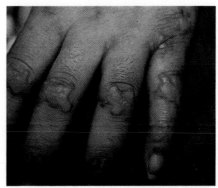

1.32. Starfish keratotic plaques on dorsum of hand (19).

Mal de Meleda

Synonym	Keratoderma palmoplantaris transgrediens
Inheritance	Autosomal recessive; secreted Ly-6/uPar related protein 1 (*SLURP1*) gene on 8qter
Prenatal Diagnosis	None
Incidence	Originally described in an inbred population on the island of Meleda in the Adriatic Sea; most cases originate from this region; M=F
Age at Presentation	After birth to first few months of life
Pathogenesis	*SLURP1* gene mutation encoding for proteins important in cell signaling and adhesion

Key Features

Skin
> **Infancy**
>> Palmoplantar erythema, scaling, thickening
>
> **After Infancy**
>> Glove-and-stocking palmoplantar keratoderma with sharp demarcation, transgrediens (extension to dorsal surface), secondary painful fissures, hyperhidrosis, maceration, fetid odor; ± constriction bands at distal phalanges
>> Hyperkeratotic plaques over elbows and knees

Nails
> Subungual hyperkeratosis; koilonychia

Differential Diagnosis	Other forms of PPK
Laboratory Data	None
Management	Referral to dermatologist—keratolytics, oral retinoids Referral to surgeon—surgical release of constriction bands Examine family members
Prognosis	Persists throughout life; normal life span

Clinical Pearls

Erythema of palms and soles at age 1–2 years often precedes hyperkeratosis...Possibility of developing contractures and pseudoainhum encourages me to periodically use oral retinoids to control hyperkeratosis. Clinical significance of commonly positive cultures for fungi is up in the air, but I am following this association carefully. *LM*

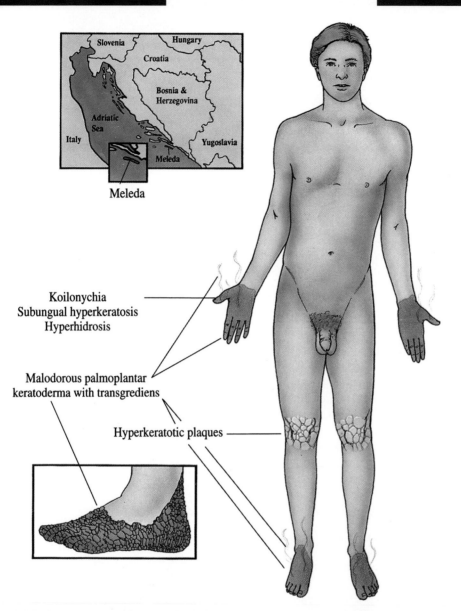

Koilonychia
Subungual hyperkeratosis
Hyperhidrosis

Malodorous palmoplantar
keratoderma with transgrediens

Hyperkeratotic plaques

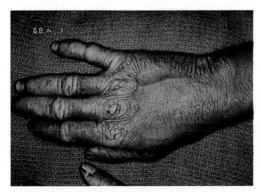

1.33. *Palmar keratoderma with transgrediens (20).*

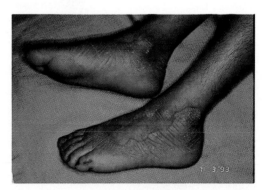

1.34. *Erythematous plantar keratoderma with transgrediens (20).*

Papillon-Lefèvre Syndrome

Synonym	Palmoplantar keratoderma with periodontosis
Inheritance	Autosomal recessive; *CTSC* gene on 11q14
Prenatal Diagnosis	None
Incidence	More than 120 case reports; M=F
Age at Presentation	Birth to 5 years old
Pathogenesis	Mutations in the *CTSC* gene encoding for cathepsin C, a lysosomal protease have been identified

Key Features

Skin
Sharply demarcated palmoplantar keratoderma with erythematous border, trangrediens (extension to dorsal surface, achilles tendon), hyperhidrosis, fetid odor; soles > palms; diffuse > punctate keratoderma
Pyogenic infections
Hyperkeratotic plaques on elbows and knees

Hair
May be sparse

Mouth
Periodontitis with severe gingivitis, alveolar bone resorption, and loss of deciduous and permanent teeth

Central Nervous System
Dural calcification at the tentorium and choroid attachments

Differential Diagnosis	Other forms of PPK
Laboratory Data	Dental films Brain CT/MRI scan Bacterial skin culture
Management	Referral to dentist—meticulous oral hygiene, regular plaque removal, oral antibiotics, extractions, dentures Referral to dermatologist—topical keratolytics, oral retinoids, antibiotics
Prognosis	Resolution of periodontitis after all teeth are shed; premature loss of teeth may lead to distortion of maxillary and mandibular bone growth; keratoderma persists throughout life

Clinical Pearls

Anecdotal reports long suggested that these patients are at high risk for cutaneous bacterial and fungal infections and for unusual systemic infections, such as hepatic abscesses. The newly identified causative gene and the importance of cathepsin C in innate immunity and neutrophil function force us to rethink the real significance of those anecdotal associations. Early mechanical and antibiotic treatment for periodontal disease is reported to save adult teeth...Keratolytics and systemic retinoids are useful for reducing keratoderma...Maybe we should consider more aggressive cutaneous antisepsis. *LM*

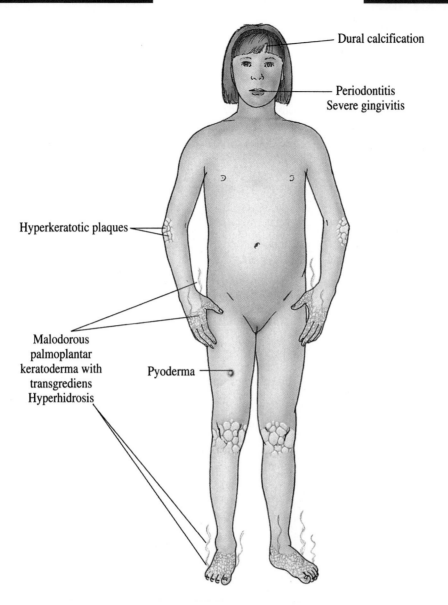

Dural calcification

Periodontitis
Severe gingivitis

Hyperkeratotic plaques

Malodorous
palmoplantar
keratoderma with
transgrediens
Hyperhidrosis

Pyoderma

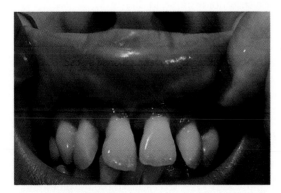

1.35. *Severe periodontitis and gingivitis (21).*

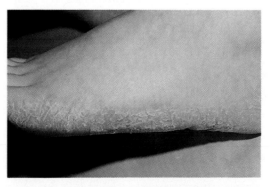

1.36. *Plantar keratoderma with transgrediens. (21).*

Richner-Hanhart Syndrome

Synonym   Tyrosinemia type II

Inheritance   Autosomal recessive; tyrosine aminotransferase gene on 16q22.1–q22

Prenatal Diagnosis

Amniocentesis: tyrosine aminotransferase assay
DNA analysis available if defect known in family

Incidence   Less than 50 cases reported; increased in patients with Italian ancestry; M=F

Age at Presentation   First few months of life (eye findings precede skin findings)

Pathogenesis   Mutations in the tyrosine aminotransferase gene on 16q leads to deficiency of the hepatic enzyme with accumulation of tyrosine in all tissues; tyrosine crystals in corneal epithelium are thought to induce an inflammatory response; tyrosine may stimulate microtubule assembly

Key Features   **Skin**
    Focal (weight-bearing plantar surfaces, hypothenar or thenar emminences, finger-tips) or diffuse palmoplantar keratoderma; with/without pain with impaired ambulation, erosions, bullae, erythema
    Hyperkeratotic plaques on elbows, knees
Eyes
    Severe keratitis with photophobia, corneal ulceration, neovascularization, and blindness
Central Nervous System
    With/without mental retardation

Differential Diagnosis   Other forms of PPK
Herpetic keratitis

Laboratory Data   Increased plasma tyrosine levels
Increased urinary tyrosine metabolites

Management   Referral to nutritionist—low phenylalanine/low tyrosine diet
Referral to dermatologist—topical therapy, oral retinoids
Referral to ophthalmologist

Prognosis   If dietetic intervention made early enough, can prevent cutaneous and ocular complications; mental retardation may not respond to diet

Clinical Pearls

Early dietary intervention is critical. Eye findings usually precede keratoderma by several years; unfortunately diagnosis may not be considered until skin findings appear...Tyrosine crystals in keratinocytes are thought to be important in pathogenesis. The mystery of why the cutaneous findings in this metabolic disease are mostly limited to palmar-plantar epidermis is deepened by a surgical success: ten years after thigh skin was transplanted to the heel it had not become hyperkeratotic, even when surrounding heel skin was.   *LM*

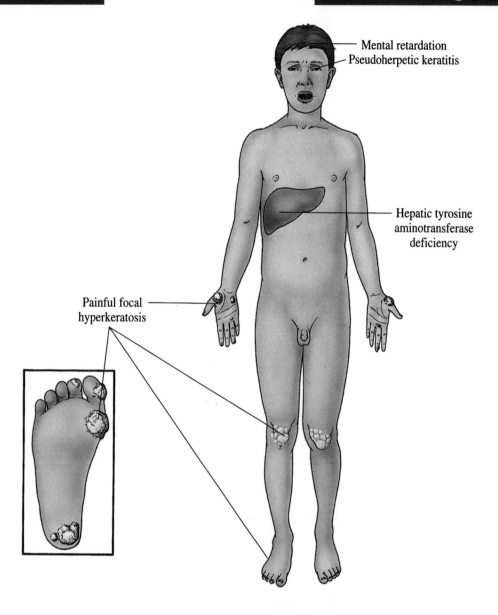

Mental retardation
Pseudoherpetic keratitis

Hepatic tyrosine aminotransferase deficiency

Painful focal hyperkeratosis

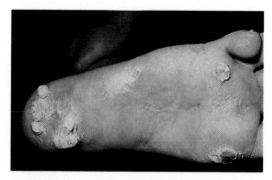

1.37. *Focal plantar keratoderma on weight-bearing surface (22).*

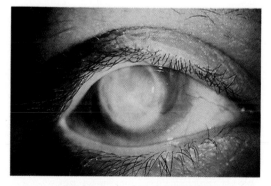

1.38. *Severe dendritic keratitis (23).*

Darier Disease

Synonym	Darier-White disease
	Keratosis follicularis
Inheritance	Autosomal dominant; *ATP2A2* gene on 12q23–24
Prenatal Diagnosis	DNA linkage analysis available
Incidence	1:55,000–1:100,000; M=F
Age at Presentation	Second decade of life; rarely in adulthood
Pathogenesis	Mutations in *ATP2A2* gene encodes SERCA2 (sarcoendoplasmic reticulum Ca^{2+}ATPase isoform 2), a Ca^{2+} pump providing increased extracellular Ca^{2+} necessary for normal epidermal differentiation and formation

Key Features

Skin
Hyperkeratotic papules coalescing to warty plaques in seborrheic distribution on trunk, face, scalp, flexures and groin; yellow-brown, greasy, malodorous, may be infected with herpes simplex virus (HSV) or bacteria, UVB sensitive
Verrucous papules on dorsum of hands (i.e., Acrokeratosis verruciformis of Hopf)
Palmoplantar punctate keratosis/pits

Nails
Red and white alternating longitudinal bands
Subungual hyperkeratosis
V-shaped nick at distal nail plate; with/without splitting

Mucous Membranes
Cobblestone papules on oral, anogenital mucosa

Central Nervous System
Schizophrenia and mental retardation reported in some families

Differential Diagnosis
Hailey-Hailey disease
Grover's disease
Pityriasis rubra pilaris
Psoriasis

Laboratory Data
Skin biopsy

Management
Referral to dermatologist
Systemic isotretinoin
Systemic acitretin
Topical retinoids, corticosteroids, emollients
Limit direct sunlight exposure—sunscreen, protective clothing
Acyclovir/antibiotics for superinfection
Referral to psychiatrist if symptomatic

Prognosis
Chronic course worsening in summer, with age; normal life span.

Clinical Pearls

Establishing a routine for these patients is tough. Avoid sun, heat, occlusion, and people with chickenpox or HSV. Recurring bacterial infection (usually *S. aureus* but watch out for rare birds) usually require systemic antibiotics...Oral retinoids are helpful, but a relative overdose can cause paradoxical worsening due to erosions. Patients with intractable disease respond to skin planning or laser ablation that removes at least some of the papillary dermis. Anecdotal reports suggest that patients with Darier disease have increased risk for depression and suicide; anyone developing a chronic disease during their teenage years deserves monitoring for psychosocial problems. *LM*

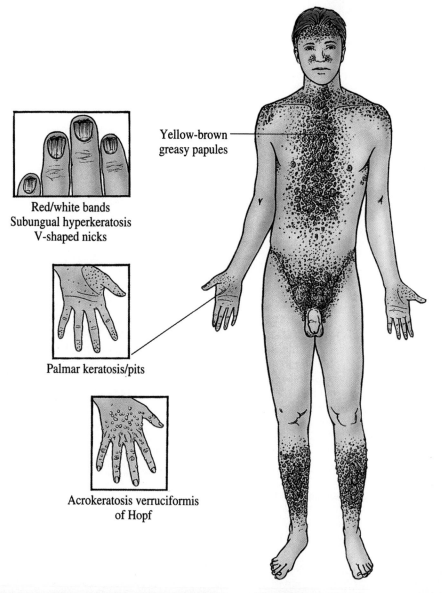

Yellow-brown greasy papules

Red/white bands
Subungual hyperkeratosis
V-shaped nicks

Palmar keratosis/pits

Acrokeratosis verruciformis
of Hopf

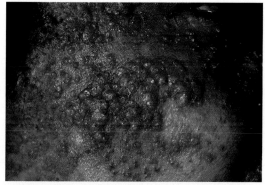

1.39. Brown, greasy, hyperkeratotic plaques on the face. (5)

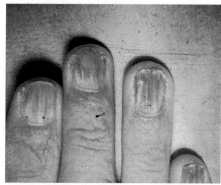

1.40. Alternating red/white longitudinal bands with v-shaped distal nicks and subungual hyperkeratosis. (5)

Epidermal Nevus Syndrome

Synonym	Ichthyosis hystrix **I**nflammatory **l**inear **v**errucous **e**pidermal **n**evus (ILVEN) Linear sebaceous nevus syndrome
Inheritance	Sporadic
Prenatal Diagnosis	None
Incidence	Over 400 cases reported; M=F
Age at Presentation	Birth to first few months of life
Pathogenesis	Thought to include many distinct genetic diseases all sharing a phenotype reflecting genetic mosaicism

Key Features

Skin
  Epidermal nevi (usually more than 2 to 3 cm in length, more than 0.5–2 cm in width)
      Nevus unius laterus: ILVEN (most common): long, linear, verrucous plaques on limbs; with/without scale, erythema
      Ichthyosis hystrix: extensive verrucous plaques in whorl-like pattern on trunk
      Linear nevus sebaceous: linear, orange-tan, waxy plaques on scalp extending onto the face
      Localized row of pigmented papillomas
Other Skin Findings
  Hemangiomas, capillary malformations, hypopigmentation, café au lait macules
Central Nervous System (associated with head and neck or extensive nevi)
  Mental retardation, seizures, spastic hemiparesis/paralysis, sensorineural deafness, cerebral hemangiomas, vascular malformations
Skeletal (associated with location of nevi)
  Hemihypertrophy, kyphoscoliosis, ankle/foot deformities, vitamin D-resistant rickets
Eyes
  Extension of nevus to lid and bulbar conjunctiva, lipodermoids, colobomas, corneal opacity, nystagmus, cortical blindness
Neoplasms (rare)
  Variety of tumors reported; syringocystadenoma papilliferum, Wilms' tumor, astrocytoma, rhabdomyosarcoma, salivary gland adenocarcinoma

Differential Diagnosis

Epidermal nevi
Proteus syndrome (p. 106)
Klippel-Trenaunay-Weber syndrome (p. 102)

Laboratory Data

Skin biopsy—rule out features of epidermolytic hyperkeratosis (EHK)
Eletroencephalogram
Brain CT/MRI
Skeletal survey
Serum calcium/phosphorus

Epidermal Nevus Syndrome *(continued)*

Management

Referral to dermatologist/dermatologic surgeon—surgical removal, dermabrasion, CO_2 laser, topical lactic acid in propylene glycol, oral retinoids
Referral to neurologist, ophthalmologist, orthopedist
Genetic counseling if at risk for EHK offspring

Prognosis

Malignancy, cerebral vascular lesion with hemorrhage, or intractable seizures may shorten life span

Clinical Pearls

This particular ENS (I'm a believer in many, distinct ENSs) has hypophosphatemia as its hallmark. Excision of the nevus or supplemental phosphate and calcitriol improve many of the biochemical abnormalities and may stall progression of bone and CNS changes. Therefore, I do the low-yield test of checking serum P on all babies with large epidermal nevi.   *LM*

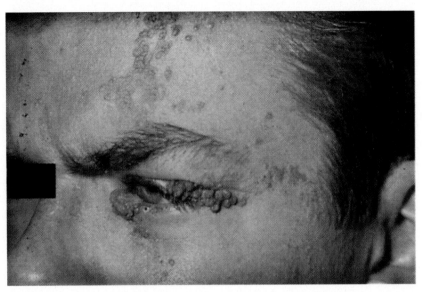

1.41. *Linear epidermal nevus involving a patient's eye (5).*

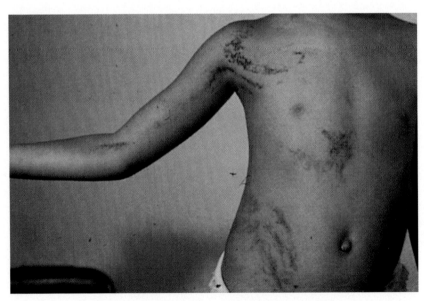

1.42. *Ichthyosis hystrix—verrucous plaques in Blaschko's lines. (5)*

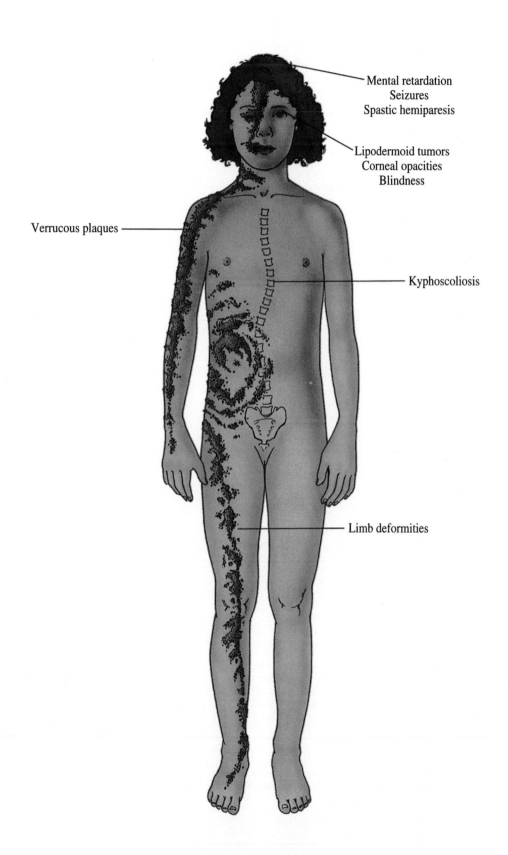

Mental retardation
Seizures
Spastic hemiparesis

Lipodermoid tumors
Corneal opacities
Blindness

Verrucous plaques

Kyphoscoliosis

Limb deformities

Suggested Reading

Ichthyosis Vulgaris

Cuevas-Covarrubias SA, Kofman-Alfaro SH, Palencia AB, et al. Accuracy of the clinical diagnosis of recessive X-linked ichthyosis vs ichthyosis vulgaris. *J Dermatol* 1996;23:594–597.

Dale BA, Sybert VP, Holbrook KA. Absence of filaggrin in patients affected with ichthyosis vulgaris. *J Invest Dermatol* 1984;82:399.

Hofmann B, Stege H, Ruzicka T, Lehmann P. Effect of topical tazarotene in the treatment of congenital ichthyoses. *Br J Dermatol* 1999;141:642–646.

Mevorah B, Marazi A, Frenk E. The prevalence of accentuated palmoplantar markings and keratosis pilaris in atopic dermatitis, autosomal dominant ichthyosis and control dermatological patients. *Br J Dermatol* 1985;112:679–685.

Nirunsuksiri W, Presland RB, Brumbaugh SG, et al. Decreased profilaggrin expression in ichthyosis vulgaris is a result of selectively impaired posttranscriptional control. *Biol Chem* 1995;270:871–876.

Okulicz JF, Schwartz RA. Hereditary and acquired ichthyosis vulgaris. *Int J Dermatol* 2003;42:95–98.

Presland RB, Boggess D, Lewis SP, et al. Loss of normal profilaggrin and filaggrin in flaky tail (ft/ft) mice: an animal model for the filaggrin-deficient skin disease ichthyosis vulgaris. *J Invest Dermatol* 2000;115:1072–1081.

Shwayder T. Disorders of keratinization: diagnosis and management. *Am J Clin Dermatol* 2004;5:17–29.

Sybert VP, Dale BA, Holbrook KA. Ichthyosis vulgaris: identification of a defect in synthesis of filaggrin correlated with an absence of keratohyaline granules. *J Invest Dermatol* 1985;84:191–194.

Wells RS, Kerr CB. Clinical features of autosomal dominant and X-linked recessive ichthyosis in an English population. *Br Med J* 1966;1:947–950.

Williams ML. Ichthyosis: mechanisms of disease. *Pediatr Dermatol* 1992;9:365–368.

Williams ML, Elias PM. Genetically transmitted, generalized disorders of cornification. The ichthyoses. *Dermatol Clin* 1987;5:155–178.

Zhong W, Cui B, Zhang Y, et al. Linkage analysis suggests a locus of ichthyosis vulgaris on 1q22. *J Hum Genet* 2003;48:390–392.

X-Linked Ichthyosis

Alperin ES, Shapiro LJ. Characterization of point mutations in patients with X-linked ichthyosis. Effects on the structure and function of the steroid sulfatase protein. *J Biol Chem* 1997;272:20756–20763.

Basler E, Grompe M, Parenti G, et al. Identification of point mutations in the steroid sulfatase gene of three patients with X-linked ichthyosis. *Am J Hum Genet* 1992;50:483–491.

Bradshaw KD, Carr BR. Placental sulfatase deficiency: maternal and fetal expression of steroid sulfatase deficiency and X-linked ichthyosis. *Obstet Gynecol Surv* 1986;41:401–413.

Costagliola C, Fabbrocini G, Illiano GM, et al. Ocular findings in X-linked ichthyosis: a survey of 38 cases. *Ophthalmologica* 1991;202:152–155.

Cuevas-Covarrubias SA, Jimenez-Vaca AL, Gonzalez-Huerta LM, et al. Somatic and germinal mosaicism for the steroid sulfatase gene deletion in a steroid sulfatase deficiency carrier. *J Invest Dermatol* 2002;119:972–975.

Elias PM, Crumrine D, Rassner U, et al. Basis for abnormal desquamation and permeability barrier dysfunction in RXLI. *J Invest Dermatol* 2004;122:314–319.

Epstein EH Jr, Krauss RM, Shackleton CHL. X-linked ichthyosis: increased blood cholesterol sulfate and electrophoretic mobility of low-density lipoprotein. *Science* 1981;214:659–660.

Jensen TG, Jensen UB, Jensen PK, et al. Correction of steroid sulfatase deficiency by gene transfer into basal cells of tissue-cultured epidermis from patients with recessive X-linked ichthyosis. *Exp Cell Res* 1993;209:392–397.

Keren DF, Canick JA, Johansen MZ, et al. Low maternal serum unconjugated estriol during prenatal screening as an indication of placental steroid sulfatase deficiency and X-linked ichthyosis. *Am J Clin Pathol* 1995;103:400–403.

Mevorah B, Krayenbuhl A, Bovey EH, et al. Autosomal dominant ichthyosis and X-linked ichthyosis: comparison of their clinical and histological phenotypes. *Acta Derm Venereol* 1991;71:431–434.

Oyama N, Satoh M, Iwatsuki K, et al. Novel point mutations in the steroid sulfatase gene in patients with X-linked ichthyosis: transfection analysis using the mutated genes. *J Invest Dermatol* 2000;114:1195–1199.

Paige DG, Emilion GG, Bouloux PM, et al. A clinical and genetic study of X-linked recessive ichthyosis and contiguous gene defects. *Br J Dermatol* 1994;131:622–629.

Shwayder T. Disorders of keratinization: diagnosis and management. *Am J Clin Dermatol* 2004;5:17–29.

Sugawara T, Shimizu H, Hoshi N, et al. PCR diagnosis of X-linked ichthyosis: identification of a novel mutation (E560P) of the steroid sulfatase gene. *Hum Mutat* 2000;15:296.

Traupe H, Happle R. Clinical spectrum of steroid sulfatase deficiency: X-linked recessive ichthyosis, birth complications and cryptorchidism. *Eur J Pediatr* 1983;140:19–21.

Valdes-Flores M, Kofman-Alfaro SH, Vaca AL, et al. Mutation report: a novel partial deletion of exons 2–10 of the STS gene in recessive X-linked ichthyosis. *J Invest Dermatol* 2000;114:591–593.

Watanabe T, Fujimori K, Kato K, et al. Prenatal diagnosis for placental steroid sulfatase deficiency with fluorescence in situ hybridization: a case of X-linked ichthyosis. *J Obstet Gynaecol Res* 2003;29:427–430.

Epidermolytic Hyperkeratosis

Bale SJ, Compton JG, DiGiovanna JJ. Epidermolytic hyperkeratosis. *Semin Dermatol* 1993;12:202–209.

Chipev CC, Yang JM, DiGiovanna JJ, et al. Preferential sites in keratin 10 that are mutated in epidermolytic hyperkeratosis. *Am J Hum Genet* 1994;54:179–190.

Compton JG, DiGiovanna JJ, Santucci SK, et al. Linkage of epidermolytic hyperkeratosis to the type II keratin gene cluster on chromosome 12q. *Nat Genet* 1992;1:301–305.

DiGiovanna JJ, Bale SJ. Clinical heterogeneity in epidermolytic hyperkeratosis. *Arch Dermatol* 1994;130:1026–1035.

DiGiovanna JJ, Robinson-Bostom L. Ichthyosis: etiology, diagnosis, and management. *Am J Clin Dermatol* 2003;4:81–95.

Ganemo A, Lindholm C, Lindberg M, et al. Quality of life in adults with congenital ichthyosis. *J Adv Nurs* 2003;44:412–419.

Leigh IM, Lane EB. Mutations in the genes for epidermal keratins in epidermolysis bullosa and epidermolytic hyperkeratosis. *Arch Dermatol* 1993;129:1571–1577.

Nazzaro V, Ermacora E, Santucci B, et al. Epidermolytic hyperkeratosis: generalized form in children from parents with systematized linear form. *Br J Dermatol* 1990;122:417–422.

Paller AS, Syder AJ, Chan YM, et al. Genetic and clinical mosaicism in a type of epidermal nevus. *N Engl J Med* 1994;331:1408.

Rothnagel JA, Dominey AM, Dempsey LD, et al. Mutations in the rod domains of keratins 1 and 10 in epidermolytic hyperkeratosis. *Science* 1992;257:1128–1130.

Rothnagel JA, Longley MA, Holder RA, et al. Prenatal diagnosis of epidermolytic hyperkeratosis by direct gene sequencing. *J Invest Dermatol* 1994;102:13–16.

Virtanen M, Smith SK, Gedde-Dahl T Jr, et al. Splice site and deletion mutations in keratin (KRT1 and KRTI0) genes: unusual phenotypic alterations in Scandinavian patients with epidermolytic hyperkeratosis. *J Invest Dermatol* 2003;121:1013–1020.

Williams ML, Elias PM. Enlightened therapy of the disorders of cornification. *Clin Dermatol* 2003;21:269–273.

Lamellar Ichthyosis

Allen DM, Esterly NB. Significant systemic absorption of tacrolimus after topical application in a patient with lamellar ichthyosis. *Arch Dermatol* 2002;138:1259–1260.

Candi E, Oddi S, Paradisi A, et al. Expression of transglutaminase 5 in normal and pathologic human epidermis. *J Invest Dermatol* 2002;119:670–677.

Choate KA, Medalie DA, Morgan JR, et al. Corrective gene transfer in the human skin disorder lamellar ichthyosis. *Nat Med* 1996;2:1263–1267.

Ganemo A, Lindholm C, Lindberg M, et al. Quality of life in adults with congenital ichthyosis. *J Adv Nurs* 2003;44:412–419.

Happle R, van de Kerkhof PC, Traupe H. Retinoids in disorders of keratinization: their use in adults. *Dermatologica* 1987;175:107–124.

Hennies HC, Kuster W, Wiebe V, et al. Genotype/phenotype correlation in autosomal recessive lamellar ichthyosis. *Am J Hum Genet* 1998;62:1052–1061.

Huber M, Limat A, Wagner E, et al. Efficient in vitro transfection of human keratinocytes with an adenovirus-enhanced receptor-mediated system. *J Invest Dermatol* 2000;114:661–666.

Huber N, Rettler I, Bernasconi K, et al. Mutations of keratinocyte transglutaminase in lamellar ichthyosis. *Science* 1995;267:525–528

Larregue M, Ottavy N, Bressieux JM, et al. Collodion baby: 32 new case reports. *Ann Derm Venereol* 1986;113:773–785.

Marulli GC, Campione E, Chimenti MS, et al. Type I lamellar ichthyosis improved by tazarotene 0.1% gel. *Clin Exp Dermatol* 2003;28:391–393.

Muramatsu S, Suga Y, Kon J, et al. A Japanese patient with a mild form of lamellar ichthyosis harbouring two missense mutations in the core domain of the transglutaminase 1 gene. *Br J Dermatol* 2004;150:390–392.

Pigg M, Gedde-Dahl T, Jr, Cox D, et al. Strong founder effect for a transglutaminase 1 gene mutation in lamellar ichthyosis and congenital ichthyosiform erythroderma from Norway. *Eur J Hum Genet* 1998;6:589–596.

Raghunath M, Hennies HC, Velten F, et al. A novel in situ method for the detection of deficient transglutaminase activity in the skin. *Arch Dermatol Res* 1998;290:621–627.

Russell LJ, DiGiovanna JJ, Rogers GR, et al. Mutations in the gene for transglutaminase 1 in autosomal recessive lamellar ichthvosis. *Nat Genet* 1995;9:279–283.

Schorderet DF, Huber M, Laurini RN, et al. Prenatal diagnosis of lamellar ichthyosis by direct mutational analysis of the keratinocyte transglutaminase gene. *Prenat Diagn* 1997;17:483–486.

Shevchenko YO, Compton JG, Toro JR, et al. Splice-site mutation in TGM1 in congenital recessive ichthyosis in American families: molecular, genetic, genealogic, and clinical studies. *Hum Genet* 2000;106:492–499.

Tok J, Garzon MC, Cserhalmi-Friedman P, et al. Identification of mutations in the transglutaminase 1 gene in lamellar ichthyosis. *Exp Dermatol* 1999;8:128–133.

Van Gysel D, Lijnen RL, Moekti SS, et al. Collodion baby: a follow-up study of 17 cases. *J Eur Acad Dermatol Venereol* 2002;16:472–475.

Williams ML, Elias PM. Heterogeneity in autosomal recessive ichthyosis: clinical and biochemical differentiation of lamellar ichthyosis and nonbullous congenital ichthyosiform erythroderma. *Arch Dermatol* 1985;121:477–488.

Yang JM, Ahn KS, Cho MO, et al. Novel mutations of the transglutaminase 1 gene in lamellar ichthyosis. *J Invest Dermatol* 2001;117:214–218.

Congenital Ichthyosiform Erythroderma

Bernhardtt M, Baden HP. Report of a family with an unusual expression of recessive ichthyosis: review of 42 cases. *Arch Dermatol* 1986;122:428–433.

Choate KA, Williams ML, Khavari PA. Abnormal transglutaminase 1 expression pattern in a subset of patients with erythrodermic autosomal recessive ichthyosis. *J Invest Dermatol* 1998;110:8–12.

DiGiovanna JJ, Peck GL. Oral synthetic retinoid treatment in children. *Pediatr Dermatol* 1983;1:77.

Hazell M, Marks R. Clinical, histologic, and cell kinetic discriminants between lamellar ichthyosis and nonbullous congenital ichthyosiform erythroderma. *Arch Dermatol* 1985;121:489–493.

Hennies HC, Kuster W, Wiebe V, et al. Genotype/phenotype correlation in autosomal recessive lamellar ichthyosis. *Am J Hum Genet* 1998;62:1052–1061.

Huber M, Rettler I, Bernasconi K, et al. Mutations of keratinocyte transglutaminase in lamellar ichthyosis. *Science* 1995;267:525–528.

Larregue M, Ottavy N, Bressieux JM, et al. Collodion baby: 32 new case reports. *Ann Dermatol Venereol* 1986;113:773–785.

Matsumoto K, Muto M, Seki S, et al: Loricrin keratoderma: A cause of congenital ichthyosiform erythroderma and collodion baby. *Br J Dermatol* 2001;145:657–660.

Shevchenko YO, Compton JG, Toro JR, et al.Splice-site mutation in TGM1 in congenital recessive ichthyosis in American families: molecular, genetic, genealogic, and clinical studies. *Hum Genet* 2000;106:492–499.

Williams ML, Elias PM. Enlightened therapy of the disorders of cornification. *Clin Dermatol* 2003;21:269–273.

Harlequin Fetus

Akiyama M, Sawamura D, Shimizu H. The clinical spectrum of nonbullous congenital ichthyosiform erythroderma and lamellar ichthyosis. *Clin Exp Dermatol*. 2003;28:235–240.

Arita K, Akiyama M. Tsuji Y, et al. Squamous cell carcinoma in a patient with non-bullous congenital ichthyosiform erythroderma. *Br J Dermatol* 2003;148:367–369.

Becker K, Csikos M, Sardy M, et al. Identification of two novel nonsense mutations in the transglutaminase 1 gene in a Hungarian patient with congenital ichthyosiform erythroderma. *Exp Dermatol* 2003;12:324–329.

Bianca S, Ingegnosi C, Bonaffini F. Harlequin foetus. *J Postgrad Med* 2003;49:81–82.

Chan YC, Tay YK, Tan LK, et al. Harlequin ichthyosis in association with hypothyroidism and juvenile rheumatoid arthritis. *Pediatr Dermatol* 2003;20:421–426.

Chua CN, Ainsworth J. Ocular management of harlequin syndrome. *Arch Ophthalmol* 2001;119:454–455.

Culican SM, Custer PL. Repair of cicatricial ectropion in an infant with harlequin ichthyosis using engineered human skin. *Am J Ophthalmol* 2002;134:442–443.

Dale BA, Holbrook KA, Fleckman P, et al. Heterogeneity in harlequin ichthyosis, an inborn error of epidermal keratinization: variable morphology and structural protein expression and a defect in lamellar granules. *J Invest Dermatol* 1990;94:6–18.

DiGiovanna JJ, Robinson-Bostom L. Ichthyosis: etiology, diagnosis, and management. *Am J Clin Dermatol* 2003;4:81–95.

Dunnwald M, Zuberi AR, Stephens K, et al. The ichq mutant mouse, a model for the human skin disorder harlequin ichthyosis: mapping, keratinocyte culture, and consideration of candidate genes involved in epidermal growth regulation. *Exp Dermatol* 2003;12:245–254.

Haftek M, Cambazard F, Dhouailly D, et al. A longitudinal study of a harlequin infant presenting clinically as non-bullous congenital ichthyosiform erythroderma. *Br J Dermatol* 1996;135:448.

Lawlor F. Progress of a harlequin fetus to nonbullous ichthyosiform erythroderma. *Pediatrics* 1988;82:870–873.

Lawlor F, Peiris S. Progress of a harlequin fetus treated with etretinate. *J R Soc Med* 1985;11:19–20.

Michel M, Fleckman P, Smith IT, et al. The calcium-activated neutral protease calpain I is present in normal foetal skin and is decreased in neonatal harlequin ichthyosis. *Br J Dermatol* 1999;141:1017–1026.

Roberts LJ. Long-term survival of a harlequin fetus. *J Am Acad Dermatol* 1989;21:335–340.

Sarkar R, Sharma RC, Sethi S, et al. Three unusual siblings with harlequin ichthyosis in an Indian family. *J Dermatol* 2000;27:609–611.

Singh S, Bhura M, Maheshwari A, et al. Successful treatment of harlequin ichthyosis with acitretin. *Int J Dermatol* 2001;40:472–473.

Smith SH, Gaunt L, Moore L, et al. De novo deletion of chromosome 18q in a baby with harlequin ichthyosis. *Am J Med Genet* 2001;102:342–345.

Vohra N, Rochelson B, Smith-Levitin M. Three-dimensional sonographic findings in congenital (harlequin) ichthyosis. *J Ultrasound Med* 2003;22:737–739.

Sjögren-Larsson Syndrome

De Laurenzi V, Rogers GR, Hamrock DJ, et al. Sjögren-Larsson syndrome is caused by mutations in the fatty aldehyde dehydrogenase gene. *Nat Genet* 1996;12:52.

DiGiovanna JJ, Robinson-Bostom L. Ichthyosis: etiology, diagnosis, and management. *Am J Clin Dermatol* 2003;4:81–95.

Fernandez-Vozmediano JM, Armario-Hita JC, Gonzalez-Cabrerizo A. Sjogren-Larsson syndrome: treatment with topical calcipotriol. *Pediatr Dermato* 2003;20:179–180.

Gomori JM, Leibovici V, Zlotogorski A, et al. Computed tomography in Sjögren-Larsson syndrome. *Neuroradiology* 1987;29:557–559.

Haddad FS, Lacour M, Harper JI, et al. The orthopaedic presentation and management of Sjögren–Larsson syndrome. *J Pediatr Orthop* 1999;19:617–619.

Jagell S, Gustayson K, Holmgren G. Sjögren-Larsson syndrome in Sweden: a clinical, genetic and epidemiological study. *Clin Genet* 1981;19:233–256.

Levisohn D, Dintiman B, Rizzo WB. Sjögren-Larsson syndrome: case reports. *Pediatr Dermatol* 1991;8:217–220.

Rizzo WB. Sjögren-Larsson syndrome. *Semin Dermatol* 1993;12:210–218.

Rizzo WB, Carney G, Lin Z. The molecular basis of Sjögren–Larsson syndrome: mutation analysis of the fatty aldehyde dehydrogenase gene. *Am J Hum Genet* 1999;65:1547–1560.

Rizzo WB, Craft DA. Sjögren–Larsson syndrome: accumulation of free fatty alcohols in cultured fibroblasts and plasma. *J Lipid Res* 2000;41:1077–1081.

Rizzo WB, Craft DA. Sjögren-Larsson syndrome. Deficient activity of the fatty aldehyde dehydrogenase component of fatty alcohol: NAD$^+$ oxidoreductase in cultured fibroblasts, *J Clin Invest* 1991;88:1643–1648.

Rizzo WB, Lin Z, Carney G. Fatty aldehyde dehydrogenase: genomic structure. expression and mutation analysis in Sjögren-Larsson syndrome. *Chem Biol Interact* 2001;130–132:297–307.

Sillen A, Holmgren G, Wadelius C. First prenatal diagnosis by mutation analysis in a family with Sjogren-Larsson syndrome. *Prenat Diagn* 1997;17:1147–1149.

Tabsh K, Rizzo WB, Holbrook K, et al. Sjögren-Larsson syndrome: technique and timing of prenatal diagnosis. *Obstet Gynecol* 1993;82:700–703.

Van Den Brink DM, Van Miert JN, Dacremont G, et al. Identification of fatty aldehyde dehydrogenase in the breakdown of phytol to phytanic acid. *Mol Genet Metab* 2004;82:33–37.

Willemsen MA, Van Der Graaf M, Van Der Knaap MS, et al. MR imaging and proton MR spectroscopic studies in Sjogren-Larsson syndrome: characterization of the leukoencephalopathy. *AJNR Am J Neuroradiol* 2004;25:649–657.

Refsum Syndrome

Bamiou DE, Spraggs PR, Gibberd FB, et al. Hearing loss in adult Refsum's disease. *Clin Otolaryngol* 2003;28:227–230.

Brown FR, Voigt R, Singh AK, et al. Peroxisomal disorders. Neurodevelopmental and biochemical aspects. *Am J Dis Child* 1993;147:617–626.

Claridge KG, Gibberd FB, Sidey MC. Refsum disease: the presentation and ophthalmic aspects of Refsum disease in a series of 23 patients. *Eye* 1992;6:371–375.

Jansen GA, Ofman R, Ferdinandusse S, et al. Refsum disease is caused by mutations in the phytanoyl-CoA hydroxylase gene. *Nat Genet* 1007;17:190–193.

Jansen GA, Ferdinandusse S, Hogenhout EM, et al. Phytanoyl-CoA hydroxylase deficiency. Enzymological and molecular basis of classical Refsum disease. *Adv Exp Med Biol* 1999;466:371–376.

Jansen GA, Waterham HR, Wanders RJ. Molecular basis of Refsum disease: sequence variations in phytanoyl-CoA hydroxylase (PHYH) and the PTS2 receptor (PEX7). *Hum Mutat* 2004;23:209–218.

Leroy BP, Hogg CR, Rath PR, et al. Clinical features & retinal function in patients with adult Refsum syndrome. *Adv Exp Med Biol* 2003;544:57–58.

Masters-Thomas A, Bailes J, Billimoria JD, et al. Heredopathia atactica polyneuritiformis (Refsum's disease): I. Clinical features and dietary management. *J Hum Nutr* 1980;34:245–250.

Mihalik SJ, Morrell JC, Kim D, et al. Identification of PAHX, a Refsum disease gene. *Nat Genet* 1997;17:185–189.

Poulos A, Pollard AX, Michell JD, et al. Patterns of Refsum's disease: phytanic acid oxidase deficiency. *Arch Dis Child* 1984;59:222–229.

Steinberg D, Herndon JH, Uhlendorf BW, et al. Refsum's disease: nature of the enzyme defect. *Science* 1967;156:1740–1742.

Straube R, Gackler D, Thiele A, et al. Membrane differential filtration is safe and effective for the long-term treatment of Refsum syndrome—an update of treatment modalities and pathophysiological cognition. *Transfus Apheresis Sci* 2003;29:85–91.

van den Brink DM, Brites P, Haasjes J, et al. Identification of PEX7 as the second gene involved in Refsum disease. *Am J Hum Genet* 2003;72:471–477.

Wanders RJ, Jansen GA, Skjeldal OH. Refsum disease, peroxisomes and phytanic acid oxidation: a review. *J Neuropathol Exp Neurol* 2001;60:1021–1031.

Conradi-Hünermann Syndrome

Becker K, Csikos M, Horvath A, et al. Identification of a novel mutation in 3beta-hydroxysterol-Delta8-Delta7-isomerase in a case of Conradi-Hünermann-Happle syndrome. *Exp Dermatol* 2001;10:286.

Curry CJ, Magenis RE, Brown M, at al. Inherited chondrodysplasia punctata due to a deletion of the terminal short arm of an X chromosome. *N Engl J Med* 1984;311:1010–1015.

Has C, Bruckner-Tuderman L, Muller D, et al. The Conradi–Hünermann–Happle syndrome (CDPX2) and emopamil binding protein: novel mutations, and somatic and gonadal mosaicism. *Hum Mol Genet* 2000;13:1951–1955.

Hoang MP, Carder KR, Pandya AG, et al. Ichthyosis and keratotic follicular plugs containing dystrophic calcification in newborns: distinctive histopathologic features of x-linked dominant chondrodysplasia punctata (Conradi-Hunermann-Happle syndrome). *Am J Dermatopathol* 2004;26:53–58.

Ikegawa S, Chashi H, Kogata T, et al. Novel and recurrent EBP mutations in X-linked dominant chondrodysplasia punctata. *Am J Med Genet* 2000;94:300–305.

Kolde G. Happle R. Histologic and ultrastructural features of the ichthyotic skin in X-linked dominant chondrodysplasia punctata. *Acta Derm Venereol* 1984;64:389.

Paltzik RL, Ente G, Panzer PH, et al. Conradi-Hünermann disease: case report and minireview. *Cutis* 1982;29:174–180.

Sheffield LJ, Danks EM, Mayne V, et al. Chondrodysplasia punctata: 23 cases of a mild and relatively common variety. *J Pediatr* 1976;89:916–923.

Shwayder T. Disorders of keratinization: diagnosis and management. *Am J Clin Dermatol* 2004;5:17–29.

Silengo MC, Luzzatti L, Silverman FN. Clinical and genetic aspects of Conradi-Hünermann disease: a report of three familial cases and review of the literature. *J Pediatr* 1908;97:911–917.

Whittock NV, Izatt L, Simpson-Dent SL, et al. Molecular prenatal diagnosis in a case of an X-linked dominant chondrodysplasia punctata. *Prenat Diagn* 2003;23:701–704.

CHILD Syndrome

Bittar M, Happle R. CHILD syndrome avant la lettre. *J Am Acad Dermatol* 2004;50:S34–S37.

Caldas H, Herman GE. NSDHL, an enzyme involved in cholesterol biosynthesis, traffics through the Golgi and accumulates on ER membranes and on the surface of lipid droplets. *Hum Mol Genet* 2003;12:2981–2991.

Enami S, Rizzo WB, Hanley KP, et al. Peroxisomal abnormality in fibroblasts from involved skin of CHILD syndrome. Case study and review of peroxisomal disorders in relation to skin disease. *Arch Dermatol* 1992;128:1213–1222.

Falek A, Heath CW, Ebbin AJ, et al. Unilateral limb and skin deformities with congenital heart disease in two siblings: a lethal syndrome. *J Pediatr* 1968;73:910–913.

Grange DK, Kratz LE, Braverman NE, et al. CHILD syndrome caused by deficiency of 3beta-hydroxysteroid-delta8, delta7-isomerase. *Am J Med Genet* 2000;90:328–335.

Happle R, Koch H, Lenz W. The CHILD syndrome. Congenital hemidysplasia with ichthyosiform erythroderma and limb defects. *Eur J Pediatr* 1980;134:27–33.

Hebert AA, Esterly NB, Holbrook KA, et al. The CHILD syndrome: histologic and ultrastructural studies. *Arch Dermatol* 1994;1:23.

Hummel M, Cunningham D, Mullett CJ, et al. Left-sided CHILD syndrome caused by a nonsense mutation in the NSDHL gene. *Am J Med Genet.* 2003;122A:246–251.

König A, Happle R, Bornholdt D, et al. Mutations in the NSDHL gene, encoding a 3β-hydroxysteroid dehydrogenase, cause CHILD syndrome. *Am J Med Genet* 2000;90:339.

Konig A, Happle R, Fink-Puches R, et al. A novel missense mutation of NSDHL in an unusual case of CHILD syndrome showing bilateral, almost symmetric involvement. *J Am Acad Dermatol* 2002;46:594–596.

Murata K, Shinkai H, Ishikiriyama S, et al. A unique point mutation in the NSDHL gene in a Japanese patient with CHILD syndrome. *J Dermatol Sci.* 2003;33:11:67–69.

Netherton Syndrome

Allen A, Siegfried E, Silverman R, et al. Significant absorption of topical tacrolimus in 3 patients with Netherton syndrome. *Arch Dermatol* 2001;137:747.

Bitoun E, Micheloni A, Lamant L, et al. LEKTI proteolytic processing in human primary keratinocytes, tissue distribution and defective expression in Netherton syndrome. *Hum Mol Genet* 2003;12:2417–2430.

Capezzera R, Venturini M, Bianchi D, et al. UVA1 phototherapy of Netherton syndrome. *Acta Derm Venereol* 2004;84:69–70.

Chavanas S, Bodemer C, Rochat A, et al. Mutations in SPINK5, encoding a serine protease inhibitor, cause Netherton syndrome. *Nat Genet* 2000;25:141–142.

Greene SL, Muller SA. Netherton's syndrome: report of a case and review of the literature. *J Am Acad Dermatol* 1985;13:329–337.

Krafchik BR. What syndrome is this? Netherton syndrome. *Pediatr Dermatol* 1992;9:157–160.

Sprecher E, Chavanas S, DiGiovanna JJ, et al. The spectrum of pathogenic mutations in SPINK5 in 19 families with Netherton syndrome: implications for mutation detection and first case of prenatal diagnosis. *J Invest Dermatol* 2001;117:179–187.

Walley AJ, Chavanas S, Moffatt MF, et al. Gene polymorphism in Netherton and common atopic disease. *Nat Genet* 2001;29:175–178.

Erythrokeratoderma Variabilis

Graham-Brown RA, Chave TA. Acitretin for erythrokeratodermia variabilis in a 9-year-old girl. *Pediatr Dermatol* 2002;19:510–512.

Luy JT, Jacobs AH, Nickoloff BJ. A child with erythematous and hyperkeratotic patches: erythrokeratodermia variabilis. *Arch Dermatol* 1988;124:1271–1272.

Macari F, Landau M, Cousin P, et al: Mutation in the gene for connexin 30.3 in a family with erythrokeratodermia variabilis. *Ana J Hum Genet* 2000;67:1296–1301.

Plantard L, Huber M, Macari F, et al. Molecular interaction of connexin 30.3 and connexin 31 suggests a dominant-negative mechanism associated with erythrokeratodermia variabilis. *Hum Mol Genet* 2003;12:3287–3294.

Richard G, Smith LG, Bailey RA, et al. Mutations in the human connexin gene GJB3 cause erythrokeratodermia variabilis. *Nat Genet* 1998;20:366–369.

Richard G, Brown N, Smith LE, et al. The spectrum of mutations in erythrokeratodermias—novel and de novo mutations in GJB3. *Hum Genet* 2000;106:321–329.

Richard G, Lin JP, Smith L, et al. Linkage studies in erythrokeratodermias: Fine mapping genetic heterogeneity, and analysis of candidate genes. *J Invest Dermatol* 1997;109:666–671.

Richard G, Smith LE, Bailey RA, et al. Mutations in the human connexin gene GJB3 Cause erythrokeratodermia variabilis. *Nat Genet* 1998;20:366–369.

Richard G, Brown N, Rouan F, et al. Genetic heterogeneity in erythrokeratodermia variabilis: novel mutations in the connexin gene GJB4 (Cx30.3) and genotype-phenotype correlations. *J Invest Dermatol* 2003;120:601–609.

Schnyder UW, Sommacal-Schopf D. Fourteen cases of erythrokeratodermia figurata variabilis within one family. *Acta Genet Statist* 1957;7:204–206.

Strober BE. Erythrokeratodermia variabilis. *Dermatol Online J* 2003;9:5.

Terrinoni A, Leta A, Pedicelli C, et al. A novel recessive connexin 31 (GJB3) mutation in a case of erythrokeratodermia variabilis. *J Invest Dermatol* 2004;122:837–839.

KID Syndrome

Caceres-Rios H, Tamayo-Sanchez L, Duran-Mckinster C, et al. Keratitis, ichthyosis and deafness (KID syndrome): review of the literature and proposal of a new terminology. *Pediatr Dermatol* 1996;13:105–113

Langer K, Konrad K, Wolff K. Keratitis, ichthyosis and deafness (KID)-syndrome: report of three cases and a review of the literature. *Br J Dermatol* 1990;122:689–697.

Madariaga J, Fromowitz F, Phillips M, et al. Squamous cell carcinoma in congenita ichthyosis with deafness and keratitis: a case report and review of the literature. *Cancer* 1986;57:2026–2029.

Morris MR, Namon A, Shaw GY, et al. The keratitis, ichthyosis, and deafness syndrome. *Otolaryngol Head Neck Surg* 1991;104:526–528.

Nazzaro V, Blanchet-Bardon C, Lorette G, et al. Familial occurrence of KID (keratitis, ichthyosis, deafness) syndrome. Case reports of a mother and daughter. *J Am Acad Dermatol* 1990;23:385–388.

Richard G, Ronan F, Willoughby CE, et al. (2002) Missense mutations in GIB2 encoding connexin-26 cause the ectodermal dysplasia keratitis-ichthyosis-deafness syndrome. *Am J Hum Genet* 2002;70:1341–1348.

Van Steensel MA, van Geel M, Nahuys M, et al. A novel connexin-26 mutation in a patient diagnosed with keratitis-ichthyosis-deafness syndrome. *J Invest Dermatol* 2002;118:724–727.

Sonoda S, Uchino L, Sonoda KH, et al. Two patients with severe corneal disease in KID syndrome. *Am J Ophthalmol* 2004;137:181–183.

Miura H, Shoda Y, Adachi J. Marked hyperkeratosis of the soles in keratitis-ichthyosis-deafness syndrome: treatment with hydrocolloid dressing. *Cutis* 2003;72:229–230.

Miteva L. Keratitis, ichthyosis, and deafness (KID) syndrome. *Pediatr Dermatol* 2002;19:513–516.

Sahoo B, Handa S, Kaur I, et al. KID syndrome: response to acitretin. *J Dermatol* 2002;29:499–502.

Szymko-Bennett YM, Russell LJ, Bale SJ, et al. Auditory manifestations of Keratitis-Ichthyosis-Deafness (KID) syndrome. Laryngoscope. 2002;112:272–280.

Yotsumoto S, Hiashiguchi T, Chen X, et al. Novel mutations in GJB2 encoding connexin-26 in Japanese patients with keratitisichthyosis-deafness syndrome. *Br J Dermatol* 2003;148:649–653.

Diffuse Palmoplantar Keratoderma

Devos SA, Delescluse J. An unusual case of palmoplantar keratoderma. *J Eur Acad Dermatol Venereol* 2003;17:68–69.

Drechsler M, Schrock E, Royer-Pokora B, et al. Keratin 9 gene mutations in epidermolytic palmoplantar keratoderma (EPPK). *Nat Genet* 1994;6:174–179.

Hatsell SJ, Eady RA, Wennerstrand L, et al. Novel splice-site mutation in keratin 1 underlies mild epidermolytic palmoplantar keratoderma in three kindreds. *J Invest Dermatol* 2001;116:606–609.

Hennies HC, Zehender D, Kunze J, et al. Keratin 9 gene mutational heterogeneity in patients with epidermolytic palmoplantar keratoderma. *Hum Genet* 1994;93:649–654.

Kelsell DP, Stevens HP, Purkis PE, et al. Fine genetic mapping of diffuse non-epidermolytic palmoplantar keratoderma to chromosome 12g11–q13: exclusion of the mapped type II keratins. *Exp Dermatol* 1999;8:388–391.

Kobayashi S, Tanaka T, Matsuyoshi N, et al. Keratin 9 point mutation in the pedigree of epidermolytic hereditary palmoplantar keratoderma perturbs keratin intermediate filament formation. *FEBS Lett* 1996;386:149–155.

Kuster W, Becker A. Indication for the identity of palmoplantar keratoderma type Unna-Thost with type Vörner: Thost's family revisited 110 years later *Acta Derm Venereol* 1992;72: 120–122.

Reis A, Hennies HC, Langbein L, et al. Keratin 9 gene mutations in epidermolytic palmoplantar keratoderma (EPPK). *Nat Genet* 1994;6:174–179.

Szalai S, Szalai C, Becker K, et al. Keratin 9 mutations in the coil 1A region in epidermolytic palmoplantar keratoderma. *Pediatr Dermatol* 1999;16:430–435.

Tsunemi Y, Hattori N, Saeki H, et al. A keratin 9 Gene mutation (Asn160Ser) in a Japanese patient with epidermolytic palmoplantar keratoderma. *J Dermatol* 2002;29:768–772.

Howel-Evans Syndrome

Harper PS, Harper RMJ, Howel-Evans AW. Carcinoma of the oesophagus with tylosis. *Q J Med* 1970;39:317–333.

Howel-Evans W, McConnell RB, Clarke CA, et al. Carcinoma of the oesophagus with keratosis palmaris et plantaris (tylosis): a study of two families. *Q J Med* 1958;27:413–429.

Kelsell DP, Risk JM, Leigh IM, et al. Close mapping of focal non-epidemolytic palmoplantar keratoderma (PPK) locus associated with oesophageal cancer (TOC). *Hum Mol Genet* 1996;5:857–860.

Risk JM, Evans KE, Jones J, et al. Characterization of a 500 kb region on 17q25 and the exclusion of candidate genes as the familial Tylosis Oesophageal Cancer (TOC) locus. *Oncogene* 2002;21:5395–5402.

Risk JM, Ruhrberg C, Hennies H. Envoplakin, a possible candidate gene for focal NEPPK/esophageal cancer (TOC): the integration of genetic and physical maps of the TOC region on 17q25. *Genomics* 1999;59:234–242.

Stevens HP, Kelsell DP, Bryant SP, et al. Linkage of an American pedigree with palmoplantar keratoderma and malignancy (palmoplantar ectodermal dysplasia type III) to 17q24: literature survey and proposed updated classification of the palmoplantar keratodermas. *Arch Dermatol* 1996;132:640–651.

von Brevern M, Holistein MC, Risk JM, et al. Loss of heterozygosity in sporadic oesophageal tumors in the tylosis oesophageal cancer (TOC) gene region of chromosome 17g. *Oncogene* 1998;17:2101–2105.

Vohwinkel Syndrome

Atabay K, Yavuzer R, Latifoglu O, Ozmen S. Keratoderma hereditarium mutilans (Vohwinkel syndrome): an unsolved surgical mystery. *Plast Reconstr Surg* 2001;108:1276–1280.

Bakirtzis G, Jamieson S, Aasen T, et al. The effects of a mutant connexin 26 on epidermal differentiation. *Cell Commun Adhes* 2003;10:359–364.

Bakirtzis G, Choudhry R, Aasen T, et al. Targeted epidermal expression of mutant Connexin 26(D66H) mimics true Vohwinkel syndrome and provides a model for the pathogenesis of dominant connexin disorders. *Hum Mol Genet* 2003;12:1737–1744.

Maestrini E, Korge BP, Ocana-Sierra J. et al. A missense mutation in connexin26, D66H, causes mutilating keratoderma with sensorineural deafness (Vohwinkel's syndrome) in three unrelated families. *Hum Mol Genet* 1999;8:1237–1243.

O'Driscoll J, Muston GC, McGrath JA, et al. A recurrent mutation in the loricrin gene underlies the ichthyotic variant of Vohwinkel syndrome. *Clin Exp Dermatol* 2002;27:243–246.

Pisoh T, Bhatia A, Oberlin C. Surgical correction of pseudo-ainhum in Vohwinkel syndrome. *J Hand Surg [Br]* 1995;20:338–341.

Reddy BS, Gupta SK. Mutilating keratoderma of Vohwinkel. *Int J Dermatol* 1983;22(9):530–533.

Richard G, White TW, Smith LE, et al. Functional defects of Cx26 resulting from a heterozygous missense mutation in a family with dominant deaf-mutism and palmoplantar keratoderma. *Hum Genet Oct* 1998;103:393–399.

Rivers JK, Duke EE, Justus DW. Etretinate: management of keratoma hereditaria mutilans in four family members. *J Am Acad Dermatol* 1985;13:43–49.

Schmuth M, Fluhr JW, Crumrine DC, et al. Structural and functional consequences of loricrin mutations in human loricrin keratoderma (vohwinkel syndrome with ichthyosis) *J Invest Dermatol* 2004;122(4):909–922.

Vohwinkel KH. Keratoma hereditarium mutilans. *Arch Derm Syph* 1929;158:354–364.

Mal de Meleda

Bergman R, Bitterman-Deutsch D, Fartasch M, et al. Mal de Meleda keratoderma with pseudo-ainhum. *Br J Dermatol* 1993;128:207–212.

Bouadjar B, Benmazouzia S, Prud'homme JF, et al. Clinical and genetic studies of 3 large, consanguineous, Algerian families with Mal de Meleda. *Arch Dermatol* 2000;136:1247–1252.

Chimienti F, Hogg RC, Plantard L, et al. Identification of SLURP-1 as an epidermal neuromodulator explains the clinical phenotype of Mal de Meleda. *Hum Mol Genet.* 2003;12:3017–3024.

Eckl KM, Stevens HP, Lestringant GG, et al. Mal de Meleda (MDM) caused by mutations in the gene for SLURP-1 in patients from Germany, Turkey, Palestine, and the United Arab Emirates. *Hum Genet* 2003;112: 50–56.

Fischer J, Bouadjar B, Heilig R, et al. Mutations in the gene encoding SLURP-1 in Mal de Meleda. *Hum Mol Genet* 2001;10:875–880.

Fischer J, Bouadjar B, Heilig R, et al. Genetic linkage of Meleda disease to chromosome 8qter. *Eur J Hum Genet* 1998;6:542–547.

Lestringant GG, Frossard PM, Adeghate E, et al. Mal de Meleda: a report of four cases from the United Arab Emirates. *Pediatr Dermatol* 1997;14:186–191.

Mastrangeli R, Donini S, Kelton CA, et al. ARS Component B: structural characterization, tissue expression and regulation of the gene and protein (SLURP-1) associated with Mal de Meleda. *Eur J Dermatol* 2003;13:560–570.

Marrakchi S, Audebert S, Bouadjar B, et al. Novel mutations in the gene encoding secreted lymphocyte antigen-6/urokinase-type plasminogen activator receptor-related protein-1 (SLURP-1) and description of five ancestral haplotypes in patients with Mal de Meleda. *J Invest Dermatol* 2003;120:351–355.

Mokni M, Charfeddine C, Ben Mously R, et al. Heterozygous manifestations in female carriers of Mal de Meleda. *Clin Genet* 2004;65:244–246.

Mozzillo N, Nunziata CA, Caraco C, et al. Melanoma Cooperative Group. Malignant melanoma developing in an area of hereditary palmoplantar keratoderma (Mal de Meleda). *J Surg Oncol* 2003;84:229–233.

Niles HD, Klumpp, MM. Mal de Meleda: review of the literature and report of four cases. *Arch Dermatol Syph* 1939;39:409–421.

Reed ML, Stanley J, Stengel F, et al. Mal de Meleda treated with 13-*cis*-retinoic acid. *Arch Dermatol* 1979;115:605–608.

Sybert VP, Dale BA, Holbrook KA. Palmar-plantar keratoderma. A clinical, ultrastructural, and biochemical study. *J Am Acad Dermatol* 1988;18:75–86.

Papillon-Lefèvre Syndrome

Allende LM, Moreno A, de Unamuno P. A genetic study of cathepsin C gene in two families with Papillon-Lefevre syndrome. *Mol Genet Metab* 2003;79:146–148.

Almuneef M, Al Khenaizan S, Al Ajaji S, Al-Anazi A. Pyogenic liver abscess and Papillon-Lefevre syndrome: not a rare association. *Pediatrics* 2003;111:e85–e88.

Battino M, Ferreiro MS, Quiles JL, et al. Alterations in the oxidation products, antioxidant markers, antioxidant capacity and lipid patterns in plasma of patients affected by Papillon-Lefèvre syndrome. *Free Radic Res* 2003;37:603–609.

de Haar SF, Jansen DC, Schoenmaker T, et al. Loss-of-function mutations in cathepsin C in two families with Papillon-Lefevre syndrome are associated with deficiency of serine proteinases in PMNs. *Hum Mutat* 2004;23:524.

Gelmetti C, Nazzaro V, Cerri D, et al. Long-term preservation of permanent teeth in a patient with Papillon-Lefèvre syndrome treated with etretinate. *Pediatr Dermatol* 1989;6:222–225.

Gorlin RJ, Sedano H, Anderson VE. The syndrome of palmar-plantar hyperkeratosis and premature periodontal destruction of the teeth: a clinical and genetic analysis of the Papillon-Lefévre syndrome. *J Pediatr* 1964;65:895–908.

Hart PS, Zhang Y, Firatli E, et al. Identification of cathepsin C mutation in ethnically diverse Papillon-Lefevre syndrome patients. *J Med Genet* 2000;37:927–932.

Hewitt C, McCormick D, Linden G, et al. The role of cathepsin C in Papillon-Lefevre syndrome, prepubertal periodontitis, and aggressive periodontitis. *Hum Mutat* 2004;23:222–228.

Kamen S, Crespi P, Eisenbud L, et al. Papillon-Lefèvre syndrome: pediatric dental management. *J Periodontol* 1986;10:356–364.

Kellum RE. Papillon-Lefèvre syndrome in four siblings treated with etretinate. A nine-year evaluation. *Int J Dermatol* 1989;28:605–608.

Laass MW, Hennies HC, Preis S, et al. Localisation of a gene for Papillon-Lefèvre syndrome to chromosome 11q14–q21 by homozygosity mapping. *Hum Genet* 1997;101:376–382.

Nakano A, Nomura K, Nakano H. Polymorphisms in the cathepsin C gene. *J Invest Dermatol* 116(2):339–343.

Noack B, Gorgens H, Hoffmann T, et al. Novel mutations in the cathepsin c gene in patients with pre-pubertal aggressive periodontitis and Papillon-Lefevre syndrome. *J Dent Res* 2004;83:368–370.

Pilger U, Hennies HC, Truschnegg A, et al. Late-onset Papillon-Lefevre syndrome without alteration of the cathepsin C gene. *J Am Acad Dermatol* 2003;49:S240–S243.

Toomes C, James J, Wood AJ, et al. Loss-of-function mutations in the cathepsin C gene result in periodontal disease and palmoplantar keratosis. *Nat Genet* 1999;23:421–424.

Ullbro C, Crossner CG, Nederfors T, et al. Dermatologic and oral findings in a cohort of 47 patients with Papillon-Lefèvre syndrome. *J Am Acad Dermatol* 2003;48:345–351.

Van Dyke TE, Taubman MA, Ebersole JL, et al. The Papillon-Lefèvre syndrome: neutrophil dysfunction with severe periodontal disease. *Clin Immunol Immunopathol* 1984;31:419.

Richner-Hanhart Syndrome

Barton DE, Yang-Feng, TL, Francke U. The human tyrosine aminotransferase gene mapped to the long arm of chromosome 16 (region 16g22–q24) by somatic cell hybrid analysis and in situ hybridization. *Hum Genet* 1986;72:221–224.

Benoldi D, Orsoni JB, Allegra F (1997) Tyrosinemia type II: a challenge for ophthalmologists and dermatologists. *Pediatr Dermatol* 1997;14:110–112.

Goldsmith LA. Tyrosinemia II: a large North Carolina kindred. *Arch Intern Med* 1985;145:1697–1700.

Farag TI. Dietetic therapy of Richner-Hanhart syndrome. *J R Soc Med* 1993;86:495.

Huhn R, Stoermer H, Klingele B, et al. Novel and recurrent tyrosine aminotransferase gene mutations in tyrosinemia type II. *Hum Genet* 1998;102:305–313.

Machino H, Miki Y, Kawatsu T, et al. Successful dietary control of tyrosinemia II. *J Am Acad Dermatol* 1983;9:533–539.

Mitchell G, Grompe M, Lambert M, et al. Hypertyrosinemia. In: Scriver CR, Beaudet A, Sly W, Valle, eds. *The metabolic and molecular bases of inherited disease.* 8th ed. New York: McGraw-Hill, 2001:1777.

Rabinowitz LG, Williams LR, Anderson CE. et al. Painful keratoderma and photophobia: hallmarks of tyrosinaemia type II. *J Pediatr* 1995;126:266–269.

Rettenmeier R, Natt E, Zentgraf H, et al. Isolation and characterization of the human tyrosine aminotransferase gene. *Nucleic Acids Res* 1990;18:3853–3861.

Sammartino A, de Crecchio G, Balato N, et al. Familial RichnerHanhart syndrome: genetic, clinical, and metabolic studies. *Ann Ophthalmol* 1984;16:1069–1074.

Tallab TM. Richner-Hanhart syndrome: importance of early diagnosis and early intervention. *J Am Acad Dermatol* 1996;35:857–859.

Darier Disease

Bashir R, Munro CS, Mason S, et at. Localisation of a gene for Darier's disease. *Hum Mol Genet* 1993;2:1937–1939.

Burge SM. Darier's disease and other dyskeratoses: response to retinoids. *Pharmacol Ther* 1989;40:75–90.

Burge S. Management of Darier's disease. *Clin Exp Dermatol* 1999;24:53.

Burge SM, Wilkinson JD. Darier-White disease: a review of the clinical features in 163 patients. *J Am Acad Dermatol* 1992;27:40–50.

Buxton RS. Yet another skin defect, Darier's disease, maps to chromosome 12q. *Hum Mol Genet* 1993;2:1763–1764.

Denicoff KD, Lehman ZA, Rubinow DR, et al. Suicidal ideation in Darier's disease. *J Am Acad Dermatol* 1990;22:196–198.

Dhitavat J, Dode L, Leslie N, et al. Mutations in the sarcoplasmic/endoplasmic reticulum Ca2+ ATPase isoform cause Darier's disease. *J Invest Dermatol* 2003;121:486–489.

Dhitavat J, Macfarlane S, Dode L, et al. Acrokeratosis verruciformis of Hopf is caused by mutation in ATP2A2: evidence that it is allelic to Darier's disease. *J Invest Dermatol* 2003;120:229–232.

Exadaktylou D, Kurwa HA, Calonje E, et al. Treatment of Darier's disease with photodynamic therapy. *Br J Dermatol* 2003;149:606–610.

Ferris T, Lamey PJ, Rennie JS. Darier's disease: oral features and genetic aspects. *Br Dent J* 1990;168:71–73.

Hulatt L, Burge S. Darier's disease: hopes and challenges. *J R Soc Med* 2003;96:439–441.

Ikeda S, Mayuzumi N, Shigihara T, et al. Mutations in ATP2A2 in patients with Darier's disease. *J Invest Dermatol* 2003;121:475–477.

Kimoto M, Akiyama M, Matsuo I. Darter's disease restricted to sun-exposed areas. *Clin Exp Dermatol* 2004;29:37–39.

Onozuka T, Sawamura D, Yokota K, et al. Mutational analysis of the ATP2A2 gene in two Darier disease families with intrafamilial variability. *Br J Dermatol* 2004;150:652–657.

Ruiz-Perez VL, Carter SA, Healey E, et al. ATP2A2 mutations in Darier's disease: variant cutaneous phenotypes are associated with missense mutations, but neuropsychiatric features are independent of mutation class. *Hum Mol Genet* 1999;8:1621–1630.

Sakuntabhai A, Burge S, Monk S, et al. Spectrum of novel ATP2A2 mutations in patients with Darier's disease. *Hum Mol Genet* 1999;8:1611.

Sakuntabhai A, Ruiz-Perez VL, Carter S, et al. Mutations in ATP2A2, encoding a Ca²+ pump, cause Darier disease. *Nat Genet* 1999;21: 271–277.

Epidermal Nevus Syndrome

Baker RS, Ross PA, Baumann RJ. Neurologic complications of the epidermal nevus syndrome. *Arch Neurol* 1987;44:227–232.

Booth TN, Rollins NK. MR imaging of the spine in epidermal nevus syndrome. *AJNR Am J Neuroradiol* 2002;23:1607–1610.

Grebe TA, Rimsza ME, Richter SF, et al. Further delineation of the epidermal nevus syndrome: two cases with new findings and literature review. *Am J Med Genet* 1993;47:24–30.

Happle R. How many epidermal nevus syndromes exist? A clinico-genetic classification. *J Am Acad Dermatol* 1991;25:550–556.

Happle R, Rogers M. Epidermal nevi. *Adv Dermatol* 2002;18:175–201.

Happle R. Epidermal nevus syndromes. *Semin Dermatol* 1995;14:111.

Ivker R, Resnick SD, Skidmore RA. Hypophosphatemic vitamin D-resistant rickets, precocious puberty, and the epidermal nevus syndrome. *Arch Dermatol* 1997;133:1557–1561.

Neumann LM, Scheer I, Kunze J, et al. Cerebral manifestations, hemihypertrophy and lymphoedema of one leg in a child with epidermal nevus syndrome (Schimmelpenning-Feuerstein-Mims). *Pediatr Radiol* 2003;33:637–640.

Paller AS. Epidermal nevus syndrome. *Neurol Clin* 1987;5:451–457.

Paller AS, Syder AJ, Chan YM, et al. Genetic and clinical mosaicism in a type of epidermal nevus. *N Engl J Med* 1994;331:1408–1415.

Rogers M, McCrossin I, Commens C. Epidermal nevi and the epidermal nevus syndrome: a review of 131 cases. *J Am Acad Dermatol* 1989;20:476–488.

Sahl WJ Jr. Familial nevus sebaceus of Jadassohn: occurrence in three generations. *J Am Acad Dermatol* 1990:22:853–854.

Zakrzewski JL, Luecke T, Bentele KH, et al. Epidermal naevus and segmental hypermelanosis associated with an intraspinal mass: overlap between different mosaic neuroectodermal syndromes. *Eur J Pediatr* 2001;160:603–606.

Zhang W, Simos PG, Ishibashi H, et al. Neuroimaging features of epidermal nevus syndrome. *AJNR Am J Neuroradiol* 2003;24:1468–1470.

Chapter 2

Disorders of Pigmentation

Clinical Pearls

Seth Orlow, M.D. (SO), Amy Paller, M.D. (AP),
Jean Bolognia M.D. (JB), and D.G.R. Evans, M.D. (DE)

Oculocutaneous Albinism Type 1 (OCA1)

Synonym	Tyrosinase-negative albinism
Inheritance	Autosomal recessive; tyrosinase (*TYR*) gene on 11q14–q21
Prenatal Diagnosis	DNA mutation analysis
Incidence	1:28,000 blacks; 1:39,000 caucasians; M=F
Age at Presentation	Birth
Pathogenesis	Mutations in the TYR gene lead to absent tyrosinase activity or lack of tyrosinase transport to melanosomes Normal number of melanocytes Unable to produce melanin in skin, hair and eyes Only stage I and II premelanosomes in melanocytes Miswiring of optic fibers

Key Features	**Skin**
	    Generalized pink-white color, solar keratoses, pink-red nevi, squamous cell cancers > basal cell cancers > melanoma
	Hair
	    Snow-white color
	Eyes
	    Blue to gray-blue irides, severe nystagmus, photophobia, impaired visual acuity (20/200 or worse), prominent red reflex throughout life, strabismus, foveal hypoplasia

Differential Diagnosis	OCA1B (yellow mutant, minimal pigment, and temperature-sensitive albinism) OCA2 (p. 58) Hermansky-Pudlak syndrome (p. 60) Chédiak-Higashi syndrome (p. 62)
Laboratory Data	DNA analysis (p. 58)
Management	See OCA2 (p. 58)
Prognosis	Skin and hair do not improve with age Vision remains stable or worsens with age

Clinical Pearls

Almost certain to get squamous cell cancer, just a matter of when . . . Some may need to be placed in special classes for the visually impaired . . . Referral to NOAH support group (see Support Groups).   *SO*

See OCA2 (p. 58)

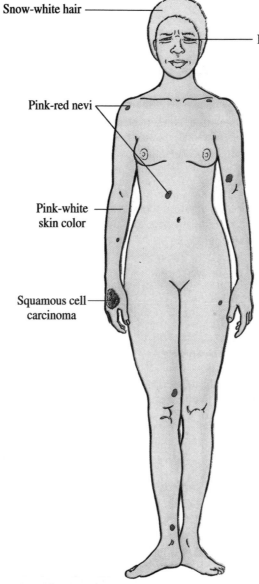

Snow-white hair

Blue to gray-blue irides
Nystagmus
Strabismus
Impaired visual acuity
Photophobia

Pink-red nevi

Pink-white
skin color

Squamous cell
carcinoma

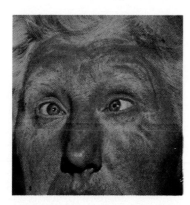

2.1. *Snow-white hair, pink skin, strabismus, and gray-blue irides in an adult.* (24)

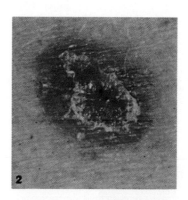

2.2. *Malignant melanoma presenting as a pink macule with crust.* (24)

Oculocutaneous Albinism Type II (OCA2)

Synonym	Tyrosinase-positive albinism
Inheritance	Autosomal recessive; P gene on 15q11.2–12
Prenatal Diagnosis	DNA linkage analysis and mutation detection available
Incidence	1:15,000 blacks; 1:37,000 whites; M=F Most common form of albinism
Age at Presentation	Birth
Pathogenesis	Mutation in P gene with decrease eumelanin synthesis; gene product thought to play a role in tyrosinase transport (+) Tyrosinase, normal number of melanocytes Decreased melanin in skin, hair, and eyes Miswiring of optic fibers

Key Features

Skin
  Generalized pink-white to cream color
  Multiple pigmented nevi, ephelides, and lentigines increase with age
  Solar keratoses, squamous cell and basal cell cancers with age
Hair
  Cream to yellow-brown color
Eyes
  Blue to yellow-brown irides (race dependent), nystagmus, photophobia, impaired visual acuity, strabismus, foveal hypoplasia

Differential Diagnosis

OCA1, OCA1B (p. 56)
Hermansky-Pudlak syndrome (p. 60)
Chédiak-Higashi syndrome (p. 62)

Laboratory Data

DNA mutation analysis

Management

Skin
  Sun avoidance (especially mid-day): broad-spectrum sunscreen, long-sleeved shirts, brim hat
  Referral to dermatologist—skin cancer screening every 6 months
Eyes
  UVB-blocking sunglasses, corrective lenses, tinted glasses/contact lenses
  Referral to ophthalmologist

Prognosis

Skin and hair pigment increases over time; eye symptomatology may improve with age

---

Clinical Pearls

Skin — More difficult problem for darker races with increased social ostracism (less than with vitiligo, however) . . . Referral to NOAH support group (see Support Groups).

Eyes — Most difficult problem for caucasians but can be equally bad for blacks depending on the level of nystagmus and severity of albinism.   *SO*

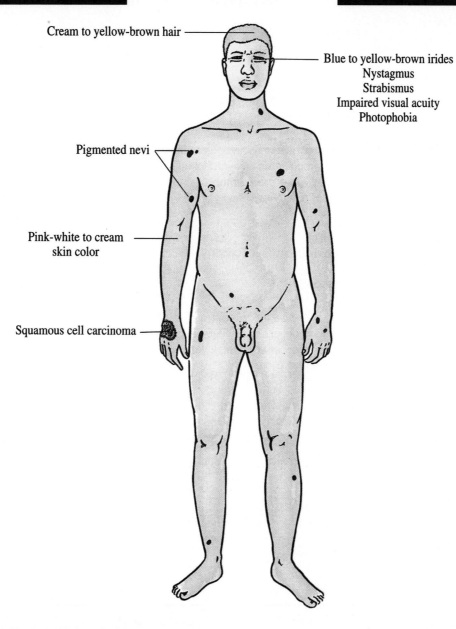

Cream to yellow-brown hair

Blue to yellow-brown irides
Nystagmus
Strabismus
Impaired visual acuity
Photophobia

Pigmented nevi

Pink-white to cream
skin color

Squamous cell carcinoma

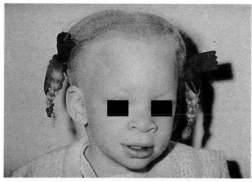

2.3. *Yellow-brown hair and pink skin in a black girl.* *(5)*

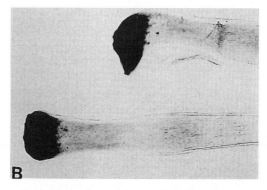

2.4. *Melanin production after hair bulb incubation test. (1)*

Hermansky-Pudlak Syndrome

Inheritance	Autosomal recessive; gene loci *HPS1* gene on 10q23 (most common, found in northwest Puerto Rico and a small village in Swiss Alps), *AP3B1* gene on 5q14.1 (HPS2); there are five other gene loci identified to date
Prenatal Diagnosis	DNA mutation analysis if defect known
Incidence	Over 200 case reports; increased frequency in Puerto Rico, Holland
Age at Presentation	Birth
Pathogenesis	Mutation in *HPS1* gene is a 16-bp duplication of the gene important in protein localization via intracellular trafficking and organelle formation *AP3B1* gene mutations cause *HPS2*—the gene encodes the β-3a subunit of AP3 adapter complex, which is thought to be important in protein packaging, vesicular formation, and membrane fusion within the cell Tyrosinase-positive Bleeding diathesis secondary to platelet storage pool defect with decreased adenosine diphosphate (ADP), adenosine triphosphate (ATP), and serotonin granules—impairs platelet aggregation Lysosomal membrane defect—accumulation of ceroid lipofuscin in macrophages within the lung and gastrointestinal tract

Key Features	**Skin**
	    Pigment dilution dependent on race
	    Pigmented nevi, solar keratoses, squamous cell cancer, basal cell cancer
	    Ecchymoses, petechiae
	Hair
	    Cream to red-brown color
	Eyes
	    Photophobia, nystagmus, decreased visual acuity, strabismus, foveal hypolasia
	Hematologic
	    Epistaxis, gingival bleeding, menorrhagia, prolonged bleeding during childbirth, dental extraction, surgery
	Lymphohistiocytic
	    Ceroid (chromolipid) deposition in macrophages in the lung (pulmonary fibrosis), gastrointestinal tract (granulomatous colitis), cardiac muscle (cardiomyopathy)

Differential Diagnosis	OCA2 (p. 58) Chédiak-Higashi syndrome (p. 62)
Laboratory Data	Bleeding time prolonged; prothrombin time/partial thromboplastin time (PT/PTT), platelet count normal Wet-mount electron microscopy—demonstrates platelets without dense granules
Management	Avoid aspirin and other prostaglandin synthesis inhibitors Baseline chest x-ray at early age Pulmonary function test and colonoscopy if symptomatic Solar protection and avoidance Referral to dermatologist, hematologist-oncologist, ophthalmologist, and symptom-specific subspecialist Educate dentist, obstetrician, and surgeon prior to dental extraction, delivery, and surgical procedure
Prognosis	Premature death secondary to hemorrhage, colitis, pulmonic disease, squamous cell cancer; otherwise normal life span

Clinical Pearls

Must first establish patient is a tyrosinase positive albino . . . Elicit country of origin; remember large Puerto Rican population in the northeast United States . . . Never give aspirin . . . Dental surgery and minor surgery may need to be done in hospital setting with platelets available . . . Approximately 33% of patients will develop symptomatic pulmonary fibrosis.   *SO*

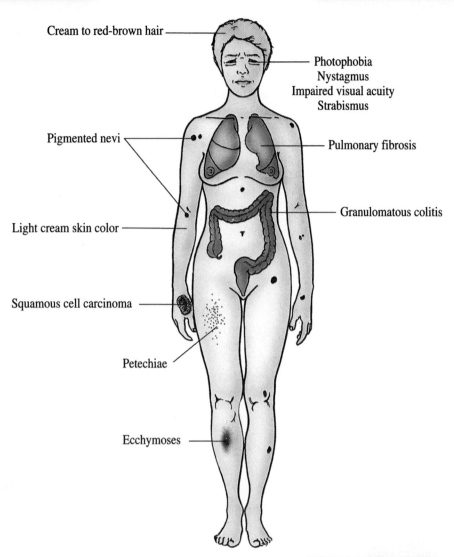

Cream to red-brown hair

Photophobia
Nystagmus
Impaired visual acuity
Strabismus

Pigmented nevi

Pulmonary fibrosis

Granulomatous colitis

Light cream skin color

Squamous cell carcinoma

Petechiae

Ecchymoses

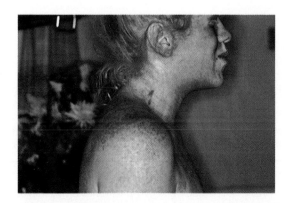

2.5. *Female with showers of petechiae and cream-colored hair and skin.* (25)

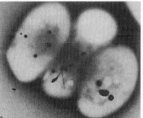

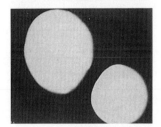

2.6. *Top: Normal platelets with dense granules. Bottom: Platelets from Hermansky-Pudlak patient with absent granules.* (26)

Chédiak-Higashi Syndrome

Inheritance	Autosomal recessive; *LYST* gene on 1q42; high consanguinity
Prenatal Diagnosis	Fetoscopy—fetal hair shafts reveal clumping of melanosomes on light microscopy; fetal blood reveals characteristic neutrophilic granules
Incidence	Rare; fewer than 100 cases reported; M=F
Age at Presentation	Birth to a few months old
Pathogenesis	*LYST* gene mutation codes for a lysosomal tracking protein that regulates microtubule-mediated lysosomal fusion/fission and protein sorting; this defect leads to accumulation of giant lysosomal granules in a variety of cells:
	Neutrophils—defective phagocytosis, decreased chemotaxis
	Melanocytes—pigmentary dilution
	Neurons—progressive neurologic deterioration
	Platelet storage pool deficiency—bleeding diathesis
	Decreased natural killer cell and antibody-dependent cell-mediated cytolysis function

Key Features

Skin
Light cream to slate-gray color, recurrent bacterial infections—*Staphylococcus aureus* most common

Hair
Light blonde color (in caucasians) with a silver sheen

Eyes
Photophobia, strabismus, nystagmus, decreased uveal pigment

Upper and Lower Respiratory Tract
Recurrent bacterial sinusitis, pneumonia

Central Nervous System
Progressive neurologic deterioration with ataxia, muscle weakness, sensory loss, seizures (rare)

Accelerated Phase (approximately 85% of patients):

Hematologic
Lymphohistiocytic proliferation with infiltration of liver, spleen, and lymph nodes; associated anemia, neutropenia, thrombocytopenia manifested as petechiae, ecchymoses, gingival bleeding, epistaxis, gastrointestinal hemorrhage, overwhelming infection

Differential Diagnosis	OCA2 (p. 58)
	Hermansky-Pudlak syndrome (p. 60)
	Chronic granulomatous disease (p. 258)
	Griscelli syndrome (p. 64)
	Elejalde syndrome
Laboratory Data	Diagnostic complete blood cell count (CBC) revealing giant granules in neutrophils
Management	Referral to pediatric hematologist-oncologist—bone marrow transplant, chemotherapy, high-dose ascorbic acid
	Antibiotics, sun protection
	Referral to dermatologist, infectious disease specialist, immunologist, neurologist, and ophthalmologist
Prognosis	Death by late childhood from overwhelming infection or hemorrhage during lymphoma-like phase; may reverse deterioration with bone marrow transplantation

Clinical Pearls	Bone marrow transplant is the treatment of choice and should be performed early on before the accelerated phase takes place . . . Lymphoma-like phase responds poorly to chemotherapy . . . Platelet storage pool defect less severe than in Hermansky-Pudlak . . . Death usually by 10 years of age. *SO*

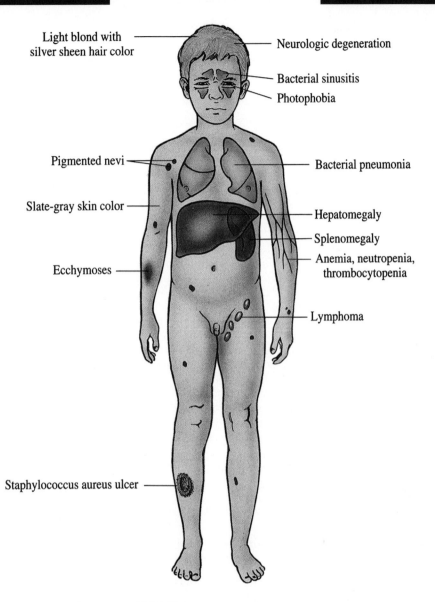

Light blond with silver sheen hair color

Neurologic degeneration

Bacterial sinusitis

Photophobia

Pigmented nevi

Bacterial pneumonia

Slate-gray skin color

Hepatomegaly

Splenomegaly

Anemia, neutropenia, thrombocytopenia

Ecchymoses

Lymphoma

Staphylococcus aureus ulcer

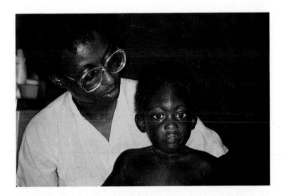

2.7. *Black child with silver-gray hair and skin.* (27)

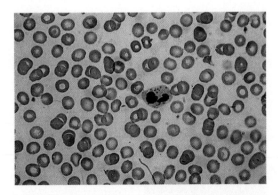

2.8. *Giant lysosomal granules in a polymorphonuclear neutrophil.* (27)

Griscelli Syndrome

Inheritance	Autosomal recessive
Prenatal Diagnosis	Fetal scalp biopsy at 21 weeks' gestation: hair evaluation; fetal blood sample: leukocyte evaluation DNA analysis
Incidence	Rare—less than 40 cases reported; M=F
Age at Presentation	First year of life
Pathogenesis	Mutations in gene encoding for myosin Va or RAB27a, proteins involved in organelle trafficking and membrane transport; melanophilin gene mutations also implicated in subset of patients

Key Features

Skin
  Pigmentary dilution; cutaneous pyogenic infections, abscesses
Hair
  Silver-gray hair, eyebrows, eyelashes
Hematologic
  Neutropenia, thrombocytopenia, without leukocyte inclusions
Immunologic
  Lymphohistiocytic infiltration leading to hepatosplenomegaly, combined T- and B-cell immunodeficiency; accelerated lymphoma-like phase (i.e., Chediak-Higashi) often occurs
Infectious Disease
  Episodic fever with/without infection, pyogenic systemic infections
Neurologic
  Progressive deterioration with hypotonia, psychomotor retardation, seizures

Differential Diagnosis	Chédiak-Higashi syndrome (p. 62) Elejalde syndrome Chronic granulomatous disease (p. 258) OCΛ2 (p. 58)
Laboratory Data	Hair—uneven clumps of melanin in medulla of hair shaft on light microscopy Complete blood count (CBC)—absent cytoplasmic inclusion bodies in neutrophils
Management	Referral to hematology-oncology-bone marrow transplant Referral to infectious disease Referral to neurologist Referral to dermatology-assist in diagnosis
Prognosis	Progressive deterioration may be aborted with bone marrow transplantation

Clinical Pearls

Patients with Griscelli syndrome caused by mutations in the *MYO5A* gene develop primary neurologic impairment (e.g., severe developmental delay) but not hemophagocytic syndrome (a phenotype similar to *dilute* mice] whereas those with *RAB27A* mutations develop a hemophagocytic syndrome and any neurologic involvement is secondary, i.e., caused by lymphocytic infiltration of the central nervous system (CNS), which is a phenotype similar to *ashen* mice.   *JB*

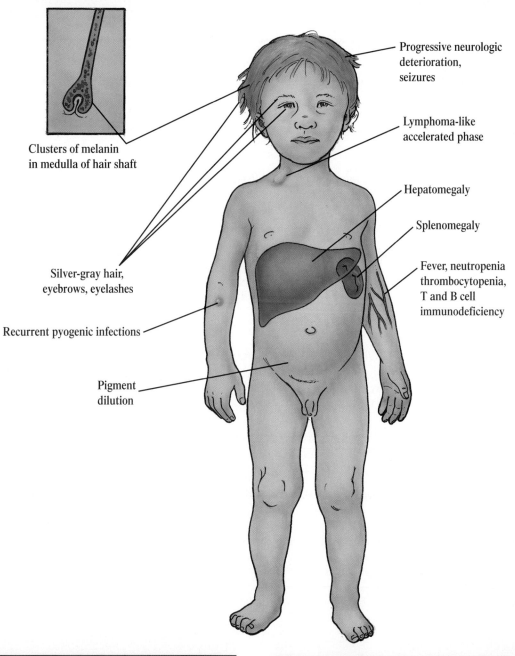

Clusters of melanin
in medulla of hair shaft

Progressive neurologic
deterioration,
seizures

Lymphoma-like
accelerated phase

Hepatomegaly

Splenomegaly

Fever, neutropenia
thrombocytopenia,
T and B cell
immunodeficiency

Silver-gray hair,
eyebrows, eyelashes

Recurrent pyogenic infections

Pigment
dilution

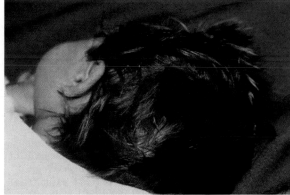

2.9. Hair with metallic silvery-gray sheen. (28)

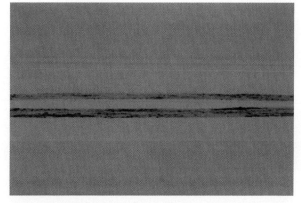

2.10. Light microscopy of hair reveals irregular, large clumps of melanin pigment. (28).

Piebaldism

Synonym	Familial white spotting
Inheritance	Autosomal dominant; mutation in c-*kit* proto-oncogene on chromosome 4q12
Prenatal Diagnosis	DNA linkage analysis and mutation detection available
Incidence	Less than 1:20,000; all races; M=F
Age at Presentation	Birth
Pathogenesis	A mutation in the c-*kit* proto-oncogene results in abnormal tyrosine kinase transmembrane receptors, decreases signal transduction, and causes abnormal melanocyte embryogenesis with defective melanoblast proliferation, migration and distribution.
Key Features	**Skin** Depigmented patches on mid-forehead, central eyebrows, neck, anterior trunk, mid-extremities; often bilateral, sparing the hands, feet, back, shoulders, hips Islands of hyperpigmented to normally pigmented patches within and at the borders of hypopigmentation **Hair** White forelock (80% to 90%) **Rare Case Reports** Hirschsprung disease, mental retardation, deafness, cerebellar ataxia
Differential Diagnosis	Waardenburg syndrome (p. 68) Vitiligo Nevus depigmentosus
Laboratory Data	Histology from depigmented area reveals decreased number or absent melanocytes and melanin
Management	Autologous cultured melanocyte grafts Sunscreen Camouflage—hair dye, Dermablend; 20% topical monobenzyl ether of hydroquinone
Prognosis	Pigmentary alteration usually stable and permanent; normal life span

Clinical Pearls

Melanocyte transplant technology not perfected yet . . . Coping mechanisms seem to be better for patients with a congenital skin defect (piebaldism) rather than an acquired skin defect (vitiligo).   *SO*

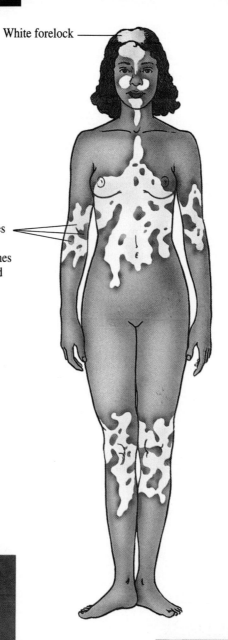

White forelock

Depigmented patches
with islands of
hyperpigmented patches
and hyperpigmented
borders

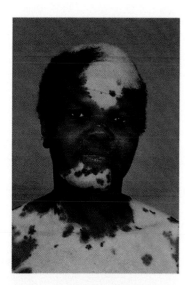

2.11. *Black female with white forelock and depigmented patches with
islands of hyperpigmentation on her
mid-face and central trunk. (29)*

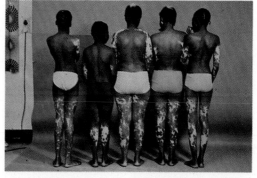

2.12. *Family of patient in Figure 2.11 with similar
cutaneous findings. (29)*

Waardenburg Syndrome

Inheritance	Autosomal dominant; *Pax3* gene on 2q35 in I and III, *MITF* gene on 13q in II, and the *SOX1O* and endothelin-3 genes on 22q13 and 20q13 respectively in IV
Prenatal Diagnosis	DNA analysis if gene defect known
Incidence	1:42,000; M=F; all races; 1% to 3% of all congenitally deaf children
Age at Presentation	Birth
Pathogenesis	Four distinct types have been defined by their unique clinical and genetic features: Types I and III are caused by mutations in PAX3, a transcription factor that controls neural crest differentiation and regulates transcription of other genes downstream including those responsible for melanoblast activation and migration, inner ear structures and facial bony and cartilaginous structures. Type II is caused by a mutation in the *MITF* gene, the melanocyte transcription factor. Three genetic etiologies involving control of neural crest development have been described for producing the phenotype seen in type IV: SOX1O transcription factor mutations, endothelin-3 signaling gene mutations and endothelin receptor gene mutations.

Key Features

Skin
  May have depigmented patches on body
Hair
  White forelock (< 50%), synophrys (70%)
Teeth
  Caries
Nose
  Broad nasal root (80%)
Eyes
  Dystopia canthorum (99% but not in II)—lateral displacement of medial canthi with normal interpupillary distance, complete or partial heterochromia irides (25%), hypopigmented fundus
Ears
  Congenital sensorineural hearing loss (20%, most common in II)
Colon
  Hirschsprung disease (< 5%, exclusively IV)
Musculoskeletal
  Cleft lip/palate (I), upper limb, and pectoral anomalies (III)

Differential Diagnosis	Piebaldism (p. 66) Vogt-Koyanagi-Harada syndrome Vitiligo Alezzandrini syndrome
Laboratory Data	Dystopia canthorum: $\dfrac{\text{inner canthal distance}}{\text{outer canthal distance}} > 0.6$
Management	Referral to audiologist, otolaryngologist, ophthalmologist Referral to gastroenterologist and surgeon if symptomatic
Prognosis	Heterochromia irides and white forelock may fade after 1 year; normal life span

Clinical Pearls

Most important, all patients must see audiologist early on to impact upon learning and phonation in the congenitally deaf . . . Benefit from hearing aids . . . Colored contacts useful for heterochromia irides . . . Watch for gastrointestinal symptomatology in newborn/infant . . . Elicit bowel habit history . . . Dermablend, hair dyes useful. *SO*

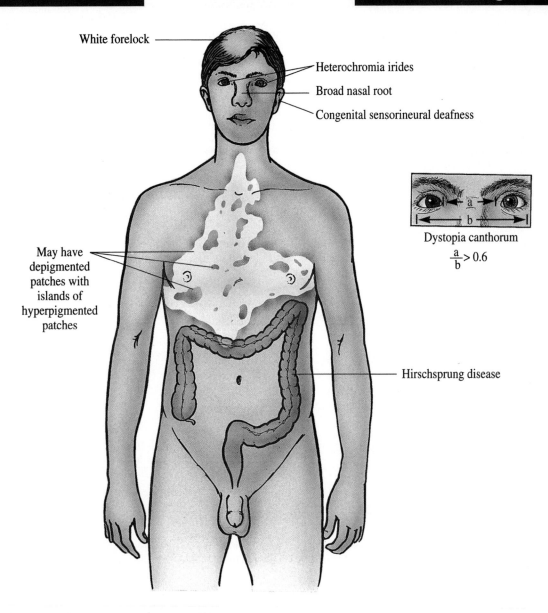

White forelock

Heterochromia irides

Broad nasal root

Congenital sensorineural deafness

May have depigmented patches with islands of hyperpigmented patches

Dystopia canthorum

$$\frac{a}{b} > 0.6$$

Hirschsprung disease

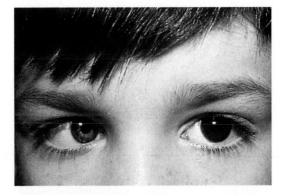

2.13. *Boy with heterochromia irides, strabismus, broad nasal root, and dystopia canthorum. (1)*

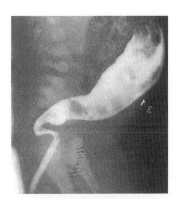

2.14. *X-ray depicting tapering of normal colon in patient with Hirschsprung disease. (30)*

Hypomelanosis of Ito

Synonym   Incontinentia pigmenti achromians

Inheritance   Not inherited; chromosomal or single gene mosaicism

Prenatal Diagnosis None

Incidence   Rare; all races; M=F

Age at Presentation Birth to 1 year old

Pathogenesis   The cutaneous phenotype reflects many different forms of genomic mosaicism

Key Features

Skin
  Unilateral and bilateral whirled marble cake hypopigmentation in Blaschko's lines
Hair
  Alopecia
Associated Findings (seen in 75% of cases):
  Central Nervous System
    Seizures, mental and motor retardation
  Eyes
    Strabismus, hypertelorism
  Musculoskeletal
    Scoliosis, limb length discrepancy
  Teeth
    Anodontia, dental dysplasia

Differential Diagnosis
Nevus depigmentosus
Tuberous sclerosis (p. 88)
Incontinentia pigmenti (p. 72)
Segmental vitiligo

Laboratory Data   None

Management   Complete physical examination by primary care physician
Referral to subspecialist if symptomatic
Camouflage cosmetics

Prognosis   Hypopigmentation may fade with time; normal life span

Clinical Pearls

Hypopigmentation is not a static finding . . . I have seen patients revert to normal pigmentation . . . Nevus depigmentosus, hypomelanosis of Ito, and linear and whorled nevoid hypermelanosis represent a spectrum of phenotype related to various mosaic genotypes.   *SO*

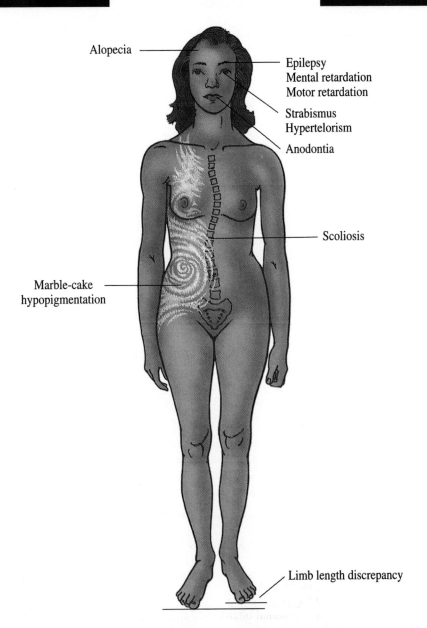

Alopecia

Epilepsy
Mental retardation
Motor retardation

Strabismus
Hypertelorism

Anodontia

Scoliosis

Marble-cake
hypopigmentation

Limb length discrepancy

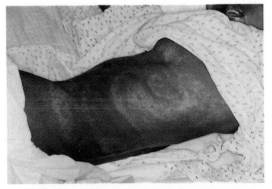

2.15. *Eighteen year-old girl with marble-cake hypopigmentation who suffered from intractable seizures, mental and motor retardation.*

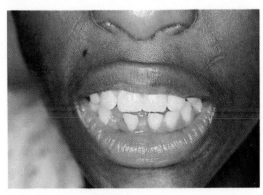

2.16. *Same patient with anodontia.*

Incontinentia Pigmenti

Synonym Bloch-Sulzberger syndrome

Inheritance X-linked dominant; rare male survivors thought to have Klinefelter syndrome; *NEMO* gene on Xq28

Prenatal Diagnosis DNA analysis if gene known in family

Incidence Over 700 cases reported; 97% female

Age at Presentation Birth to first few weeks of life

Pathogenesis Mutation in *NEMO* (NF-κB essential modulator) gene leads to defective NF-κB activation (80% have identical mutation secondary to gene rearrangement in paternal meiosis). NF-κB is a transcription factor essential for several inflammatory, immune and apoptotic pathways

Key Features

Skin
  Stage I
    Vesicular (birth to 1 to 2 weeks): vesicles and bullae in a linear arrangement on extremities, trunk, and scalp; erythematous macules and papules
  Stage II
    Verrucous (2 to 6 weeks): streaks of hyperkeratotic papules, pustules, and papules on extremities
  Stage III
    Hyperpigmentation (3 to 6 months): whorls and swirls of hyperpigmentation along Blaschko's lines
  Stage IV
    Hypopigmentation (second to third decade): hypopigmented whorls and swirls replacing hyperpigmentation; with/without follicular atrophy
Hair
  Scarring alopecia (30%)
Nails
  Dystrophic changes (5% to 10%)
Teeth
  Anodontia, peg/conical teeth (66%); deciduous and permanent affected
Eyes (25% to 35%)
  Strabismus, cataracts, optic atrophy, retinal vascular changes with secondary blindness, retrolental mass
Central Nervous System (30%)
  Seizures, mental retardation, spastic paralysis

Incontinentia Pigmenti *(continued)*

Differential Diagnosis

Neonate
- Epidermolysis bullosa (p. 200)
- Impetigo
- Herpes simplex virus
- Epidermolytic hyperkeratosis (p. 6)
- Congenital syphilis

Childhood
- Hypomelanosis of Ito (p. 70)

Laboratory Data

Skin biopsy in vesicular stage—abundant eosinophils
Complete blood count—peripheral eosinophilia in infancy

Management

Referral to dermatologist—diagnosis, topical care
Referral to dentist at 1 year old
Referral to ophthalmologist at time of diagnosis
Referral to neurologist if symptomatic

Prognosis

Normal life span

Clinical Pearls

Dentist can provide dentures, prosthodontics for correction of dysfunctional teeth . . . Refer to ophthalmologist to fix strabismus, cataracts, and retrolental-fibroplasia-like ocular disease . . . I let the clinical exam dictate my work-up of other systems . . . Genetic counseling extremely important . . . Affected women may have a very difficult time conceiving and an increased rate of miscarriages . . . Always examine Mom. *SO*

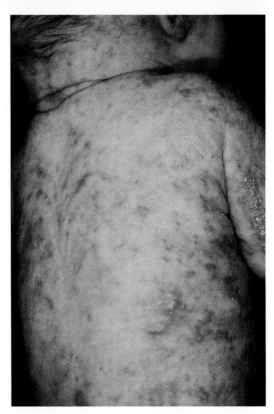

2.17. *Bullae and verrucous papules along Blaschko's lines on infant's trunk and extremity. (4)*

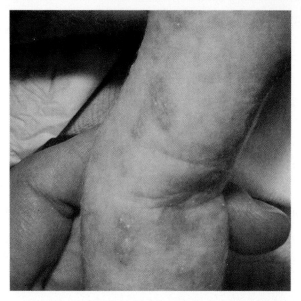

2.18. *Close-up of bullae in a linear distribution on infant's arm. (1)*

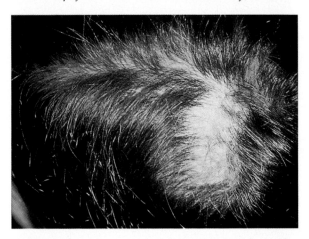

2.20. *Scarring alopecia in a patient with incontinentia pigmenti. (1)*

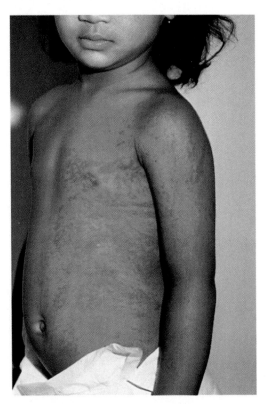

2.19. *Whorls and swirls of hyperpigmentation in Blaschko's lines. (1)*

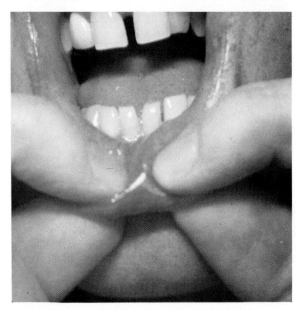

2.21. *Pegged teeth in mother of an affected infant. (1)*

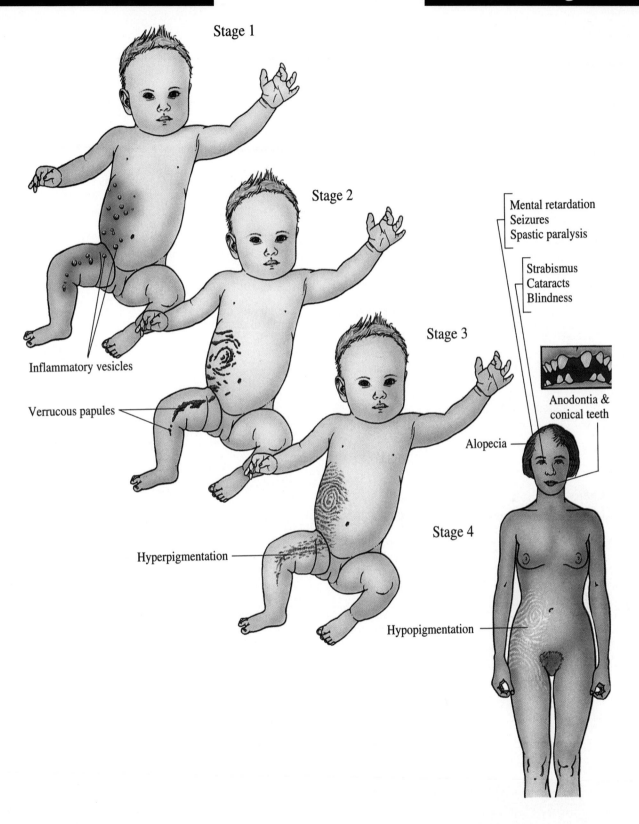

Stage 1

Stage 2

Inflammatory vesicles

Verrucous papules

Stage 3

Hyperpigmentation

Mental retardation
Seizures
Spastic paralysis

Strabismus
Cataracts
Blindness

Anodontia &
conical teeth

Alopecia

Stage 4

Hypopigmentation

LEOPARD Syndrome

Synonym	Multiple lentigines syndrome
Inheritance	Autosomal dominant; *PTPN11* gene on 12q24
Prenatal Diagnosis	DNA analysis if defect known
Incidence	Over 70 cases reported; M=F
Age at Presentation	Lentigines begin at birth or first few months of life; abundant by 4 to 5 years old
Pathogenesis	A mutation in *PTPN1 1*, a gene encoding the nonreceptor protein tyrosine phosphatase *SHP2* and implicated in Noonan syndrome, has been isolated in nine patients evaluated with the LEOPARD phenotype.

Key Features

Skin
Generalized multiple **L**entigines; mucous membranes spared
Café noir spots
Café au lait spots
Cardiovascular
Electrocardiographic (ECG) conduction defects
Pulmonic stenosis, aortic stenosis, obstructive cardiomyopathy
Craniofacial
Ocular hypertelorism
Triangular facies
Genitourinary
Abnormal genitalia—hypospadias, cryptorchidism
Musculoskeletal
Growth **R**etardation
Pectus excavatum or carinatum
Central Nervous System
Sensorineural **D**eafness
Mild mental retardation (rare)

Differential Diagnosis	Carney Complex (p. 78) Peutz-Jeghers syndrome (p. 186) Noonan syndrome (p. 354) Premature aging and multiple nevi
Laboratory Data	Skin biopsy
Management	Thorough cutaneous examination by dermatologist Complete physical examination by primary care physician Referral to cardiologist, audiologist, urologist Evaluate first-degree family member
Prognosis	Normal life span; pulmonic stenosis rarely disabling Speech difficulties secondary to deafness if not diagnosed early on

Clinical Pearls

Patients with multiple lentigines should always be sent for cardiac evaluation if this diagnosis is being considered . . . It is often difficult to assess genitalia abnormalities and sensorineural deafness accurately during infancy/early childhood . . . Once diagnosis is made, it is critical to evaluate for deafness in order to prevent difficulties with phonation and learning . . . Skin biopsy may be necessary to help differentiate lentigines from nevi and ephelides. *SO*

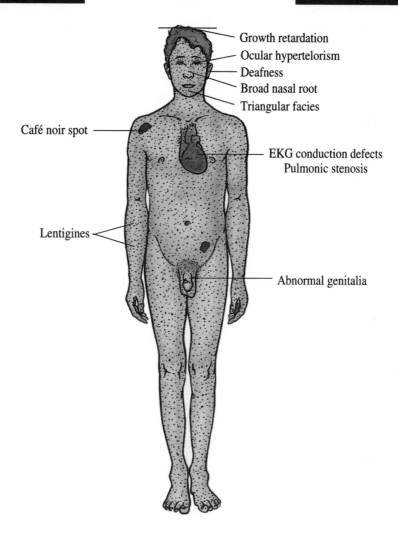

Growth retardation
Ocular hypertelorism
Deafness
Broad nasal root
Triangular facies
Café noir spot
EKG conduction defects
Pulmonic stenosis
Lentigines
Abnormal genitalia

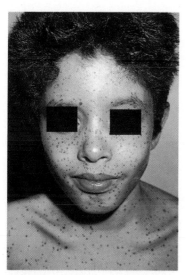

2.22. *Affected boy with multiple lentigines, triangular facies, and hypertelorism. (31)*

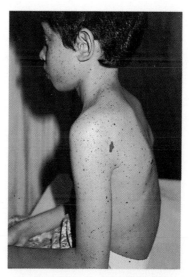

2.23. *Same patient with café noir spot and lentigines on trunk. (31)*

Carney Complex

Synonym	NAME syndrome, LAMB syndrome
Inheritance	Autosomal dominant; *PRKAR1A* gene on 17q23, almost all other cases on 2p16
Prenatal Diagnosis	DNA mutation analysis if defect known
Incidence	Rare; increased in Jewish population; M=F
Age at Presentation	Birth to first few years of life
Pathogenesis	A mutation in *PRKAR1A*, a tumor suppressor gene encoding the regulatory subunit type 1A of protein kinase A has been isolated in half the cases

Key Features

Skin
Lentigines, blue **N**evi, melanocytic **N**evi, **E**phelides (can involve mucosa)
Myxomas
Cardiac
Atrial myxomas
Secondary embolization and congestive heart failure (CHF) may occur
Endocrine
Pigmented nodular adrenocortical disease—Cushing syndrome
Pituitary adenoma—acromegaly
Genitourinary Tract
Testicular tumors (large-cell calcifying Sertoli tumor, Leydig cell tumor)—sexual precocity
Nervous System
Psammomatous melanotic schwannomas

Differential Diagnosis	LEOPARD syndrome (p. 76) Peutz-Jeghers syndrome (p. 186)
Laboratory Data	Skin biopsy Echocardiogram
Management	Referral to dermatologist—excision of myxoma or pigmented lesions for cosmesis or diagnosis; may recur Referral to cardiologist/cardiac surgeon—excision of atrial myxomas Referral to endocrinologist once diagnosis is made Examination of first-degree relatives
Prognosis	Complications of cardiac myxomas may shorten life span

Clinical Pearls

Lentigines and ephelides usually begin after birth and increase in number with age . . . Nevi are often congenital . . . Adults are more likely to have cutaneous and cardiac myxomas or endocrine disease . . . Atrial myxomas must be excised . . . Adrenal and pituitary function tests should be done once the diagnosis is made.
SO

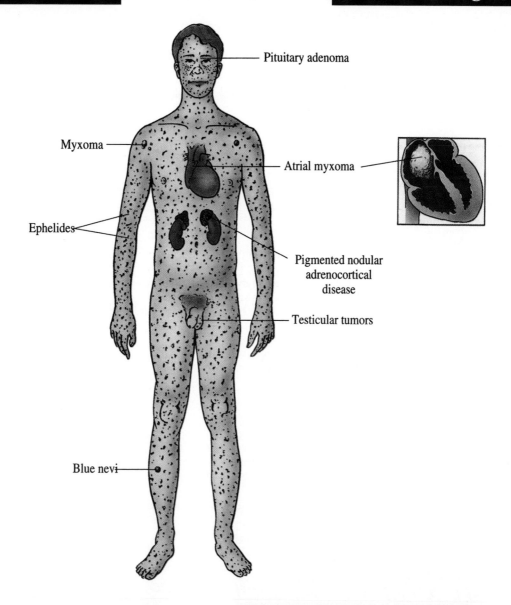

Pituitary adenoma

Myxoma

Atrial myxoma

Ephelides

Pigmented nodular
adrenocortical
disease

Testicular tumors

Blue nevi

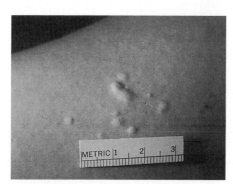

2.24. *Cutaneous myxomas in clusters. (32)*

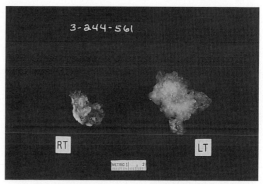

3-244-561

RT   LT

2.25. *Gross appearance of excised left and right atrial
myxomas. (32)*

McCune-Albright Syndrome

Synonym	Albright syndrome
Inheritance	Sporadic; postzygotic somatic mutations in *GNAS1* gene on 20q13.2
Prenatal Diagnosis	None
Incidence	Rare; M=F
Age at Presentation	Birth to first few months of life
Pathogenesis	Mosaic for mutations in the *GNAS1* gene encoding for the α subunit of the stimulatory G proteins that regulates adenylate cyclase

Key Features	**Skin**
	    Large, segmental café au lait macule(s) with "coast of Maine" border
	Bone
	    Polyostotic fibrous dysplasia—long bones and facial bones commonly affected, often occurs beneath café au lait macule
	    Recurrent fractures, bowing of limbs, limb length discrepancies
	    Diffuse sclerosis at base of skull
	Endocrine
	    Precocious puberty—females > males
	    Hyperthyroidism—(20% to 30%)

Differential Diagnosis	Neurofibromatosis I (p. 82)
Laboratory Data	Skeletal x-rays Serum alkaline phosphatase (elevated) Urinary luteinizing hormone, estrogen, 17-hydroxycorticoid, 17-ketosteroid levels (may be elevated in affected females) Thyroid function tests
Management	Referral to orthopedist—surgical correction Referral to endocrinologist
Prognosis	Normal life span

Clinical Pearls

I would investigate radiologically the bone corresponding to the site of the segmental café au lait macule . . . Bone fractures are the most common orthopedic problem . . . Referral to orthopedist and endocrinologist once the diagnosis is confirmed.
SO

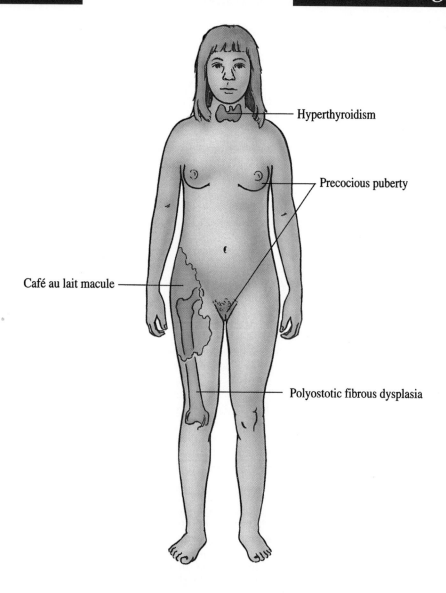

Hyperthyroidism

Precocious puberty

Café au lait macule

Polyostotic fibrous dysplasia

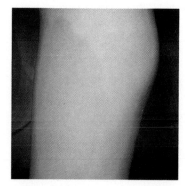

2.26. *Large café au lait macule. (1)*

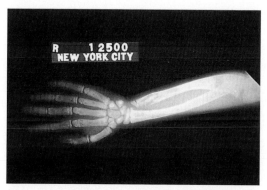

2.27. *Polyostotic fibrous dysplasia—bone lucencies and bowing of the ulna and radius in McCune's original patient. (33)*

Neurofibromatosis I

Synonym	von Recklinghausen disease; NF-1
Inheritance	Autosomal dominant; gene locus 17q11.2; spontaneous mutation in 50% of cases
Prenatal Diagnosis	DNA mutation analysis if defect known
Incidence	1:3000; M=F; all races Most common form of neurofibromatosis—85% of all cases
Age at Presentation	Birth to early childhood
Pathogenesis	Neurofibromin, the NF-1 gene product, is a tumor suppressor that dampens products of *ras* proto-oncogenes and its loss may contribute to tumor progression when gene mutation occurs

Key Features

Skin (See Diagnostic Criteria)
  Café au lait macules—increase in number and size in first 5 years of life
  Greater than 6 suggests NF-1
  Freckling in axillary or inguinal folds
  Neurofibromas
    Dermal, subcutaneous—appear at puberty, increase in number with age and during pregnancy, prominent on trunk
    Plexiform-congenital, progressive growth, with/without hyperpigmentation, hypertrichosis
    Pruritus-overlying a growing neurofibroma

Eyes (see Diagnostic Criteria)
  Lisch nodules-iris hamartomas, seen in more 90% patients older than 6 years old, increase in number with age, asymptomatic
  Congenital glaucoma
  Choroidal nevi

Neoplasia
  Central Nervous System
    Optic glioma (see Diagnostic Criteria)—approximately 66% asymptomatic, may cause blindness if untreated; other astrocytomas, meningioma, vestibular schwannoma (acoustic neuroma), ependymoma
  Non-Central Nervous System
    Neurofibrosarcoma, rhabdomyosarcoma, pheochromocytoma, Wilms' tumor, nonlymphocytic childhood leukemia, visceral neurofibromas

Skeletal (See Diagnostic Criteria)
  Sphenoid wing dysplasia, macrocephaly, scoliosis (± cervical-thoracic kyphosis), vertebral disc dysplasia, pseudoarthrosis of tibia, short stature

Central Nervous System
  Seizures, learning disability with speech defects and nonspecific incoordination, hydrocephalus, headache

Vascular
  Vascular dysplasia with cerebral, GI, and renal involvement; secondary infarction, renovascular hypertension

Gastrointestinal
  Constipation

Psychiatric
  Heavy psychosocial burden, particularly during adolescence

Differential Diagnosis
Neurofibromatosis II (p. 86)
Other forms of NF (3–9)
McCune-Albright syndrome (p. 80)
Watson syndrome—an allelic variant
Noonan syndrome (p. 354)—may occur simultaneously
Proteus syndrome (p. 106)

NIH Consensus Criteria for Diagnosis—1987

Need Two or More Features
Six or more café au lait macules over 5 mm in greatest diameter in prepubertal individuals and over 15 mm in greatest diameter in postpubertal individuals
Two or more neurofibromas of any type **-or-** one plexiform neurofibroma
Freckling in the axillary or inguinal regions
Optic glioma
Two or more Lisch nodules
A distinctive osseous lesion such as sphenoid dysplasia or thinning of long bone cortex with or without pseudoarthrosis
A first-degree relative with NF-1 by the above criteria

Laboratory Data
Baseline magnetic resonance imaging (MRI) of brain and spinal cord

Management
Complete history and physical examination
Baseline ophthalmologic examination
Regular follow-up with pediatrician, internist, ophthalmologist, neurologist, dermatologist
Referral to orthopedist, audiologist, psychiatrist, surgeon, neurosurgeon, oncologist if symptomatic
Examine first-degree relatives

Prognosis
May have shortened life span secondary to neurofibrosarcoma, pheochromocytoma, vascular disease complications, CNS tumor complications; great variation in severity of disease

Clinical Pearls

It is important that children with café au lait spots have an annual opththalmologic examination for the first 5 to 6 years then every 2 to 3 years. I do not routinely obtain a baseline MRI, but offer that option to parents . . . Always evaluate other family members for the presence of cutaneous lesions to consider if a sporadic mutation or if a parent is affected, even with a mosaic form. This information is important in counseling about the risk for future siblings. Ophthalmologic examinations may be helpful if the diagnosis is equivocal. . . Always check blood pressure; if elevated in child, consider renal artery stenosis; if elevated in adult, consider pheochromocytoma. . . Precocious puberty may suggest CNS tumor. Multiple juvenile xanthogranuloma (JXG) may be associated with nonlymphocytic leukemia in a child with café au lait spots. If these xanthogranulomas are present, obtain a CBC, but recognize that the likelihood of finding evidence of leukemia is small. It is important to follow a child with serial head circumference measurements because of the risk of hydrocephalus and the frequency of macrocephaly without hydrocephalus. Always palpate the skin carefully, especially under large café au lait spots, because they may overlie a plexiform neurofibroma. . . Refer to NF support group. *AP*

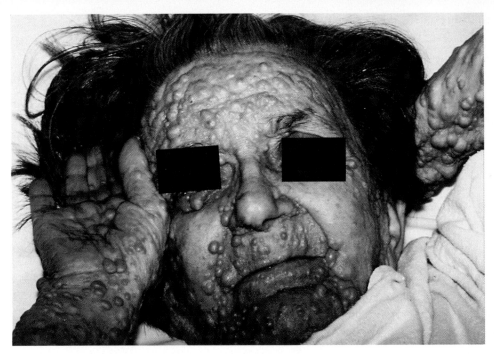

2.28. *Generalized neurofibromas on face and arms. (34)*

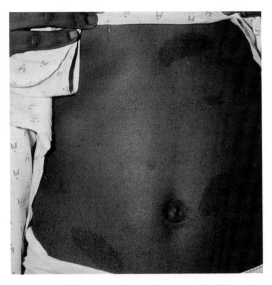

2.29. *Multiple café au lait macules on trunk. (35)*

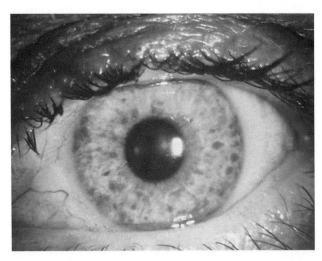

2.30. *Lisch nodules studding the iris. (1)*

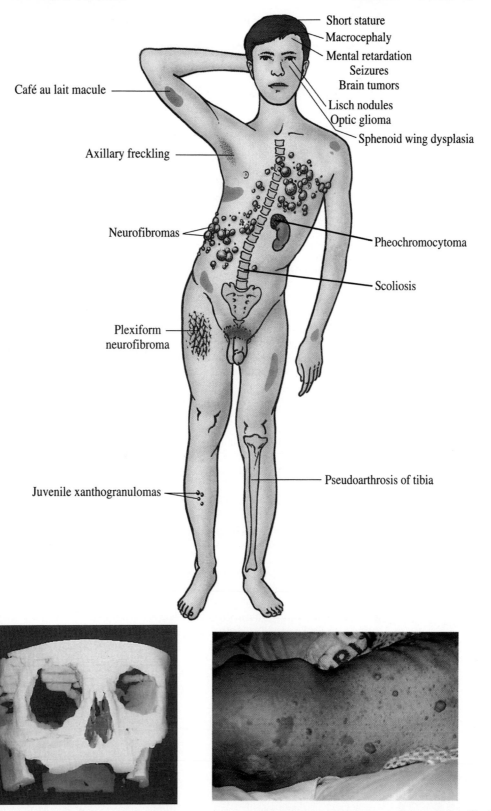

Short stature
Macrocephaly
Mental retardation
Seizures
Brain tumors
Lisch nodules
Optic glioma
Sphenoid wing dysplasia

Café au lait macule

Axillary freckling

Neurofibromas

Pheochromocytoma

Scoliosis

Plexiform
neurofibroma

Juvenile xanthogranulomas

Pseudoarthrosis of tibia

2.31. *Three-dimensional CT reformation highlighting sphenoid wing dysplasia in patient's right orbit.* (36)

2.32. *Malignant schwannoma eroding overlying skin.* (1)

Neurofibromatosis II

Synonym	Bilateral acoustic neurofibromatosis; central neurofibromatosis
Inheritance	Autosomal dominant; mutation in *SCH* gene on 22q11–13.1; spontaneous mutation in 50% of cases
Prenatal Diagnosis	DNA mutation analysis if defect known
Incidence	1:35,000; M=F; all races
Age at Presentation	Symptoms frequently appear at 15 to 25 years of age
Pathogenesis	A defect in schwannomin/merlin, the NF-2 gene product, may affect tumor suppressor activity at the cell membrane level

Key Features

Skin
Neurofibromas (less common than in NF-1)
Three Types
Subcutaneous with overlying pigment and hair (most common)
Subcutaneous spherical tumor associated with palpable nerve
Intradermal (i.e., NF-1)
Café au lait macules—large, pale, 1 to 2 lesions (less common than in NF-1)

Central Nervous System
Bilateral vestibular schwannomas (acoustic neuromas)
Schwannomas of other cranial nerves
Meningiomas—intracranial and spinal
Astrocytomas, ependymomas
Tumors may be complicated by deafness, tinnitus, poor balance, headache, muscular wasting, underwater disorientation

Eyes
Juvenile posterior subcapsular lenticular opacity

Differential Diagnosis	NF-1 and other forms of NF (3–9) (p. 82)
Laboratory Data	Brain MRI
NIH Consensus Criteria for Diagnosis—1987	Bilateral eighth nerve masses (visualized with CT or MRI) *-or-* First-degree relative with NF-2 *-and either-* Unilateral eighth nerve mass *-or-* Any two of the following: neurofibroma, meningioma, spinal glioma, schwannoma, juvenile posterior subcapsular lenticular opacity
Management	Referral to neurologist/neurosurgeon—surgical debulking of tumors Referral to ENT specialist/audiologist, ophthalmologist, dermatologist Examine first-degree relatives
Prognosis	Progressive deterioration with loss of hearing, ambulation, and sight; death resulting from CNS tumors approximately 20 years after onset of symptomatology

Clinical Pearls

Patients must never swim alone and must avoid going under water . . . Surgical intervention may add to morbidity . . . Normal intelligence . . . Offspring of affected individuals should have an ophthalmologic examination at birth because cataracts may be present very early on.   *DE*

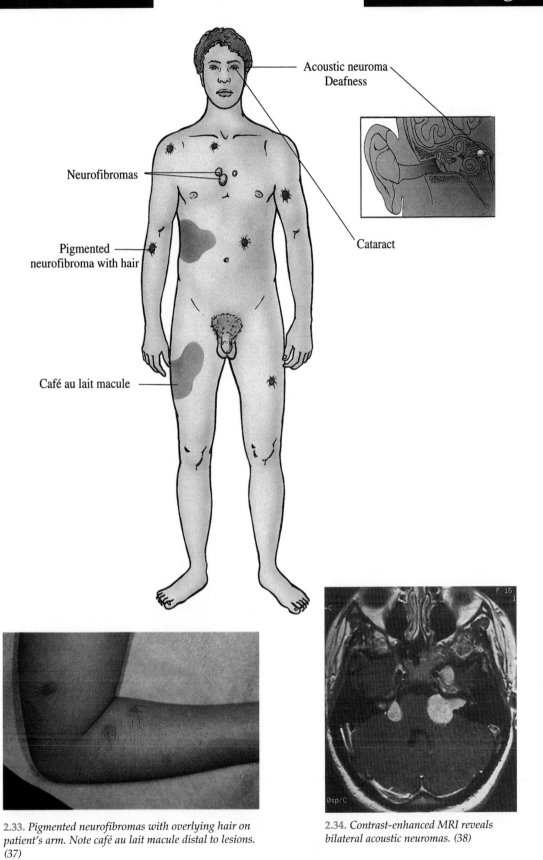

Acoustic neuroma
Deafness

Neurofibromas

Pigmented
neurofibroma with hair

Café au lait macule

Cataract

2.33. *Pigmented neurofibromas with overlying hair on patient's arm. Note café au lait macule distal to lesions.* (37)

2.34. *Contrast-enhanced MRI reveals bilateral acoustic neuromas.* (38)

Tuberous Sclerosis

Synonym	Bourneville's syndrome; epiloia
Inheritance	Autosomal dominant; *TSC1* gene on 9q34, *TSC2* gene on l6pl3 Up to 66% may be spontaneous mutations
Prenatal Diagnosis	Fetal echocardiogram revealing rhabdomyoma DNA analysis if mutation known
Incidence	1:10,000; M=F; all races
Age at Presentation	Birth
Pathogenesis	Mutations in either *TSC1* encoding hamartin or *TSC2* encoding tuberin lead to tumor suppression and interact to regulate GTPase activity of rap 1 GAP family genes. *TSC2* (tuberin) with renal cysts may be associated with deletion in contiguous polycystic kidney gene (*PKD1*)

Key Features

Skin
Hypopigmented macules: **ash-leaf**—earliest finding, most characteristic; **polygonal**—most common, **confetti**—pretibial
Shagreen patch—connective tissue nevus
Facial angiofibromas—"adenoma sebaceum"
Periungual fibromas
Fibrous plaque of face
Café au lait macule

Central Nervous System
Infantile spasms, tonic–clonic seizures, hypsarrhythmia, mental retardation, cortical tumors, paraventricular calcification, subependymal nodules with or without obstructive hydrocephalus, astrocytomas

Eyes
Retinal hamartomas (phakomas)

Kidney
Angiomyolipoma, cysts

Cardiac
Rhabdomyoma

Oral
Enamel pits, gingival fibromas

Musculoskeletal
Phalangeal cysts, periosteal thickening

Lungs
Lymphangiomyomatosis

Differential Diagnosis

Nevus depigmentosus
Nevus anemicus
Vitiligo
Idiopathic guttate hypomelanosis
Hypomelanosis of Ito (p. 70)

Laboratory Data   Wood's light examination, transfontanelle ultrasound, CT scan/MRI of brain, electroencephalogram (EEG), fundoscopic examination, renal ultrasound, echocardiogram in infancy

Management   Complete physical examination with routine follow-up by primary care physician
Referral to neurosurgeon/neurologist—neurosurgical removal of brain tumors, anti-convulsant medications, shunting of obstructive hydrocephalus
Referral to laser specialist—CO_2 or copper vapor laser excision of facial angiofibromas
Referral to ophthalmologist
Referral to other specialists if symptomatic
Careful cutaneous and general examination of first-degree relatives

Prognosis   Premature death may occur secondary to cardiovascular complications early on with brain, renal, pulmonary and seizure morbidity contributing to mortality later in life

Clinical Pearls

Angiofibromas can be a tremendous cosmetic problem for patients. . . Remember, 0.2% to 0.3% of normal neonates have hypopigmented macules. . . Rhabdomyomas are common in infancy and regress spontaneously with age. . . Echocardiagram is nice test to do in infancy if diagnosis is equivocal. . . Approximately 40% of patients have normal intelligence. . . I prefer MRI to CT scan of the brain given lack of radiation and increased sensitivity; ultrasound through the fontanelle may be performed in neonates and young infants.   *AP*

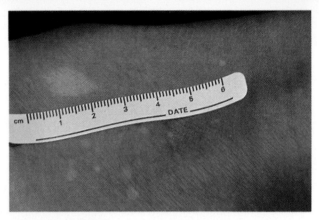

2.35. *Ash-leaf and polygonal hypopigmented macules.* (1)

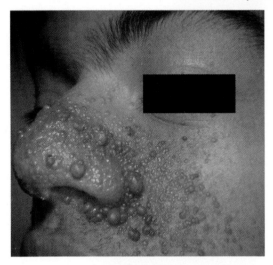

2.36. *Angiofibromas ("adenoma sebaceum").* (1)

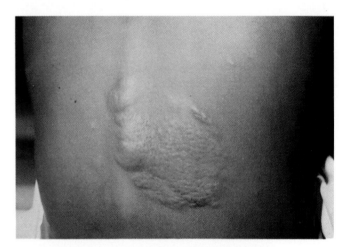

2.37. *Shagreen patch overlying lumbosacral region.* (1)

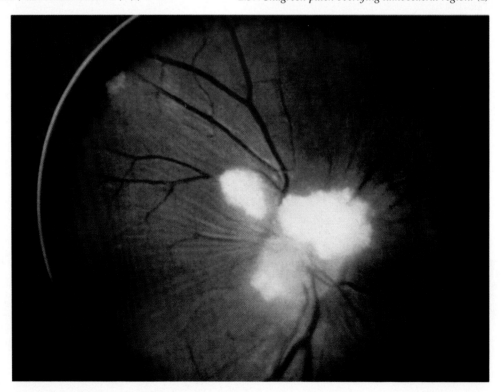

2.38. *Astrocytic hamartomas of the retina and optic nerve.* (39)

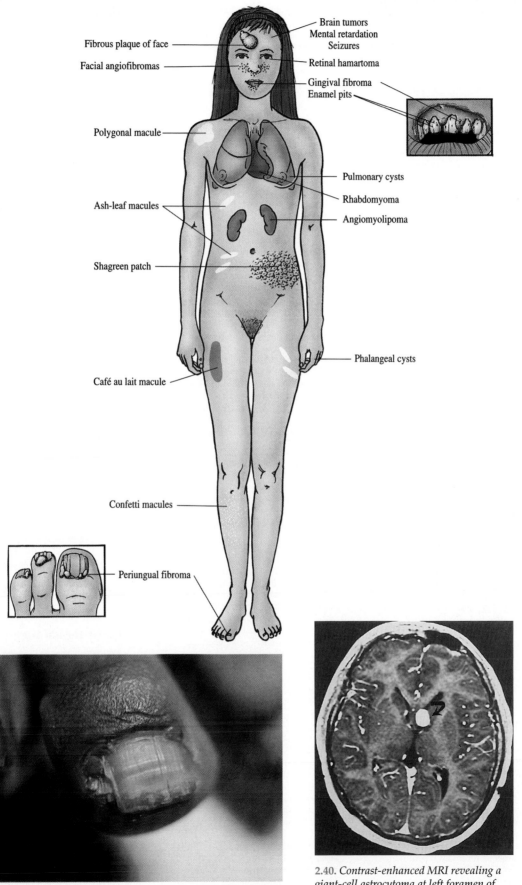

Fibrous plaque of face

Facial angiofibromas

Polygonal macule

Ash-leaf macules

Shagreen patch

Café au lait macule

Confetti macules

Periungual fibroma

Brain tumors
Mental retardation
Seizures

Retinal hamartoma

Gingival fibroma
Enamel pits

Pulmonary cysts

Rhabdomyoma

Angiomyolipoma

Phalangeal cysts

2.39. *Periungual fibromas. (1)*

2.40. *Contrast-enhanced MRI revealing a giant-cell astrocytoma at left foramen of Monro. (36)*

Suggested Reading

OCA1

Camand O, Marchant D, Boutboul S, et al. Mutation analysis of the tyrosinase gene in oculocutaneous albinism. *Hum Mutat* 2001;17:352.

Gershoni-Baruch R, Rosenmann A, Droetto S, et al. Mutations of the tyrosinase gene in patients with oculocutaneous albinism from various ethnic groups in Israel. *Am J Hum Genet* 1994;54:586–594.

Nakamura E, Miyamura Y, Matsunaga J, et al. A novel mutation of the tyrosinase gene causing oculocutaneous albinism type 1 (OCA1). *J Dermatol Sci* 2002;28:102–105.

Oetting WS. The tyrosinase gene and oculocutaneous albinism type 1 (OCA1): a model for understanding the molecular biology of melanin formation. *Pigment Cell Res* 2000;13:320.

Oetting WS, Fryer JP, Shriram S, King RA. Oculocutaneous albinism type 1: the last 100 years. *Pigment Cell Res* 2003;16:307–311.

Oetting WS, King RA. Molecular basis of albinism: mutations and polymorphisms of pigment genes associated with albinism. *Hum Mutat* 1999;13:99.

Oetting WS, Brilliant MH, King RA. The clinical spectrum of albinism in humans. *Mol Med Today* 1996;2:330–335.

Pehamberger H, Honisgmann H, Wolff K. Dysplastic nevus syndrome with multiple primary amelanotic melanomas in oculocutaneous albinism. *J Am Acad Dermatol* 1984;11:731–735.

Perry PK, Silverberg NB. Cutaneous malignancy in albinism. *Cutis* 2001;67:427–430.

Spritz RA, Strunk KM, Giebel LB, et al. Detection of mutations in the tyrosine gene in a patient with type IA oculocutaneous albinism. *N Engl J Med* 1990;322:1724–1728.

Summers CG, Oetting WS, King RA. Diagnosis of oculocutaneous albinism with molecular analysis. *Am J Ophthalmol* 1996;724–726.

Toyofuku K, Wada I, Spritz RA, et al. The molecular basis of oculocutaneous-albinism type 1 (OCA1): sorting failure and degradation of mutant tyrosinases results in a lack of pigmentation. *Biochem J* 2001;355:259–269.

OCA2

Akiyama M, Shimizu H, Sugiura M, et al. Do pigmented naevi in albinism provide evidence of tyrosinase positivity? *Br J Dermatol* 1992;127:649–653.

Bloom KE. Advances in inherited disorders of hypopigmentation: comparisons of mice and men. *Curr Opin Pediatr* 1993;5:458–463.

Brilliant MH. The mouse p (*pink-eyed dilution*) and human P genes, oculocutaneous albinism type 2 (OCA2), and melanosomal pH. *Pigment Cell Res* 2001;14:86.

Ihn H, Nakamura K, Abe M, et al. Amelanotic metastatic melanoma in a patient with oculocutaneous albinism. *J Am Acad Dermatol* 1993;28:895–900.

Kato A, Fukai K, Oiso N, et al. A novel P gene missense mutation in a Japanese patient with oculocutaneous albinism type II (OCA2). *J Dermatol Sci* 2003;31:189–192.

Kerr R, Stevens G, Manga P, et al. Identification of P gene mutations in individuals with oculocutaneous albinism is sub-Saharan Africa. *Hum Mutat* 2000;15:166–172.

Manga P, Orlow SJ. (1999) The pink-eyed dilution gene and the molecular pathogenesis of tyrosinase-positive albinism (OCA2). J Dermatol 1999;26:738–747.

Oetting WS, Gardner JM, Fryer JP, et al. Mutations of the human P gene associated with Type II oculocutaneous albinism (OCA2). Mutations in brief no. 205. Online. *Hum Mutat* 1998;12:434.

Ramsay M, Colman MA, Stevens G, et al. The tyrosinase-positive oculocutaneous albinism locus maps to chromosome 15q11. 2–q12. *Am J Hum Genet* 1992;51:879–884.

Toyofuku K, Valencia JC, Kushimoto T, et al. The etiology of oculocutaneous albinism (OCA) type II: the pink protein modulates the processing and transport of tyrosinase [published erratum appears in *Pigment Cell Res* 2002t;15:400]. *Pigment Cell Res* 2002;15:217–224.

Hermansky-Pudlak Syndrome

Anderson PD, Huizing M, Claassen DA, et al. Hermansky Pudlak syndrome type 4 (HPS-4): clinical and molecular characteristics. *Hum Genet* 2003;113:10–17.

Avila NA, Brantly M, Premkumar A, et al. Hermansky-Pudlak syndrome: radiography and CT of the chest compared with pulmonary function tests and genetic studies. *AJR Am J Roentgenol* 2002;179:887–892.

Bachli EB, Brack T, Eppler E, et al. Hermansky-Pudlak syndrome type 4 in a patient from Sri Lanka with pulmonary fibrosis. *Am J Med Genet* 2004;127A:201–207.

Chiang PW, Oiso N, Gautam R, et al. The Hermansky-Pudlak syndrome 1 (HPS1) and HPS4 proteins are components of two complexes, BLOC-3 and BLOC-4, involved in the biogenesis of lysosome-related organelles. *J Biol Chem* 2003;278:20332–20337.

Clark RH, Stinchcombe JC, Day A, et al. Adaptor protein 3-dependent microtubule-mediated movement of lytic granules to the immunological synapse. *Nat Immunol* 2003;4:1111–1120.

Corral J, Gonzalez-Conejero R, Pujol-Moix N, et al. Mutation analysis of HPS1, the gene mutated in Hermansky-Pudlak syndrome, in patients with isolated platelet dense-granule deficiency. *Haematologica* 2004;89:325–329.

Dell'Angelica EC, Shotelersuk V, Aguilar RC, et al. Altered trafficking of lysosomal proteins in Hermansky–Pudlak syndrome due to mutations in the beta 3A subunit of the AP-3 adaptor. *Mol Cell* 1999;3:11–21.

Di Pietro SM, Falcon-Perez JM, Dell'Angelica EC. Characterization of BLOC-2, a complex containing the Hermansky-Pudlak syndrome proteins HPS3, HPS5 and HPS6. *Traffic* 2004;5:276–283.

Gahl WA, Brantly M, Kaiser-Kupfer MI, et al. Genetic defects and clinical characteristics of patients with a form of oculocutaneous albinism (Hermansky-Pudlak syndrome). *N Engl J Med* 1998;338:1258–1264.

Garay SM, Gardella JE, Fazzini EP, et al. Hermansky-Pudlak syndrome: pulmonary manifestations of a ceroid storage disorder. *Am J Med* 1979;66:737–747.

Hermansky F, Pudlak P. Albinism associated with hemorrhagic diathesis and unusual pigmented reticular cells in the bone marrow: report of two cases with histochemical studies. *Blood* 1959;14:162–169.

Huizing M, Anikster Y, Gahl WA. Hermansky-Pudlak syndrome and related disorders of organelle formation. *Traffic* 2000;1:823–835.

Huizing M, Boissy RE, Gahl WA. Hermansky-Pudlak syndrome: vesicle formation from yeast to man. *Pigment Cell Res* 2002;15:405–419.

Mahadeo R, Markowitz J, Fisher S, et al. Hermansky-Pudlak syndrome with granulomatous colitis in children. *J Pediatr* 1991;118:904–906.

Schachne JP, Glaser N, Lee SH, et al. Hermansky-Pudlak syndrome: case report and clinicopathologic review *J Am Acad Dermatol* 1990;22:926–932.

Toro J, Turner M, Gahl WA. Dermatologic manifestations of Hermansky–Pudlak syndrome in patients with and without a 16-base pair duplication in the HPS1 gene. *Arch Dermatol* 1999;135:774–780.

Chédiak-Higashi Syndrome

Ahluwalia J, Pattari S, Trehan A, et al. Accelerated phase at initial presentation: an uncommon occurrence in Chediak-Higashi syndrome. *Pediatr Hematol Oncol* 2003;20:563–567.

Anderson LL, Paller AS, Malpass D, et al. Chédiak-Higashi syndrome in a black child. *Pediatr Dermatol* 1992;9:31–36.

Barton LM, Roberts P, Trantou V, et al. Chediak-Higashi syndrome. *Br J Haematol* 2004;125:2.

Blume RS, Wolff SM. The Chédiak-Higashi syndrome: studies in four patients and a review of the literature. *Medicine* 1972;51:247–280.

Certain S, Barrat F, Pastural E, et al. Protein truncation test of *LYST* reveals heterogeneous mutations in patients with Chédiak-Higashi syndrome. Blood 2000;95:979–983.

Filipovich AH. Bone marrow transplantation from unrelated donors for congenital immunodeficiencies. *Bone Marrow Transplant* 1993;11:78–80.

Harfi HA, Malik SA. Chédiak-Higashi syndrome: clinical, hematologic, and immunologic improvement after splenectomy. *Ann Allergy* 1992;69:147–150.

Introne W, Boissy RE, Gahl WA. Clinical, molecular, and cell biological aspects of Chédiak-Higashi syndrome. *Mol Genet Metab* 1999;68:283–303.

Karim MA, Suzuki K, Fukai K, et al: Apparent genotype-phenotype correlation in childhood, adolescent, and adult Chédiak-Higashi syndrome. *Am J Med Genet* 2002;108:16–22.

Masui N, Nishikawa T, Takagi Y, et al. The rat lysosomal trafficking regulator (Lyst) gene is mapped on the telomeric region of chromosome 17. *Exp Anim* 2003;52:89–91.

Nagle DL, Karim MA, Woolf EA, et al. Identification and mutation analysis of the complete gene for Chédiak-Higashi syndrome. *Nat Genet* 1996;14:307–311.

Sayanagi K, Fujikado T, Onodera T, et al. Chediak-Higashi syndrome with progressive visual loss. *Jpn J Ophthalmol* 2003;47:304–306.

Scheinfeld NS. Syndromic albinism: a review of genetics and phenotypes. *Dermatol Online J* 2003;9:5.

Stinchcombe JC, Page LJ, Griffiths GM, et al. Secretory lysosome biogenesis in cytotoxic T lymphocytes from normal and Chédiak-Higashi syndrome patients. *Traffic* 2000;1:435–444.

Stolz W, Graubner U, Gerstmeier J, et al. Chédiak-Higashi syndrome approaches in diagnosis and treatment. *Curr Probl Dermatol* 1989;18:93–100.

Griscelli Syndrome

Anikster Y, Huizing M, Anderson PD, et al. Evidence that Griscelli syndrome with neurological involvement is caused by mutations in RAB27A, not MYO5A [published erratum appears in *Am J Hum Genet* 2002;71:1007]. *Am J Hum Genet* 2002;71:407–414.

Arico M, Zecca M, Santoro N, et al. Successful treatment of Griscelli syndrome with unrelated donor allogeneic hematopoietic stem cell transplantation. *Bone Marrow Transplant* 2002;29:995–998.

Bahadoran P, Busca R, Chiaverini C, et al. Characterization of the molecular defects in Rab27a, caused by RAB27A missense mutations found in patients with Griscelli syndrome. *J Biol Chem* 2003;278:11386–11392.

Dolman KM, Revesz T, Niemeyer CM, et al. Myelodysplastic Features in Griscelli Syndrome. *J Pediatr Hematol Oncol* 2004;26:275–276.

Izumi T, Gomi H, Kasai K, et al. The roles of Rab27 and its effectors in the regulated secretory pathways. *Cell Struct Funct* 2003;28:465–474.

Menasche G, Fischer A, de Saint Basile G. Griscelli syndrome types 1 and 2. *Am J Hum Genet* 2002;71:1237–1238; author reply 1238.

Menasche G, Ho CH, Sanal O, et al. Griscelli syndrome restricted to hypopigmentation results from a melanophilin defect (GS3) or a MYO5A F-exon deletion (GS1). *J Clin Invest* 2003;112:450–456.

Menasche G, Pastural E, Feldmann J, et al. (2000) Mutations in RAB27A cause Griscelli syndrome associated with haemophagocytic syndrome. *Nat Genet* 2000;25:173–176.

Pastural E, Ersoy F, Yalman N, et al. (2000) Two genes are responsible for Griscelli syndrome at the same 15g21 locus. Genomics 2000;63:299–306.

Rath S, Jain V, Marwaha RK, et al. Griscelli syndrome. *Indian J Pediatr* 2004;71:173–175.

Stein MP, Dons J, Wandinger-Ness A. Rab proteins and endocytic trafficking: potential targets for therapeutic intervention. *Adv Drug Deliv Rev* 2003;55:1421–1437.

Piebaldism

Bloom KE. Advances in inherited disorders of hypopigmentation: comparisons of mice and men. *Curr Opin Pediatr* 1993;5:458–463.

Garg T, Khaitan BK, Manchanda Y. Autologous punch grafting for repigmentation in piebaldism. *J Dermatol* 2003;30:849–850.

Guerra L, Primavera G, Raskovic D, et al. Permanent repigmentation of piebaldism by erbium:YAG laser and autologous cultured epidermis. *Br J Dermatol* 2004;150:715–721.

Kaplan P, de Chaderevian JP. Piebaldism-Waardenburg syndrome: histopathologic evidence for a neural crest syndrome. *Am J Med Genet* 1988;31:679–688.

Spritz RA. Piebaldism, Waardenburg syndrome, and related disorders of melanocyte development. *Semin Cutan Med Surg* 1997;16:15–23.

Spritz RA, Ho L, Strunk KM. Inhibition of proliferation of human melanocytes by a KIT antisense oligodeoxynucleotide: implications for human piebaldism and mouse dominant white spotting (W). *J Invest Dermatol* 1994;103: 148–150.

Spritz RA, Holmes SA, Berg SZ, et al. A recurrent deletion in the KIT (mast/stem cell growth factor receptor) protooncogene is a frequent cause of human piebaldism. *Hum Mol Genet* 1993;2(9):1499–1500.

Spritz RA., Itin PH, Gutmann DH. Piebaldism and neurofibromatosis type 1: horses of very different colors. *J Invest Dermatol* 2004;122:xxxiv–xxxv.

Syrris P, Heathcote K, Carrozzo R, et al. Human piebaldism: six novel mutations of the proto-oncogene KIT. *Hum Mutat* 2002;20:234.

Tomita Y. The molecular genetics of albinism and piebaldism. *Arch Dermatol* 1994;130:355–358.

Winship I, Young K, Martell R, et al. Piebaldism: an autonomous autosomal dominant entity. *Clin Genet* 1991;39:330–337.

Waardenburg Syndrome

Boudurand N, Pingault V, Goerich DE, et al. Interaction among SOX10, PAX3 and MITF, three genes altered in Waardenburg syndrome. *Hum Mol Genet* 2000;9:1907–1917.

Delleman JW, Hageman MJ. Ophthalmological findings in 34 patients with Waardenburg syndrome. *J Pediatr Ophthalmol Strabismus* 1978;15:341–345.

Hill RE, Hanson IM. Molecular genetics of the Pax gene family. *Curr Opin Cell Biol* 1992;4:967–972.

Hoth CF, Milunsky A, Lipsky N, et al. Mutations in the paired domain of the human PAX3 gene cause Klein-Waardenburg syndrome (WS-III) as well as Waardenburg syndrome type I (WS-I). *Am J Hum Genet* 1993;52:455–462.

Lalwani AK, Brister JR, Fex J, et al. Further elucidation of the genomic structure of PAX3, and identification of two different point mutations within the PAX3 homeobox that cause Waardenburg syndrome type 1 in two families. *Am J Hum Genet* 1995;56:75–83.

Lang D, Epstein JA. Sox10 and Pax3 physically interact to mediate activation of a conserved c-RET enhancer. *Hum Mol Genet* 2003;12:937–945.

Nobukuni Y, Watanabe A, Takeda K, et al. (1996) Analyses of loss-of-function mutations of the MITF gene suggest that haploinsufficiency is a cause of Waardenburg syndrome type 2A. *Am J Hum Genet* 1996;59:76–83.

Pignault V, Bondurand N, Lemort N, et al. A heterozygous endothelin 3 mutation in Waardenburg-Hirschsprung disease: is there a dosage effect of EDN3/EDNRB gene mutations on neurocristopathy phenotypes? *J Med Genet* 2001;38:205–209.

Pingault V, Bondurand N, Kuhlbrodt K, et al. SOX10 mutations in patients with Waardenburg-Hirschsprung disease. *Nat Genet* 1998;18:171–173.

Read AP, Newton VE. Waardenburg syndrome. *J Med Genet* 1997;34:656–665.

Tachibana M, Kobayashi Y, Matsushima Y. Mouse models for four types of Waardenburg syndrome. *Pigment Cell Res* 2003;16:448–454.

Wollnik B, Tukel T, Uyguner O, et al. Homozygous and heterozygous inheritance of PAX3 mutations causes different types of Waardenburg syndrome. *Am J Med Genet.* 2003;122A:42–45.

Hypomelanosis of Ito

Chitayat D, Friedman JM, Johnston MM. Hypomelanosis of Ito—a nonspecific marker of somatic mosaicism. *Am J Med Genet* 1990;35:422.

Donnai D, Read AP, McKeown C, Andrews T. Hypomelanosis of Ito: a manifestation of mosaicism or chimerism. *J Med Genet* 1988;25:809–818.

Happle R. Mosaicism in human skin. Understanding the patterns and mechanisms. *Arch Dermatol* 1993;129:1460–1470.

Kuster W, Konig A. Hypomelanosis of Ito: no entity, but a cutaneous sign of mosaicism. *Am J Med Genet* 1999;85:346.

Loomis CA. Linear hypopigmentation and hyperpigmentation including mosaicism. *J Cutan Med Surg* 1997;16:44.

Meyer CH, Freyschmidt-Paul P, Happle R, et al. Unilateral linear hyperpigmentation of the skin with ipsilateral sectorial hyperpigmentation of the retina. *Am J Med Genet* 2004;126A:89–92.

Nehal KS, PeBenito R, Orlow SJ. Analysis of 54 cases of hypopigmentation and hyperpigmentation along the lines of Blaschko. *Arch Dermatol* 1996;132:1167–1170.

Pascual-Castroviejo I, Lopez-Rodriguez L, de la Cruz-Medina M, et al. Hypomelanosis of Ito: neurological complications in 34 cases. *Can J Neurol Sci* 1988;15:124–129.

Ruiz-Maldonado R, Toussaint S, Tamayo L, et al. Hypomelanosis of Ito: diagnostic criteria and report of 41 cases. *Pediatr Dermatol* 1992;9:1–10.

Sybert VA, Pagon RA, Donian M, et al. Pigmentary abnormalities and mosaicism for chromosomal aberration: association with clinical features similar to hypomelanosis of Ito. *J Pediatr* 1990;116:581–586.

Incontinentia Pigmenti

Bell S, Degitz K, Quirling M, et al. Involvement of NF-kappaB signalling in skin physiology and disease. *Cell Signal* 2003;15:1–7.

Berlin AL, Palter AS, Chan LS. Incontinentia pigmenti: a review and update on the molecular basis of pathophysiology. *J Am Acad Dermatol* 2002;47:169–187; quiz 188–190.

Bodak N, Hadj-Rabia S, Hamel-Teillac D, et al. Late recurrence of inflammatory first-stage lesions in incontinentia pigmenti: an unusual phenomenon and a fascinating pathologic mechanism. *Arch Dermatol* 2003;139:201–204.

Cannizzaro LA, Hech F. Gene for incontinentia pigmenti maps to band Xp11 with an (X;10) (p11;q22) translocation. *Clin Genet* 1987;32:66–69.

Carney RG, Jr. Incontinentia pigmenti: a world statistical analysis. *Arch Dermatol* 1976;112:535–542.

Carney RG, Carney RG Jr. Incontinentia pigmenti. *Arch Dermatol* 1970;102:157–162.

Chan YC, Happle R, Giam YC. Whorled scarring alopecia: a rare phenomenon in incontinentia pigmenti? *J Am Acad Dermatol* 2003;49:929–931.

Doruk C, Bicakci AA, Babacan H. Orthodontic and orthopedic treatment of a patient with incontinentia pigmenti. *Angle Orthod* 2003;73:763–768.

Fiorillo L, Sinclair DB, O'Byrne ML, et al. Bilateral cerebrovascular accidents in incontinentia pigmenti. *Pediatr Neurol* 2003;29:66–68.

Hadj-Rabia S, Froidevaux D, Bodak N, et al. Clinical study of 40 cases of incontinentia pigmenti. *Arch Dermatol* 2003;139:1163–1170.

Happle R. A fresh look at incontinentia pigmenti. *Arch Dermatol* 2003;139:1206–1208.

International Incontinentia Pigmenti Consortium. Genomic rearrangement in NEMO impairs NF-kappaB activation and is a cause of incontinentia pigmenti. *Nature* 2000;405:466–472.

Jouet M, Stewart H, Landy S et al. Linkage analysis in 16 families with incontinentia pigmenti. *Eur J Hum Genet* 1997;5:168–170.

Landy SJ, Donnai D. Incontinentia pigmenti (Bloch-Sulzberger syndrome). *J Med Genet* 1993;30:53–59.

Mirowski GW, Caldemeyer KS. Incontinentia pigmenti. *J Am Acad Dermatol* 2000;43:517–518.

Montes CM, Maize JC, Guerry-Force ML. Incontinentia pigmenti with painful subungual tumors: a two-generation study. *J Am Acad Dermatol* 2004;50:S45–S52.

Rosenfeld SI, Smith ME. Ocular findings in incontinentia pigmenti. *Ophthalmology* 1985;92:543–546.

Shah SN, Gibbs S, Upton CJ, et al. Incontinentia pigmenti associated with cerebral palsy and cerebral leukomalacia: a case report and literature review. *Pediatr Dermatol* 2003;20:491–494.

Shastry BS. Recent progress in the genetics of incontinentia pigmenti (Bloch-Sulzberger syndrome). *J Hum Genet* 2000;45:323–326.

Smahi A, Courtois G, Rabia SH, et al. The NF-kappaB signalling pathway in human diseases: from incontinentia pigmenti to ectodermal dysplasias and immune-deficiency syndromes. *Hum Mol Genet* 2002;11:2371–2375.

LEOPARD Syndrome

Chen B, Bronson RT, Klaman LD, et al. Mice mutant for Egfr and Shp2 have defective cardiac semilunar valvulogenesis. *Nat Genet* 2000;24:296–299.

Chong WS, Klanwarin W, Giam YC. Generalized lentiginosis in two children lacking systemic associations: case report and review of the literature. *Pediatr Dermatol* 2004;21:139–145.

Conti E, Dottorini T, Sarkozy A, et al. A novel PTPN11 mutation in LEOPARD syndrome. *Hum Mutat* 2003;21:654.

Coppin BD, Temple IK. Multiple lentigines syndrome (LEOPARD syndrome or progressive cardiomyopathic lentiginosis). *J Med Genet* 1997;34:582–586.

Dechert U, Duncan AMV, Bastien L, et al. Protein-tyrosine phosphatase SH-PTP2 (PTPN11) is localized to 12q24.1–24.3. *Hum Genet* 1995;96:609–615.

Digilio MC, Conti E, Sarkozy A, et al. Grouping of multiple-lentigines/LEOPARD and Noonan syndromes on the PTPN11 gene. *Am J Hum Genet* 2002;71:389–394.

Digilio MC, Pacileo G, Sarkozy A, et al. Familial aggregation of genetically heterogeneous hypertrophic cardiomyopathy: a boy with LEOPARD syndrome due to PTPN11 mutation and his nonsyndromic father lacking PTPN11 mutations. *Birth Defects Res Part A Clin Mol Teratol* 2004;70:95–98.

Gorlin RJ, Anderson RC, Slaw ME. Multiple lentigines syndrome: complex comprising multiple lentigines, electrocardiographic conduction abnormalities, ocular hypertelorism, pulmonary stenosis, abnormalities of genitalia, retardation of growth, sensorineural deafness, and autosomal dominant hereditary pattern. *Am J Dis Child* 1969;117:652–662.

Kontoes PP, Vlachos SP, Marayiannis KV. Intense pulsed light for the treatment of lentigines in LEOPARD syndrome. *Br J Plast Surg* 2003;56:607–610.

Legius E, Schrander-Stumpel C, Schollen E, et al. PTPN 11 mutations in LEOPARD syndrome. *J Med Genet* 2002;39:571–574.

Moynahan EJ. Progressive cardiomyopathic lentiginosis: first report of autopsy findings in a recently recognized inheritable disorder (autosomal dominant). *Proc R Soc Med* 1974;63:448–451.

Seuanez H, Mane-Garzon F, Kolski R. Cardiocutaneous syndrome (the "LEOPARD" syndrome): review of the literature and a new family. *Clin Genet* 1976;9:266–276.

Torres J, Russo P, Tobias JD. Anaesthetic implications of LEOPARD syndrome. *Paediatr Anaesth* 2004;14:352–356.

Yagubyan M, Panneton JM, Lindor NM, et al. LEOPARD syndrome: a new polyaneurysm association and an update on the molecular genetics of the disease. *J Vasc Surg* 2004;39:897–900.

Carney Complex

Amano J, Kono T, Wada Y, et al. Cardiac myxoma: its origin and tumor characteristics. *Ann Thorac Cardiovasc Surg* 2003;9:215–221.

Aspres N, Bleasel NR, Stapleton KM. Genetic testing of the family with a Carney-complex member leads to successful early removal of an asymptomatic atrial myxoma in the mother of the patient [published erratum appears in *Australas J Dermatol* 2003;44:508]. *Australas J Dermatol* 2003;44:121–122.

Atherton DJ, Pitcher DW, Wells RS, et al. A syndrome of various cutaneous pigmented lesions, myxoid neurofibromata and atrial myxoma: the NAME syndrome. *Br J Dermatol* 1980;103:421–429.

Carney JA, Gordon H, Carpenter PC, et al. The complex of myxomas, spotty pigmentation, and endocrine overactivity. *Medicine* 1985;64:270–283.

Carney JA, Headington JT, Su WP. Cutaneous myxomas: a major component of the complex of myxomas, spotty pigmentation, and endocrine overactivity. *Arch Dermatol* 1986;122:790–798.

Groussin L, Kirschner LS, Vincent-Dejean C, et al. Molecular analysis of the cyclic AMP-dependent protein kinase A (PKA) regulatory subunit 1A (PRKAR1A) gene in patients with Carney complex and primary pigmented nodular adrenocortical disease (PPNAD) reveals novel mutations and clues for pathophysiology: augmented PKA signaling is associated with adrenal tumorigenesis in PPNAD. *Am J Hum Genet* 2002;71:1433–1442.

Koopman RJ, Happle R. Autosomal dominant transmission of the NAME syndrome (nevi, atrial myxoma, mucinosis of the skin and endocrine overactivity). *Hum Genet* 1991;86:300–304.

Proppe KH, Scully RE. Large-cell calcifying Sertoli cell tumor of the testis. *Am J Clin Pathol* 1980;74:607–619.

Robinson-White A, Handley TR, Shiferaw M, et al. Protein kinase-A activity in PRKAR1A-mutant cells, and regulation of mitogen-activated protein kinases ERK1/2. *Hum Mol Genet* 2003;12:1475–1484.

Stergiopoulos SG, Stratakis CA. Human tumors associated with Carney complex and germline PRKARIA mutations: a protein kinase A disease. *FEBS Lett* 2003;546:59–64.

Stratakis CA. Clinical genetics of multiple endocrine neoplasias, Carney complex and related syndromes. *J Endocrinol Invest* 2001;24:370–383.

Stratakis CA, Kirschner LS, Carney JA. Clinical and molecular features of Carney complex: diagnostic criteria and recommendations for patient evaluation. *J Clin Endocrinol Metab* 2001;86:4041–4046.

Young WF, Carney JA, Musa BU, et al. Familial Cushing's syndrome due to primary pigmented nodular adrenocortical disease: reinvestigation 50 years later. *N Engl J Med* 1989;321:1659–1678.

McCune-Albright Syndrome

Akintoye SO, Chebli C, Booher S, et al. Characterization of gsp-mediated growth hormone excess in the context

of McCune-Albright syndrome. *J Clin Endocrinol Metab* 2002;87:5104–5112.

Cavanah SF, Dons RF. McCune-Albright syndrome: how many endocrinopathies can one patient have? *South Med J* 1993;86:364–367.

Cohen MM Jr, Howell RE. Etiology of fibrous dysplasia and McCune-Albright syndrome. *Int J Oral Maxillofac Surg* 1999;28:366–371.

De Sanctis C, Lala R, Matarazzo P, et al. McCune-Albright syndrome: a longitudinal clinical study of 32 patients. *J Pediatr Endocrinol Metab* 1999;12:817–826.

Esterly NF, Baselga E, Drolet BA. Polyostotic fibrous dysplasia (McCune-Albright syndrome). In: Nordlund JJ, Boissy RE, Hearing VJ, et al., eds. *The pigmentary system: physiology and pathophysiology*. New York: Oxford University Press, 1998:748.

Kim IS, Kim ER, Nam HJ, at al. Activating mutation of GSa in McCune-Albright syndrome causes skin pigmentation by tyrosinase gene activation on affected melanocytes. *Horm Res* 1999;52:235–240.

Lee PA, Van Dop C, Migeon CAJ. McCune-Albright syndrome: long-term follow-up. *JAMA* 1986;256:2980–2984.

Levine MA. Clinical implications of genetic defects in G proteins: oncogenic mutations in Gαs as the molecular basis for the McCune-Albright syndrome [review]. *Arch Med Res* 1999;30:522–531.

Pohlenz J, Ahrens W, Hiort O. A new heterozygous mutation (L338N) in the human Gsalpha (GNAS1) gene as a cause for congenital hypothyroidism in Albright's hereditary osteodystrophy. *Eur J Endocrinol* 2003;148:463–468.

Riminucci M, Fisher LW, Majolagbe A, et al. A novel GNAS1 mutation, R201G, in McCune-albright syndrome. *J Bone Miner Res* 1999;14:1987–1989.

Ringel MD, Schwindinger WF, Levine MA. Clinical implications of genetic defects in G proteins. The molecular basis of McCune-Albright syndrome and Albright hereditary osteodystrophy. *Medicine (Baltimore)* 1996;75:171–184.

Roth JG, Esterly NB. McCune-Albright syndrome with multiple bilateral cafe au fait spots. *Pediatr Dermatol* 1991;8:35–39.

Schwindinger WF, Francomano CA, Levine MA. Identification of a mutation in the gene encoding the alpha subunit of the stimulatory G-protein of adenylyl cyclase in McCune Albright syndrome. *Proc Nat Acad Sci USA* 1992;89:5152–5156.

Shenker A, Weinstein LS, Moran A, et al. Severe endocrine and nonendocrine manifestations of the McCune-Albright syndrome associated with activating mutations of stimulatory G protein GS. *J Pediatr* 1993;123:509–518.

Neurofibromatosis 1

Ackerman CD, Cohen BA. Juvenile xanthogranuloma and

neurofibromatosis. *Pediatr Dermatol* 1991;8:339–340.

Akbarnia BA, Gabriel KR, Beckman E, et al. Prevalence of scoliosis in neurofibromatosis. *Spine* 1992;17:S244–S248.

Astrup J. Natural history and clinical management of optic pathway glioma. *Br J Neurosurg* 2003;17:327–335.

Barker D, Wright E, Nguyen K, et al. Gene for von Recklinghausen neurofibromatosis is in the pericentric region of chromosome 17. *Science* 1987;236:1100–1102.

Bilgic B, Ates LE, Demiryont M, et al. Malignant peripheral nerve sheath tumors associated with neurofibromatosis type 1. *Pathol Oncol Res* 2003;9:201–205.

Cohen MM Jr. Further diagnostic thoughts about the Elephant Man. *Am J Med Genet* 1988;29:777–782.

Crawford AH, Schorry EK. Neurofibromatosis in children: the role of the orthopaedist. *J Am Aced Orthop Surg* 1999;7:217–230.

Cutting LE, Koth CW, Denckla MB. How children with neurofibromatosis type 1 differ from "typical" learning disabled clinic attenders: nonverbal learning disabilities revisited. *Dev Neuropsychol* 2000;17:29–47.

Dasgupta B, Dugan LL, Gutmann DH. The neurofibromatosis 1 gene product neurofibromin regulates pituitary adenylate cyclase-activating polypeptide-mediated signaling in astrocytes. *J Neurosci* 2003;23:8949–8954.

Drappier JC, Khosrotehrani K, Zeller J, et al. Medical management of neurofibromatosis 1: a cross-sectional study of 383 patients. *J Am Acad Dermatol* 2003;49:440–444.

Durrani AA, Crawford AH, Chouhdry SN, et al. (2000) Modulation of spinal deformities in patients with neurofibromatosis type 1. 2000;25:69–75.

Guttman DH, Aylsworth A, Carey JC, et al. The diagnostic evaluation and multidisciplinary management of neurofibromatosis 1 and neurofibromatosis 2. *JAMA* 1997;278:51–57.

Gutmann DH, James CD, Poyhonen M, et al. Molecular analysis of astrocytomas presenting after age 10 in individuals with NF 1. *Neurology* 2003;61:1397–1400.

Imes RK, Hoyt WF. Magnetic resonance imaging signs of optic nerve gliomas in neurofibromatosis 1. *Am J Ophthalmol* 1991;111:729–734.

Karadimas P, Hatzispasou E, Bouzas EA. Retinal vascular abnormalities in neurofibromatosis type 1. *J Neuroophthalmol* 2003;23:274–275.

Kluwe L, Siebert R, Gesk S, et al. Screening 500 unselected neurofibromatosis 1 patients for deletions of the NF1 gene. *Hum Mutat* 2004;23:111–116.

Lacaze E, Kieffer V, Streri A, et al. Neuropsychological outcome in children with optic pathway tumours when first-line treatment is chemotherapy. *Br J Cancer* 2003;89:2038–2044.

Listernick R, Louis DN, Packer RJ, et al. Optic pathway gliomas in children with neurofibromatosis 1: consensus statement from the NF1 Optic Pathway Glioma Task Force. *Ann Neurol* 1997;41:143–149.

Lubs ME, Bauer MS, Formas ME, et al. Lisch nodules in neurofibromatosis type 1. *N Engl J Med* 1991;324:1264–1266.

Messiaen LM, Callens T, Monier G, et al. Exhaustive mutation analysis of the NF1 gene allows identification of 95% of mutations and reveals a high frequency of unusual splicing defects. *Hum Mutat* 2000;15:541–555.

Mulvihill JJ, Parry DM, Sherman JL, et al. NIH conference. Neurofibromatosis 1 (Recklinghausen disease) and neurofirbromatosis 2 (bilateral acoustic neurofibromatosis). *Ann Intern Med* 1990;113:39–52.

Nichols JC, Amato JE, Chung SM. Characteristics of Lisch nodules in patients with neurofibromatosis type 1. *J Pediatr Ophthalmol Strabismus* 2003;40:293–296.

NIH Consensus Development Conference. Neurofibromatosis: conference statement. *Arch Neurol* 1988;45:575–578.

Pinsk I, Dukhno O, Ovnat A, et al. Gastrointestinal complications of von Recklinghausen's disease: two case reports and a review of the literature. *Scand J Gastroenterol* 2003;38:1275–1278.

Serra E, Rosenbaum T, Winner U, et al. Schwann cells harbor the somatic NF1 mutation in neurofibromas: evidence of two different schwann cell subpopulations. *Hum Mol Genet* 2000;9:3055–3064.

Sorensen SA, Mulvihill JJ, Nielsen A. Long-term follow-up on von Recklinghausen neurofibromatosis: survival and malignant neoplasms. *N Engl J Med* 1986;314:1010–1015.

Stern HJ, Sall HM, Lee JS, et al. Clinical variability of type 1 neurofibromatosis: is there a neurofibromatosis-Noonan syndrome? *J Med Genet* 1992;29:184–187.

Thiagalingam S, Flaherty M, Billson F, et al. Neurofibromatosis type 1 and optic pathway gliomas: follow-up of 54 patients. *Ophthalmology* 2004;111:568–577.

Truhan AP, Filipek PA. Magnetic resonance imaging. Its role in the neuroradiologic evaluation of neurofibromatosis, tuberous sclerosis, and Sturge-Weber syndrome. *Arch Dermatol* 1993;129:219–226.

Upadhyaya M, Han S, Consoli C, et al. Characterization of the somatic mutational spectrum of the neurofibromatosis type 1 (NF1) gene in neurofibromatosis patients with benign and malignant tumors. *Hum Mutat* 2004;23:134–146.

Venturin M, Guarnieri P, Natacci F, et al. Mental retardation and cardiovascular malformations in NF1 microdeleted patients point to candidate genes in 17q11.2. *J Med Genet* 2004;41:35–41.

Waye JS, Greig G, Leinwand L, et al. Gene for von Recklinghausen neurofibromatosis is in the pericentromeric region of chromosome 17. *Science* 1987;236:1100–1102.

Xu G, O'Connell P, Viskochil D, et al. The neurofibromatosis type 1 gene encodes a protein related to GAP. *Cell* 1990;62:599–608.

Neurofibromatosis II

Baser ME, Kuramoto L, Joe H, et al. Genotype-phenotype correlations for cataracts in neurofibromatosis 2. *J Med Genet* 2003;40:758–760.

Bouzas EA, Freidlin V, Parry DM, et al. Lens opacities in neurofibromatosis 2: further significant correlations. *Br J Ophthalmol* 1993;77:354–357.

Evans DGR, Huson SM, Donnai D, et al. A clinical study of type 2 neurofibromatosis. *Q J Med* 1992;84:603–618.

Evans DGR, Huson SM, Donnai D, et al. A genetic study of type 2 neurofibromatosis in the United Kingdom. II. Guidelines for genetic counselling. *J Med Genet* 1992;29:847–852.

Evans DG, Trueman L, Wallace A et al. Genotype/phenotype correlations in type 2 neurofibromatosis (NF2): evidence for more severe disease associated with truncating mutations. *J Med Genet* 1998;35:450–455.

Glasscock ME III, Hays JW, Minor LB, et al. Preservation of hearing in surgery for acoustic neuromas. *J Neurosurg* 1993;78:864–870.

Kinzler KW, Vogelstein B. Cancer. A gene for neurofibromatosis 2 news; comment. *Nature* 1993;363:495–496.

Kissil JL, Wilker EW, Johnson KC, et al. Merlin, the product of the Nf2 tumor suppressor gene, is an inhibitor of the p21-activated kinase, Pak1. *Mol Cell* 2003;12:841–849.

MacCollin M, Ramesh V, Jacoby LB, et al. Mutational analysis of patients with neurofibromatosis 2. *Am J Hum Genet* 1994;55:314–320.

Martuza RL, Eldridge R. Neurofibromatosis 2 (bilateral acoustic neurofibromatosis). *N Engl J Med* 1988;318:684–688.

Mulvihill JJ, Parry DM, Sherman JL, et al. NIH conference. Neuro-fibromatosis 1 (Recklinghausen disease) and neurofibromatosis 2 (bilateral acoustic neurofibromatosis). An update. *Ann Intern Med* 1990;113:39–52.

NIH Consensus Development Conference. Neurofibromatosis: conference statement. *Arch Neurol* 1988;45:475–578.

Nunes F, MacCollin M. Neurofibromatosis 2 in the pediatric population. *J Child Neurol* 2003;18:718–724.

Otsuka G, Saito K, Nagatani T, et al. Age at symptom onset and long-term survival in patients with neurofibromatosis Type 2. *J Neurosurg* 2003;99:480–483.

Parry DM, Eldridge R, Kaiser-Kupfer MI, et al. Neurofibromatosis 2 (NF2): clinical characteristics of 63 affected individuals and clinical evidence for heterogeneity. *Am J Med Genet* 1994;52:450–461.

Parry DM, MacCollin MM, Kaiser-Kupfer MI, et al. Germline mutations in the neurofibromatosis 2 gene: correlation with disease severity and retinal abnormalities. *Am J Hum Genet* 1996;59:529–539.

Pastores GM, Michels VV, Jack CR Jr. Early childhood diagnosis of acoustic neuromas in presymptomatic individuals at risk for neurofibromatosis 2. *Am J Med Genet* 1991;41:325–329.

Rouleau GA, Merel P, Lutchman, et al. Alteration in a new gene encoding a putative membrane-organizing protein causes neurofibromatosis type 2. *Nature* 1993;363:515–521.

Schwartz MS, Otto SR, Brackmann DE, et al. Use of a multichannel auditory brainstem implant for neurofibromatosis type 2. *Stereotact Funct Neurosurg* 2003;81:110–114.

Shaw RJ, McClatchey AL, Jacks T. Localization and functional domains of the neurofibromatosis type II tumor suppressor, merlin. *Cell Growth Differ* 1998;9:287–296.

Surace EL, Haipek CA, Gutmann DH. Effect of merlin phosphorylation on neurofibromatosis 2 (NF2) gene function. *Oncogene* 2004;15;23:580–587.

Tang BH. Vestibular schwannoma growth. *J Neurosurg* 2004;100:734–735; author reply 735.

Trofatter JA, MacCollin MM, Rutter JL, et al. A novel moezin-, ezrin-, radixin-like gene1993 andidate for the neurofibromatosis 2 tumor suppressor. *Cell* 1993;72:791–800.

Wagner LM, Zhou H, Brockmeyer DL, et al. Spinal cord schwannomas mimicking drop metastases in a patient with intramedullary ependymoma and neurofibromatosis 2. *J Pediatr Hematol Oncol* 2004;26:56–59.

Xiao GH, Chernoff J, Testa JR. NF2: the wizardry of merlin. *Genes Chromosomes Cancer* 2003;38:389–399.

Tuberous Sclerosis

Ariyurek Y, Lecuwen IL, Spruit L, et al. Large deletions in the polycystic kidney disease 1 (PKD1) gene. *Hum Mutat* 2004;23:99.

Au KS, Rodriguez JA, Finch JL, et al. Germ-line mutational analysis of the TSC2 gene in 90 tuberous-sclerosis patients. *Am J Hum Genet* 1998;62:286–294.

Bader RS, Chitayat D, Kelly E, et al. Fetal rhabdomyoma: prenatal diagnosis, clinical outcome, and incidence of associated tuberous sclerosis complex. *J Pediatr* 2003;143:620–624.

Bernauer T, Mirowski GW, Caldemeyer KS. Tuberous sclerosis. Part II. Musculoskeletal and visceral findings. *J Am Acad Dermatol* 2001;45:450–452.

Caldemeyer K, Mirowski G. Tuberous sclerosis. Part I. Clinical and central nervous system findings. *J Am Acad Dermatol* 2001;45:448.

Dabora SL, Jozwiak S, Franz DN, et al. Mutational analysis in a cohort of 224 Tuberous Sclerosis patients indicates increased severity of TSC2, compared with TSC1, disease in multiple organs. *Am J Hum Genet* 2001;68:64–80.

Feng JH, Yamamoto T, Nanba E, et al. Novel TSC2 mutations and decreased expression of tuberin in cultured tumor cells with an insertion mutation. *Hum Mutat* 2004;23:397.

Fesslova V, Villa L, Rizzuti T, et al. Natural history and long-term outcome of cardiac rhabdomyomas detected prenatally. *Prenat Diagn* 2004;24:241–248.

Fricke BL, Donnelly LF, Casper KA, et al. Frequency and imaging appearance of hepatic angiomyolipomas in pediatric and adult patients with tuberous sclerosis. *AJR Am J Roentgenol* 2004;182:1027–1030.

Fryer AE, Osborne JP, Schutt W. Forehead plaque: a presenting skin sign in tuberous sclerosis. *Arch Dis Child* 1987;62:292–304.

Giacoia GP. Fetal rhabdomyoma: a prenatal echocardiographic marker of tuberous sclerosis. *Am J Perinatol* 1992;9:111–114.

Harabayashi T, Shinohara N, Katano H, et al. Management of renal angiomyolipomas associated with tuberous sclerosis complex. *J Urol* 2004;171:102–105.

Henske EP, Wessner LL, Golden J, et al. Loss of tuberin in both subependymal giant cell astrocytomas and angiomyolipomas supports a two-hit model for the pathogenesis of tuberous sclerosis tumors. *Am J Pathol* 1997;151:1639–1647.

Hodges AK, Li S, Maynard J, et al. Pathological mutations in TSC1 and TSC2 disrupt the interaction between hamartin and tuberin. *Hum Mol Genet* 2001;10:2899–2905.

Hunt A. Tuberous sclerosis: a survey of 97 cases: II: physical findings. *Dev Med Child Neurol* 1983;25:350–352.

Hyman MH, Whittemore VH. National Institutes of Health Consensus Conference: tuberous sclerosis complex. *Arch Neurol* 2000;57:662–665.

Jansen FE, Van Nieuwenhuizen O, Van Huffelen AC. Tuberous sclerosis complex and its founders. *J Neurol Neurosurg Psychiatry* 2004;75:770.

Jarrar RG, Buchhalter JR, Raffel C. Long-term outcome of epilepsy surgery in patients with tuberous sclerosis. *Neurology* 2004;62:479–481.

Jones KA, Jiang X, Yamamoto Y, et al. Tuberin is a component of lipid rafts and mediates caveolin-1 localization: role of TSC2 in post-Golgi transport. *Exp Cell Res* 2004;295:512–524.

Jozwiak S, Kwiatkowski D, Kotulska K, et al. Tuberin and hamartin expression is reduced in the majority of subependymal giant cell astrocytomas in tuberous sclerosis complex consistent with a two-hit model of pathogenesis. *J Child Neurol* 2004;19:102–106.

Kaminaga T, Takeshita T, Kimura I. Role of magnetic resonance imaging for evaluation of tumors in the cardiac region. *Eur Radiol* 2003;13:L1–L10.

Kandt RS. Tuberous sclerosis complex and neurofibromatosis type 1: the two most common neurocutaneous diseases. *Neurol Clin* 2003;21:983–1004.

Knowles MA, Habuchi T, Kennedy W, et al. Mutation spectrum of the 9q34 tuberous sclerosis gene TSC1 in transitional cell carcinoma of the bladder. *Cancer Res* 2003;63:7652–7656.

Krymskaya VP. Tumour suppressors hamartin and tuberin: intracellular signalling. *Cell Signal* 2003;15:729–739.

Kwiatkowski DJ, Short MP. Tuberous sclerosis. *Arch Dermatol* 1994;130:348–354.

Laass MW, Spiegel M, Jauch A, et al. Tuberous sclerosis and polycystic kidney disease in a 3-month-old infant. *Pediatr Nephrol* 2004;19:602–608.

Lazarowski A, Lubieniecki F, Camarero S, et al. Multidrug resistance proteins in tuberous sclerosis and refractory epilepsy. *Pediatr Neurol* 2004;30:102–106.

Lewis JC, Thomas HV, Murphy KC, et al. Genotype and psychological phenotype in tuberous sclerosis. *J Med Genet* 2004;41:203–207.

Marantz P, Guerchicoff M, Villa A, et al. Diagnosis and follow-up of fetal cardiac tumors. *Echocardiography* 2004;21:212.

Martignoni G, Bonetti F, Pea M, et al. Renal disease in adults with TSC2/PKD1 contiguous gene syndrome. *Am J Surg Pathol* 2002;26:198–205.

Narayanan V. Tuberous sclerosis complex: genetics to pathogenesis. *Pediatr Neurol* 2003;29:404–409.

Nellist M, van Slegtenhorst MA, Goedbloed M, et al. Characterization of the cytosolic tuberin-hamartin complex. Tuberin is a cytosolic chaperone for hamartin. *J Biol Chem* 1999;274:35647–35652.

Roach ES, Smith M, Huttenlocher P. Diagnostic criteria: tuberous sclerosis complex. Report of the Diagnostic Criteria Committee of the National Tuberous Sclerosis Association. *J Child Neurol* 1992;7:221–224.

Roach ES, DiMario FJ, Kandt RS, et al. Tuberous Sclerosis Consensus Conference: recommendations for diagnostic evaluation. National Tuberous Sclerosis Association. *J Child Neurol* 1999;14:401.

Sampson JR. TSC1 and TSC2: genes that are mutated in the human genetic disorder tuberous sclerosis. *Biochem Soc Trans* 2003;31:592–596.

Sampson JR, Attwood D, Al Mughery AS, et al. Pitted enamel hypoplasia in tuberous sclerosis. *Clin Genet* 1992;42:50–52.

Sampson JR, Maheshwar MM, Aspinwall R, et al. Renal cystic disease in tuberous sclerosis: role of the polycystic kidney disease 1 gene. *Am J Hun Genet* 1997;61:843–851.

Smolarek TA, Wessner LL, McCormack FX, et al. Evidence that lymphangiomyomatosis is caused by TSC2 mutations: chromosome 16p13 loss of heterozygosity in angiomyolipomas and lymph nodes from women with lymphangiomyomatosis. *Am J Hum Genet* 1998;62:810–815.

Tee AR, Manning BD, Roux PP, et al. Tuberous sclerosis complex gene products, Tuberin and Hamartin, control mTOR signaling by acting as a GTPase-activating protein complex toward Rheb. *Curr Biol* 2003;13:1259–1268.

Truhan AP, Filipek PA. Magnetic resonance imaging. Its role in the neuroradiologic evaluation of neurofibromatosis, tuberous sclerosis, and Sturge-Weber syndrome. *Arch Dermatol* 1993;129:219–226.

Vanderhooft SL, Francis JS, Pagon RA, et al. Prevalence of hypopigmented macules in a healthy population. *J Pediatr* 1996;129:355–361.

van Slegtenhorst M, de Hoogt R, Hermans C, et al: Identification of the tuberous sclerosis gene TSC1 on chromosome 9q34. *Science* 1997;277:805–808.

Webb DW, Thomas RD, Osborne JP. Cardiac rhabdomyomas and their association with tuberous sclerosis. *Arch Dis Child* 1993;68:367–370.

Chapter 3

Disorders of Vascularization

Clinical Pearls

Amy Paller, M.D. (AP), Kurt Hirschhorn, M.D. (KH), Judith Willner, M.D. (JW), and Ilona Frieden, M.D. (IF)

Sturge-Weber Syndrome

Synonym	Encephalotrigeminal angiomatosis
Inheritance	Sporadic
Prenatal Diagnosis	None
Incidence	Rare; 2% to 11% of children with facial capillary malformation (0.3% to 0.6% of infants are born with facial capillary malformation) approximately 10% with V_1 distribution; M=F
Age at Presentation	Birth; seizures at 1 to 2 years old
Pathogenesis	Defect in morphogenesis within the cephalic neural crest with subsequent abnormal vasculature in the upper facial dermis, choroid, and pia-arachnoid (mesoectodermal tissue); may be an autosomal lethal mutation surviving by mosaicism

Key Features

Skin
  Facial capillary malformation
    Trigeminal nerve distribution ($V_1 \pm V_2, V_3$)
    Unilateral more common than bilateral
    Progressive soft tissue and skeletal hypertrophy beneath malformation
Central Nervous System
  Cerebral atrophy
  Capillary, venous, and arteriovenous malformations ipsilateral to skin malformation in leptomeninges
  Tram-track calcification in temporal and occipital cortex beneath leptomeningeal malformation
  Seizures(> 70%), intellectual impairment (50%), hemiparesis, headache
Eyes
  Choroid malformation
  Ipsilateral glaucoma with secondary buphthalmos, visual loss

Differential Diagnosis	Periorbital hemangioma Salmon patch
Laboratory Data	Magnetic resonance imaging (MRI) with gadolinium; computed tomography (CT) with contrast Less than 6 months: positron emission tomography/single-photon emission computed tomography (PET/SPECT) scan may be useful EEG (if above positive)
Management	Referral to dermatologist—laser treatment of capillary malformation Referral to ophthalmologist—at presentation to detect and manage glaucoma, preserve vision Referral to neurologist—seizure control Referral to orthodontist/oral surgeon-treat complications of maxillary hypertrophy (occlusion deformity, cross-bite), gingival hypertrophy
Prognosis	If seizures are difficult to control, there is an increased frequency of intellectual impairment over time; visual impairment if glaucoma left untreated; normal life span

Clinical Pearls

Having a port wine stain in the distribution of the first branch of the trigeminal nerve is not uncommon; the minority will have Sturge-Weber syndrome . . . We only perform an MRI scan if the neonate or young infant shows evidence of neurologic disorder, most commonly seizure activity . . . Atrophic changes may be detected prior to calcifications on MRI . . . If MRI is initially normal and there is suspicion, I would repeat the scan at 2 to 3 years of age . . . I get an ophthalmologic examination . . . Seizures are often controlled at least partially with anticonvulsants, but may require hemispherectomy . . . Pulsed dye laser can be initiated early for the facial port wine stains.   *AP*

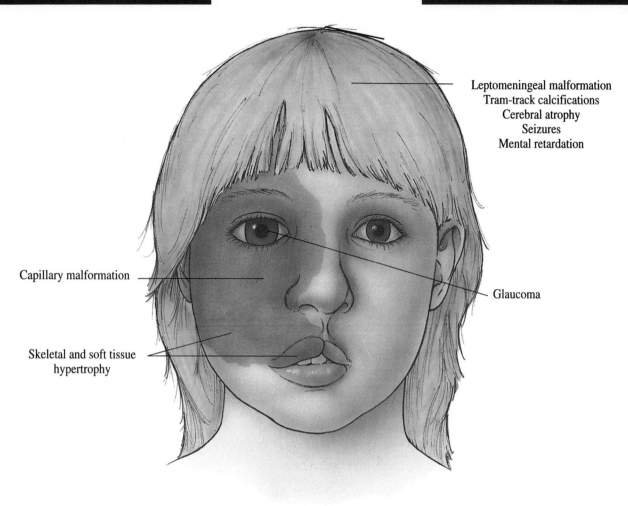

Leptomeningeal malformation
Tram-track calcifications
Cerebral atrophy
Seizures
Mental retardation

Capillary malformation

Glaucoma

Skeletal and soft tissue hypertrophy

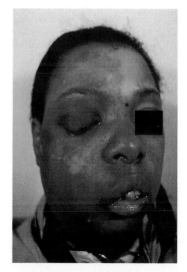

3.1. *Unilateral facial capillary malformation overlying marked soft tissue and bony hypertrophy. (1)*

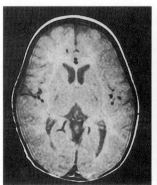
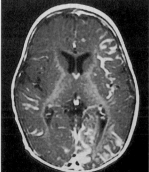

3.2. *MRI with gadolinium revealing leptomeningeal malformation. (5)*

Klippel-Trenaunay Syndrome

Synonym	Angio-osteohypertrophy syndrome
Inheritance	Sporadic
Prenatal Diagnosis	None
Incidence	M > F
Age at Presentation	Birth; capillary malformation first sign
Pathogenesis	Increased vascular supply hypothesized as cause of limb hypertrophy

Key Features

Skin
Capillary malformation involving lower extremity (95%), upper extremity (5%), or combined (15%); unilateral in 85%

Musculoskeletal
Soft tissue, muscle and bony hypertrophy below cutaneous malformation with increased limb length and/or girth; rarely hypotrophic limb, polydactyly, syndactyly

Vascular
Superficial venous varicosities, phleboliths, deep venous malformation, arteriovenous fistulas (Parkes–Weber variant), superficial thrombophlebitis, deep vein thrombosis complicated by pulmonary embolism (rare)

Lymphatic
Lymphatic malformation with/without lymphedema

Differential Diagnosis

Proteus syndrome (p. 106)
Neurofibromatosis I (p. 82)
Maffucci syndrome (p. 118)
Capillary malformation

Laboratory Data

Doppler ultrasound in childhood
MRI, magnetic resonance angiography (MRA), venography, lymphography

Management

Compression wraps (young infant), stockings, pump
Routine measurement of limb length and circumference
Referral to orthopedist—correction of limb length discrepancy
Referral to vascular surgeon—treatment of symptomatic varicosities, arteriovenous fistulas
Referral to laser specialist—pulsed dye laser correction of capillary malformation

Prognosis

Progressive limb hypertrophy after birth-degree of hypertrophy dependent on extent of malformation, lymphedema and presence of A-V fistulas
High-output cardiac failure if A-V fistula untreated

Clinical Pearls

Probably the most useful intervention is the use of a compression garment once hypertrophy and varicosities begin to develop . . . Practically speaking, compression may be very difficult when you are treating a child wearing diapers . . . If we see a leg length discrepancy > 1 cm, we will consider a leg lift . . . Doppler imaging is very useful for following patients, particularly if an A-V fistula is present . . . Distal foot bacterial infections, paronychias, and warts are very common in a lymphedematous leg . . . May be confused with Proteus syndrome.   *AP*

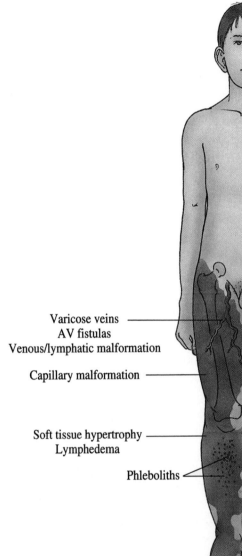

Varicose veins
AV fistulas
Venous/lymphatic malformation

Capillary malformation

Bone hypertrophy
Limb lengthening

Soft tissue hypertrophy
Lymphedema

Phleboliths

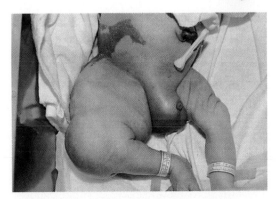

*3.3. Unilateral capillary malformation overlying
massive venous-lymphatic malformation in a
newborn. (35)*

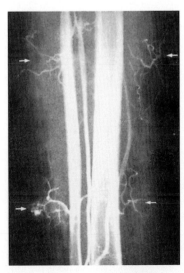

*3.4. Angiography reveals discrete
areas of arteriovenous malformation
(arrows) in the calf of a patient. (40)*

Cobb Syndrome

Synonym	Cutaneomeningospinal angiomatosis
Inheritance	Sporadic
Prenatal Diagnosis	None
Incidence	Rare; spinal arteriovenous malformations (AVMs) more common without skin involvement, M=F
Age at Presentation	Birth; neurologic complications develop in early adulthood
Pathogenesis	Unknown

Key Features

Skin
Posterior thoracic/lumbar/limb vascular lesion in a dermatomal distribution overlying a corresponding segment of spinal cord

Central Nervous System
Fast-flow vascular malformation within the intramedullary (most common) spinal cord with secondary compression/anoxia-secondary pain, weakness, muscle atrophy, and sensation loss below the level of compression; bladder and sphincter dysfunction if malformation extensive; subarachnoid hemorrhage; malformation may involve vertebral body

Differential Diagnosis	Capillary malformation overlying a meningoencephalocele, spinal dysraphism, tethered spinal cord
Laboratory Data	MRI, MRA Spinal angiography
Management	Referral to neurologist—complete neurologic examination Referral to neurosurgeon—extirpation of lesion, embolization
Prognosis	Dependent on degree of symptomatology prior to intervention—may be irreversible

Clinical Pearls

MRI is my imaging technique of choice at time of presentation . . . Spinal malformations are particularly difficult to approach surgically . . . Embolization is feasible in certain cases. *AP*

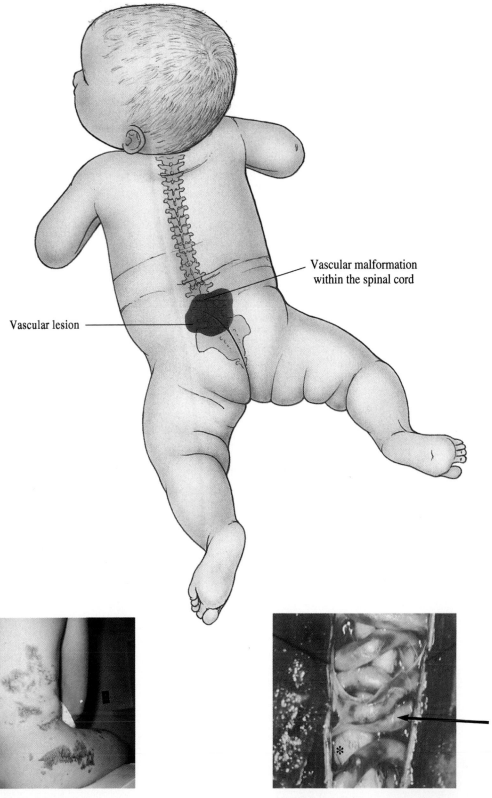

Vascular malformation
within the spinal cord

Vascular lesion

3.5. *Extensive capillary malformation extending to involve the lumbosacral spine. (41)*

3.6. *Arteriovenous malformation (arrow) within the spinal cord (*). (42)*

Proteus Syndrome

Synonym	Most likely includes Riley-Smith and Bannayan syndromes
Inheritance	Sporadic
Prenatal Diagnosis	None
Incidence	Rare; M=F
Age at Presentation	Birth; may develop over time
Pathogenesis	Mosaicism for an autosomal lethal mutation in the PTEN tumor suppressor gene has been reported in some patients

Key Features

Skin
Soft, subcutaneous masses (likely lymphatic and venous-lymphatic malformations), lipomas, capillary malformations, linear epidermal nevi, plantar/palmar hyperplasia, varicose veins

Musculoskeletal
Macrocephaly, facial asymmetry, skull hyperostoses, frontal bossing, syndactyly, asymmetric soft tissue and bony hypertrophy of hands, feet, limbs; kyphoscoliosis
Reports of cataracts, strabismus, microphthalmos, blindness, testicular tumors, penile hypertrophy

Differential Diagnosis
Klippel-Trenaunay-Weber syndrome (p. 102)
Maffucci syndrome (p. 118)
Neurofibromatosis I (p. 82)

Laboratory data
Bone x-rays/MRI

Management
Referral to plastic surgeon, orthopedic surgeon, physiatrist
Referral to symptom-specific subspecialist

Prognosis
Potential for gross deformity and debilitation exists; malignant potential unknown

Clinical Pearls

It is well documented that Joseph Merrick, the "Elephant Man," had Proteus syndrome rather than neurofibromatosis . . . The striking plantar hyperplasia is distinct for this syndrome . . . The malformations can be so extensive that surgical correction is very difficult. *KH, JW*

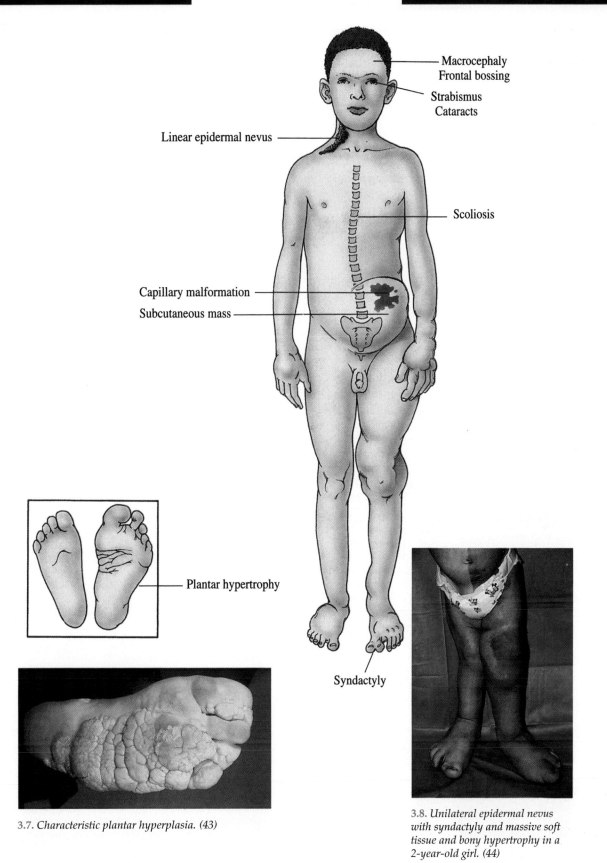

Macrocephaly
Frontal bossing

Strabismus
Cataracts

Linear epidermal nevus

Scoliosis

Capillary malformation

Subcutaneous mass

Plantar hypertrophy

Syndactyly

3.7. *Characteristic plantar hyperplasia.* (43)

3.8. *Unilateral epidermal nevus with syndactyly and massive soft tissue and bony hypertrophy in a 2-year-old girl.* (44)

Beckwith-Wiedemann Syndrome

Synonym	Exomphalos-macroglossia-gigantism (EMG) syndrome
Inheritance	Most cases are sporadic; variety of transmissions described; p57 (*KIP2*) gene on 11p15.5
Prenatal Diagnosis	Ultrasound—macrosomia, visceromegaly, omphalocele visualized DNA analysis in familial cases
Incidence	Unknown; M=F
Age at Presentation	Birth
Pathogenesis	Mutation in the p57 (KIP2) gene, a cyclin-dependent kinase inhibitor gene acting as a negative regulator of cell proliferation, leads to overgrowth of organs and increased susceptibility to malignancies

Key Features

Skin
Capillary malformation on mid-forehead, glabella, and upper eyelids extending to nose and upper lip in some cases

Mouth
Macroglossia

Ears
Linear earlobe crease, circular depressions on rim of posterior helices

Viscera
Hepatomegaly, splenomegaly, nephromegaly, pancreatomegaly, cardiomegaly
Omphalocele
Intestinal malrotation

Endocrine
Neonatal hypoglycemia with secondary neurologic sequelae if unrecognized

Musculoskeletal
Somatic gigantism—birth weight and length greater than 90th percentile
Hemihypertrophy (33%)

Neoplasms (10%)
Wilms' tumor > hepatoblastoma > adrenal cortical carcinoma, rhabdomyosarcoma; increased in patients with hemihypertrophy

Differential Diagnosis	Down syndrome (p. 346) Mucopolysaccharidoses (p. 318) Congenital hypothyroidism
Laboratory Data	Blood glucose level Abdominal and renal ultrasound at 3-month intervals through early childhood Serum alpha-fetoprotein levels (screen for hepatoblastoma)
Management	Monitor blood glucose in the neonate Complete physical examination Referral to pediatric surgeon Referral to appropriate subspecialist as necessary
Prognosis	Normal intellect as long as hypoglycemia well controlled in the neonate; typically large (approximately 2 standard deviations above the mean) adults leading normal lives; may have shortened life span secondary to neoplasm

Clinical Pearls

The phenotype is quite variable . . . The clinical diagnosis may be difficult in a preemie who lacks macrosomia . . . Severe neurologic sequelae may result from undetected hypoglycemia . . . Macroglossia can be surgically reduced if respiratory complications ensue . . . Ultrasound every 3 months in the first few years, every 6 months thereafter to rule out embryonic tumors linked to mutations in a paternally imprinted region on chromosome 11p.   *KH, JW*

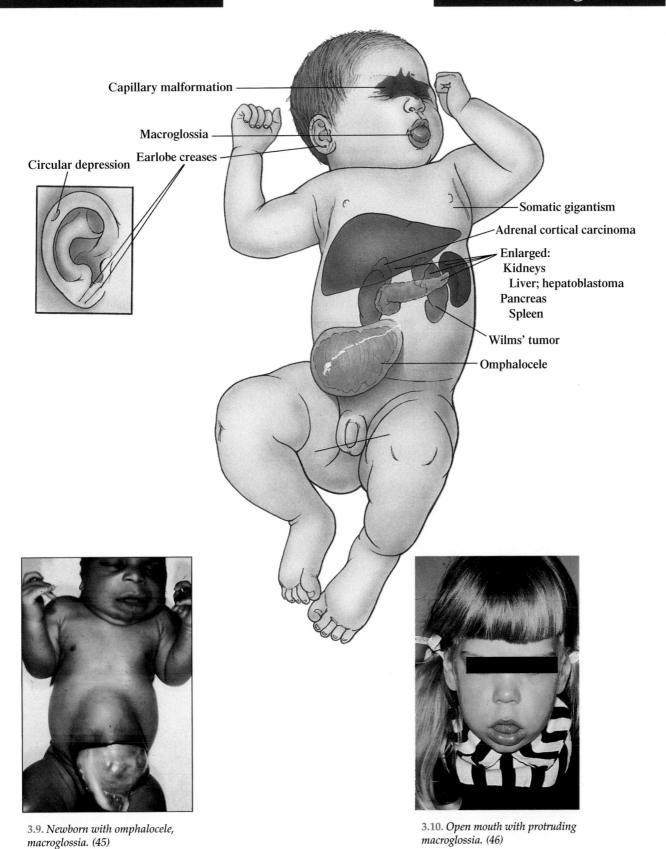

Capillary malformation

Macroglossia

Circular depression

Earlobe creases

Somatic gigantism

Adrenal cortical carcinoma

Enlarged:
  Kidneys
    Liver; hepatoblastoma
  Pancreas
    Spleen

Wilms' tumor

Omphalocele

3.9. *Newborn with omphalocele, macroglossia. (45)*

3.10. *Open mouth with protruding macroglossia. (46)*

Von Hippel-Lindau Syndrome

Inheritance	Autosomal dominant; *VHL* gene on 3p26–p25
Prenatal Diagnosis	DNA linkage analysis or mutation detection
Incidence	1:50,000–60,000; M=F
Age at Presentation	Usually by the fourth decade of life
Pathogenesis	Mutation in the *VHL* tumor suppressor gene leads to phenotype

Key Features

Eyes
Retinal hemangioblastomas with secondary visual impairment, blindness if untreated

Central Nervous System
Cerebellar > medullary, spinal cord hemangioblastomas with secondary signs of increased intracranial pressure (i.e., headache, vomiting, vertigo, ataxia, mental changes) or spinal cord compression (loss of sensation, proprioception, spastic paraparesis)

Kidneys
Renal-cell carcinoma, cysts

Endocrine
Pheochromocytoma, pancreatic cysts, adrenal carcinoma

Skin (< 5%)
Capillary malformation—head and neck

Hematologic
Polycythemia secondary to cerebellar hemangioblastoma and renal cell carcinoma production of erythropoietin

Differential Diagnosis
Cerebellar tumors

Laboratory Data
CT/MRI scan of brain/spinal cord
Abdominal CT/MRI scan
Urinary vanillylmandelic acid (VMA) level screen
Serum catecholamine level screen
Complete blood cell count

Management
Referral to ophthalmologist—photocoagulation or cryocoagulation of tumor
Referral to neurosurgeon/neurologist—surgical removal
Referral to urologist—surgical removal
All first-degree relatives: annual retinal examination, neurologic examination, regular screening with brain and abdominal scans, VMA and catecholamine screens

Prognosis
Premature death secondary to progressive growth of central nervous system (CNS) hemangioblastomas or metastatic renal cell carcinoma

Clinical Pearls

This is a progressive, universally fatal disease with death by the fourth decade . . . Hematuria is a common presenting sign . . . We screen with a sonogram of the belly, MRI and CT of the brain (to pick up both cerebellar tumors and calcifications), and an eye examination . . . DNA testing for mutations in the *VHL* gene is available and indicated for appropriate screening in children of affected patients and for confirmation of diagnosis . . . Angiography usually performed preoperatively . . . If kidney involvement, these patients may be candidates for renal transplantation. *KH, JW*

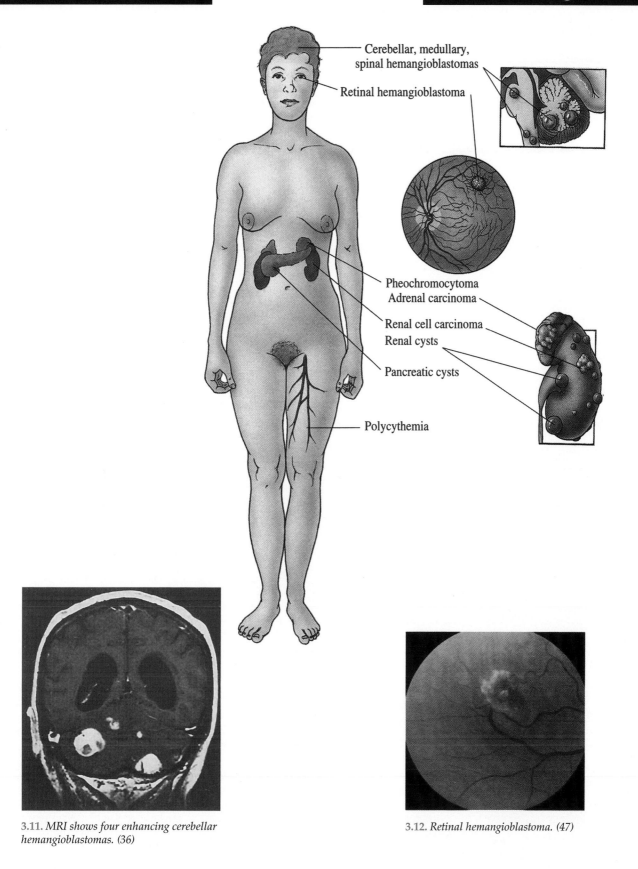

Cerebellar, medullary,
spinal hemangioblastomas

Retinal hemangioblastoma

Pheochromocytoma
Adrenal carcinoma

Renal cell carcinoma
Renal cysts

Pancreatic cysts

Polycythemia

3.11. *MRI shows four enhancing cerebellar hemangioblastomas. (36)*

3.12. *Retinal hemangioblastoma. (47)*

Ataxia-Telangiectasia

Synonym Louis-Bar syndrome

Inheritance Autosomal recessive; Ataxia-telangiectasia mutated (*ATM*) gene on 11q22–23

Prenatal Diagnosis Amniocentesis: chromosomal breaks in amniocytes
Maternal serum: elevated alpha-fetoprotein levels
Molecular DNA analysis

Incidence 1:30,000–100,000 live births; M=F

Age at Presentation Ataxia presents initially in second or third year of life when child begins to walk; telangiectasias by 3 to 6 years old

Pathogenesis ATM gene codes for protein important in DNA repair, especially after ionizing radiation exposure; activates (via phosphorylation) repair mechanism utilizing a p53-dependent pathway that regulates apoptosis and cell cycle arrest; defective cellular and humoral immunity
Progressive depletion of Purkinje cells in the cerebellum

Key Features
Skin
Telangiectasias—bulbar conjunctiva first with subsequent ear, eyelid, cheeks, neck, upper chest, and flexor forearms involvement; progeric facies with decreased sub-cutaneous fat, atrophy, sclerosis; granulomas, café au lait macules
Hair
Canities
Central Nervous System
Cerebellar ataxia, progressive nystagmus, slurred speech, oculomotor apraxia, growth retardation, intellectual impairment
Sinopulmonary
Recurrent viral or bacterial infections, progressive respiratory impairment
Endocrine
Ovarian dysgenesis, insulin-resistant diabetes
Neoplasms
Lymphoreticular, breast carcinoma (heterozygotes)

Differential Diagnosis Hereditary Hemorhagic Telangiectasia Syndrome (p. 114)
Generalized essential telangiectasia
Bloom syndrome (p. 234)

Laboratory Data Increased T-suppressor cells, decreased T-helper cells
Alpha-fetoprotein (AFP) elevated
Immunoglobulin (Ig) A, IgG2, IgE decreased or absent

Management Evaluate family members for carriers of ATM mutation-increased incidence of breast cancer and lymphoid malignancies (dominant negative missense mutations most closely associated with carrier morbidity)
Referral to hematologist—oncologist-intravenous γ-globulin, malignancy management
Referral to pulmonologist/infectious disease specialist
Referral to neurologist
Avoid x-rays, radiotherapy, bleomycin
Sun avoidance, sunscreen may help prevent progeric changes

Prognosis Most patients confined to wheelchair by 10 years of age; premature death secondary to lymphoreticular malignancy or infection in the second decade of life

Clinical Pearls

Major caretaker is the neurologist . . . While patients usually present to neurology initially, I follow a wheelchair-bound 20-year-old patient who developed telangiec-tasias in the first years of life and did not develop ataxia until 8 years old . . . While x-irradiation is a problem, patients seem to be UV sensitive as well . . . We tend to cover them with sunscreen and protective clothing . . . If radiotherapy used to treat lymphoma, one must use very small fractionated doses . . . Family members who are carriers are at increased risk of developing malignancies, and may show chromoso-mal breaks after irradiation . . . Risk of breast cancer in female heterozygotes is 5 times that of the normal population . . . Ultrasound and good physical examination are theoretically safer than mammograms for screening these women. *AP*

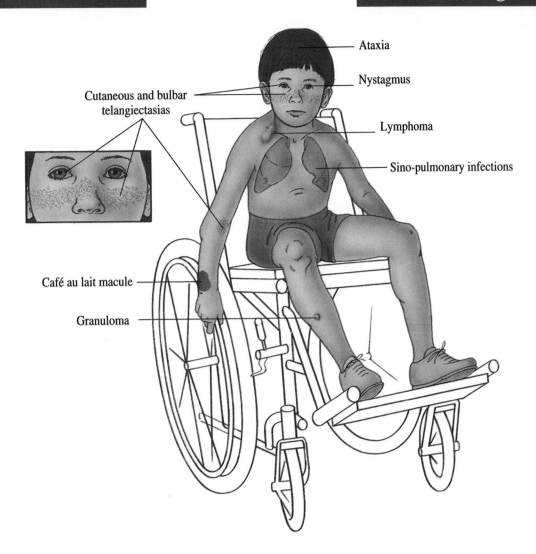

Ataxia

Nystagmus

Cutaneous and bulbar telangiectasias

Lymphoma

Sino-pulmonary infections

Café au lait macule

Granuloma

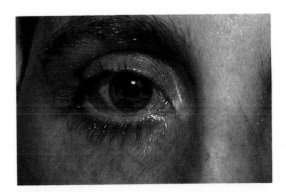

3.13. *Telangiectasias involving bulbar conjunctiva and cheek. (1)*

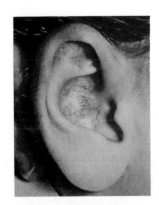

3.14. *Telangiectasias on external ear. (48)*

Hereditary Hemorrhagic Telangiectasia Syndrome

Synonym

Osler-Weber-Rendu syndrome

Inheritance

Autosomal dominant—HHT1: endoglin gene on 9q33–34
Autosomal dominant—HHT2: *ALK1* gene on chromosome 12

Prenatal Diagnosis

DNA linkage analysis or mutation detection

Incidence

1–2:100,000; M=F; all races, most common in whites

Age at Presentation

Early childhood to young adulthood with epistaxis in 50% of patients
Cutaneous, gastrointestinal telangiectasias usually begins in the third to fourth decade

Pathogenesis

HHT1: Mutation in endoglin gene on chromosome 9q33–34, a transforming growth factor (TGF)-β–binding protein on endothelial cells essential for angiogenesis
HHT2: Mutation on chromosome 12 encoding for activin receptor-like kinase 1 (ALK1) expressed on endothelial cells

Key Features

Skin
   Telangiectasias on face, palms, soles, subungual region
Mucous Membranes
   Telangiectasias on vermillion, oral and nasopharyngeal mucosa, conjunctiva
Ear-Nose-Throat
   Epistaxis—recurrent in more than 80% of patients
Gastrointestinal
   Telangiectasias with secondary hemorrhage; hepatic AVMs
Pulmonary
   Arteriovenous fistulas complicated by hemorrhage, cerebral abscesses

Differential Diagnosis

CREST syndrome
Generalized essential telangiectasia
Ataxia-telangiectasia (p. 112)
Fabry disease (p. 306)

Laboratory Data

Chest x-ray screen, follow-up MRI if positive
Complete blood count (CBC)
Guaiac stool screen
Endoscopy—if symptomatic

Management

Referral to otolaryngologist—cautery, packing, estrogen, septal dermoplasty for recurrent epistaxis; transfusions, iron supplementation
Referral to gastroenterologist if symptomatic
Referral to thoracic surgeon—excision, embolization of A-V fistula
Referral to dermatologist—pulsed dye laser for telangiectasias

Prognosis

HHT1 families have increased incidence of pulmonary A-V fistulaes
HHT2 families with increase in hepatic AVMs

Clinical Pearls

Pulmonary A-V shunts are the most serious potential problem facing these patients . . . Shunts are best treated surgically . . . Ability to treat gastrointestinal bleeds with Nd:YAG laser dependent upon accessibility of lesion . . . Pulsed dye or argon laser may be useful to treat telangiectasias, but they will reform . . . Estrogens can be used if telangiectasias are recalcitrant. *AP*

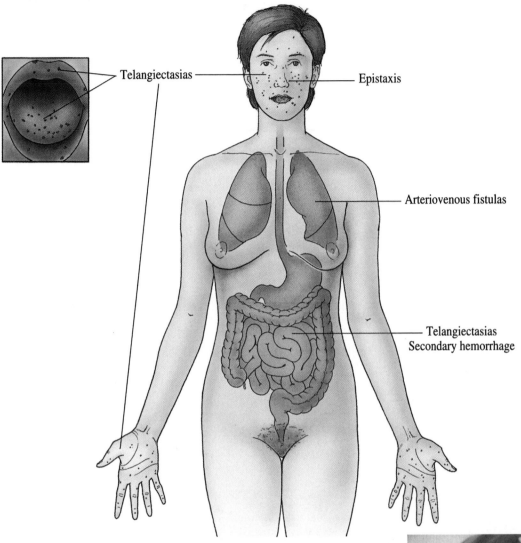

Telangiectasias

Epistaxis

Arteriovenous fistulas

Telangiectasias
Secondary hemorrhage

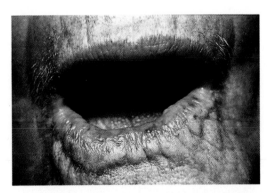

3.15. Multiple telangiectasias on vermillion border. (5)

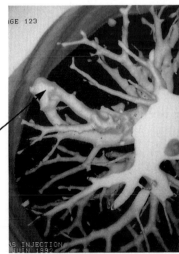

3.16. Three-dimensional CT reconstruction of a pulmonary arteriovenous malformation (arrow). (48a)

115

Cutis Marmorata Telangiectatica Congenita

Inheritance	Sporadic; some familial reports
Prenatal Diagnosis	None
Incidence	Rare—approximately 1:3,000 neonates; M=F
Age at Presentation	Birth
Pathogenesis	May be an autosomal lethal mutation with ability to survive only in a mosaic state
Key Features	**Skin** 　Atrophic, reticulated vascular patches on extremities > trunk > face; localized, segmental, or generalized with rare ulceration; phlebectasias, capillary malformation **Associated findings** 　Seen in 50% of cases, more common in generalized cutis marmorata telangiectatica congenita 　**Musculoskeletal** 　　Ipsilateral hemiatrophy or hemihypertrophy of extremity (limb length and circumference discrepancy) 　**Cardiovascular** 　　Patient ductus arteriosus, arterial stenosis 　**Eyes** 　　Glaucoma (with periocular involvement only) 　**Central Nervous System** 　　Mental retardation
Differential Diagnosis	Capillary malformation Physiologic cutis marmorata Neonatal lupus erythematosus Rothmund-Thomson syndrome (p. 238)
Laboratory Data	None
Management	Complete physical examination Regular interval measurements of limb length and circumference Referral to ophthalmologist if periocular involvement
Prognosis	Skin lesion often fades within the first few years of life; limb length or circumference discrepancy may improve with time

Clinical Pearls

The most common problem is atrophy of soft tissue and leg length discrepancy . . . The quoted 50% of patients with associated findings is high . . . Some people have a reticulated form of nevus flammeus that is misdiagnosed as CMTC; the reticulated pattern is not as coarse and the affected areas do not ulcerate. *AP*

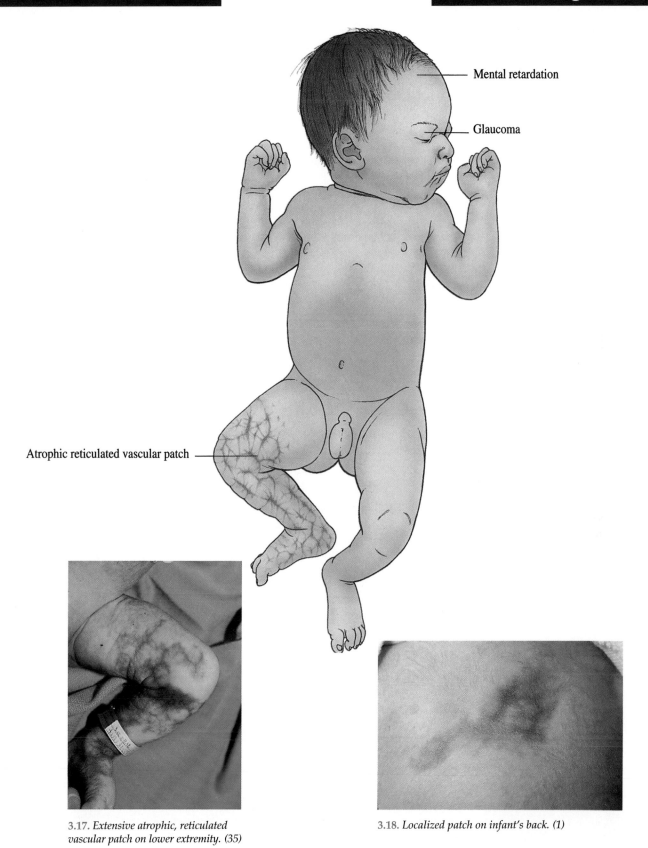

Mental retardation

Glaucoma

Atrophic reticulated vascular patch

3.17. *Extensive atrophic, reticulated vascular patch on lower extremity.* (35)

3.18. *Localized patch on infant's back.* (1)

Maffucci Syndrome

Inheritance	Sporadic
Prenatal Diagnosis	None
Incidence	Rare; at least 100 cases reported; M=F
Age at Presentation	Birth to early childhood
Pathogenesis	May reflect an autosomal lethal mutation surviving in a mosaic state

Key Features

Skin
Superficial and deep venous malformations—increased on hands and feet but can occur anywhere; asymmetric
Venous-lymphatic malformations—less common

Bone
Enchondromas—benign, cartilaginous tumors; increased on phalanges, long bones but can occur anywhere; asymmetric; secondary fractures, limb length discrepancy, bowing of limbs
Cranial and vertebral enchondromas can lead to severe neurologic sequelae
Short stature

Neoplasm
Chondrosarcoma (15% to 20%)—occurs within enchondromas
Less common: angiosarcoma, fibrosarcoma, osteosarcoma, lymphangiosarcoma

Differential Diagnosis
Ollier disease (enchondromatosis without venous malformations)
Blue rubber bleb nevus syndrome (p. 120)
Proteus syndrome (p. 106)

Laboratory Data
X-ray
Bone biopsy of changing enchondroma

Management
Regular physical examination
Regular radiographic evaluation
Referral to orthopedist on presentation
Referral to dermatologist/plastic surgeon

Prognosis
Progression of skin and bone lesions ceases by second to third decade
If no malignant degeneration, normal life span

Clinical Pearls

The orthopedist is usually the primary physician following these patients . . .
Swimming and other low-stress activity should be recommended . . .
The angiosarcomas, regardless of treatment, are often fatal. *AP*

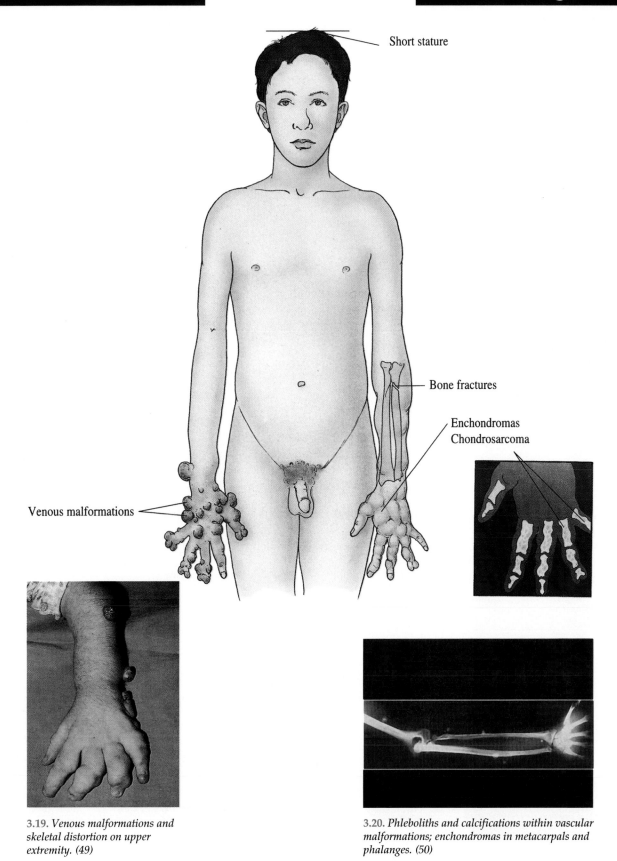

Short stature

Bone fractures

Enchondromas
Chondrosarcoma

Venous malformations

3.19. *Venous malformations and
skeletal distortion on upper
extremity. (49)*

3.20. *Phleboliths and calcifications within vascular
malformations; enchondromas in metacarpals and
phalanges. (50)*

Blue Rubber Bleb Nevus Syndrome

Inheritance	Sporadic; rare reports of autosomal dominant transmission
Prenatal Diagnosis	None
Incidence	Rare; M=F
Age at Presentation	Birth to early childhood
Pathogenesis	Unknown
Key Features	**Skin**
	Multiple venous malformations—soft, dark blue, compressible, 0.1 to 5.0 cm nodules on trunk and extremities; with/without pain, with/without increased sweat over lesion; increase in size and number with age; may have combined lymphatic-venous malformation
	Gastrointestinal
	Venous malformations (especially in small intestine) with secondary hemorrhage, anemia
	Other Viscera
	Case reports of venous malformations in most organ systems with associated complications
Differential Diagnosis	Maffucci syndrome (p. 118)
	Diffuse neonatal hemangiomatosis (p. 124)
	Fabry Disease (p. 306); multiple angiokeratomas
	Multiple glomus tumors
Laboratory Data	Endoscopy
	MRI to evaluate gastrointestinal lesions
	CBC
	Stool guaiacs
Management	Surgical excision/CO_2 laser of skin lesions if symptomatic or for cosmesis
	Screening of gastrointestinal tract with stool guaiac test
	Anemia controlled with iron supplementation, tranfusions, endoscopic cauterization or bowel resection, if necessary
	Referral to dermatologist, gastroenterologist, surgeon
Prognosis	Normal life span if bleeding controlled; venous malformations persist throughout life

Clinical Pearls

May be very difficult to differentiate from multiple glomus tumors . . . If lesions are superficial, they may improve somewhat with pulsed dye laser, but surgical excision is usually needed . . . Must warn patients that lesions tend to recur after surgical excision . . . May not see gastrointestinal lesions with MRI or x-ray . . . Gastrointestinal involvement may be complicated by intussusception that requires surgical intervention if not easily reduced . . . One may find other organ involvement, particularly the CNS. *AP*

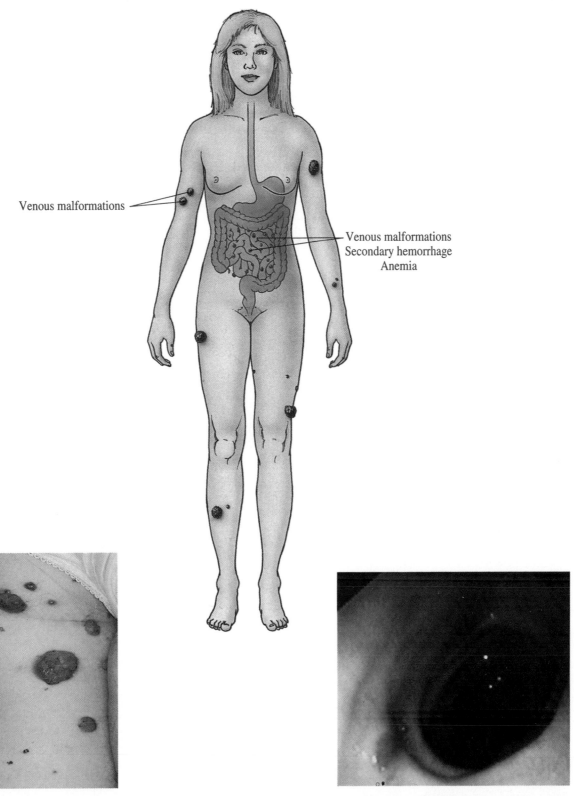

Venous malformations

Venous malformations
Secondary hemorrhage
Anemia

3.21. *Multiple venous malformations of varying size on thigh.* (51)

3.22. *Venous malformation on the mucosal surface of the small intestine.* (52)

Kasabach-Merritt Syndrome

Inheritance	Sporadic
Prenatal Diagnosis	None
Incidence	Over 175 cases reported in medical literature in English; F:M = 2–3:1
Age at Presentation	Birth to first few weeks old (median age, 5 weeks old)
Pathogenesis	Consumption coagulopathy within a kaposiform hemangioendothelioma or tufted angioma

Key Features

Skin
Large, rapidly growing, tender, bruising reddish-purple soft-tissue, vascular mass with purpura; most common vascular tumors include kaposiform hemangioendotheliomas or tufted angiomas; may occur with a lymphatic malformation; petechiae, ecchymoses; tumor usually leaves residual stain, fibrotic plaque, papules, swelling

Hematologic
Thrombocytopenia, microangiopathic hemolytic anemia, disseminated intravascular coagulation
Acute hemorrhage—gastrointestinal, pleural, pulmonic, CNS

Cardiac
Congestive heart failure (CHF)

Differential Diagnosis	Hemangioma with secondary sepsis, disseminated intravascular coagulation (DIC)
Laboratory Data	Complete blood cell count Prothrombin (PT)/activated partial thromboplastin time (aPTT) prolonged; fibrinogen level decreased; fibrin degradation products increased
Management	Prednisone Vincristine Interferon-α Referral to pediatric hematologist—transfusions, infusions of fibrinogen and fresh frozen plasma; platelet transfusions only if active bleeding (may enlarge mass and worsen condition) Referral to pediatric surgeon—embolization, surgical excision Referral to pediatric cardiologist—management of CHF
Prognosis	Up to 20% mortality secondary to hemorrhage, infection, or iatrogenic causes

Clinical Pearls

Now known to be associated with vascular tumors that are not hemangiomas of infancy, particularly tufted angiomas and hemangioendotheliomas . . . Once diagnosis is established we start the patient on prednisolone 2 to 3 mg/kg per day . . . Many now use vincristine as an alternative or adjunctive to the prednisolone because of the risk of spastic diplegia in young infants treated with interferon-α . . . Prednisone is tapered to every-other-day dose as soon as we can . . . Depending on the degree of DIC, anticoagulant therapy may also be started.   *AP*

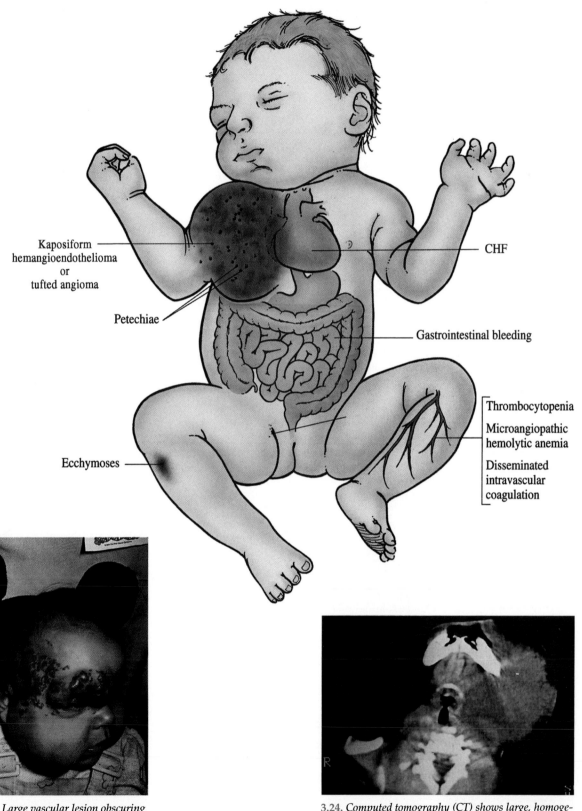

Kaposiform hemangioendothelioma or tufted angioma

Petechiae

Ecchymoses

CHF

Gastrointestinal bleeding

Thrombocytopenia

Microangiopathic hemolytic anemia

Disseminated intravascular coagulation

3.23. *Large vascular lesion obscuring the infant's right side of the face. (1)*

3.24. *Computed tomography (CT) shows large, homogenous mass in a patient with facial vascular tumor and Kasabach-Merritt syndrome (53)*

Diffuse Neonatal Hemangiomatosis

Synonym
Multiple neonatal hemangiomatosis
Benign neonatal hemangiomatosis (skin only)

Inheritance
Sporadic

Prenatal Diagnosis
None

Incidence
Rare; F:M=2–3:1

Age at Presentation
Birth to first few months old

Pathogenesis
Unknown

Key Features
Skin
Multiple 0.2 to 2.0 cm hemangiomas; generalized distribution
Viscera
Hemangiomas involving any organ; most commonly in liver > lungs, gastrointestinal tract, CNS
Liver hemangiomas may be complicated by hepatomegaly, obstructive jaundice, portal hypertension, hemorrhage, thrombocytopenia, anemia, high-output CHF
Cardiac
High-output CHF; may occur with or without visceral involvement

Differential Diagnosis
Blue rubber bleb nevus syndrome (p. 120)
Fabry disease (p. 306)
Multiple glomus tumors

Laboratory Data
Skin biopsy if necessary
Liver ultrasound
Abdominal, head, chest CT/MRI
Chest x-ray
CBC/coagulation studies
Stool guaiacs
Urinalysis-hematuria

Management
Prednisone 2 to 3 mg/kg per day if symptomatic
Vincristine
Interferon-α if symptomatic
Digoxin, diuretics if CHF
Hepatic artery ligation/embolization, liver transplant if unresponsive to systemic therapy
Close follow-up with pediatrician
Referral to pediatric gastroenterologist, cardiologist if symptomatic
Referral to surgeon—excision, embolization
Referral to dermatologist
Referral to pediatric ophthalmologist (periocular involvement)

Prognosis
High mortality if visceral and/or liver involvement secondary to congestive heart failure, hemorrhage, or infection; hemangiomas undergo spontaneous regression by early childhood

Clinical Pearls

Every child with even a single hemangioma deserves a complete, thorough physical examination . . . With multiple hemangiomas (>6), we get a history, do a complete physical examination, and check stool and urine for blood . . . Many also obtain a hepatic ultrasound, but the rest of the evaluation is based on changes found on physical examination . . . I do not treat cutaneous lesions unless in a problematic location, breaking down, bleeding, or in the groin area where there will be long-term friction and increase in ulceration.   *AP*

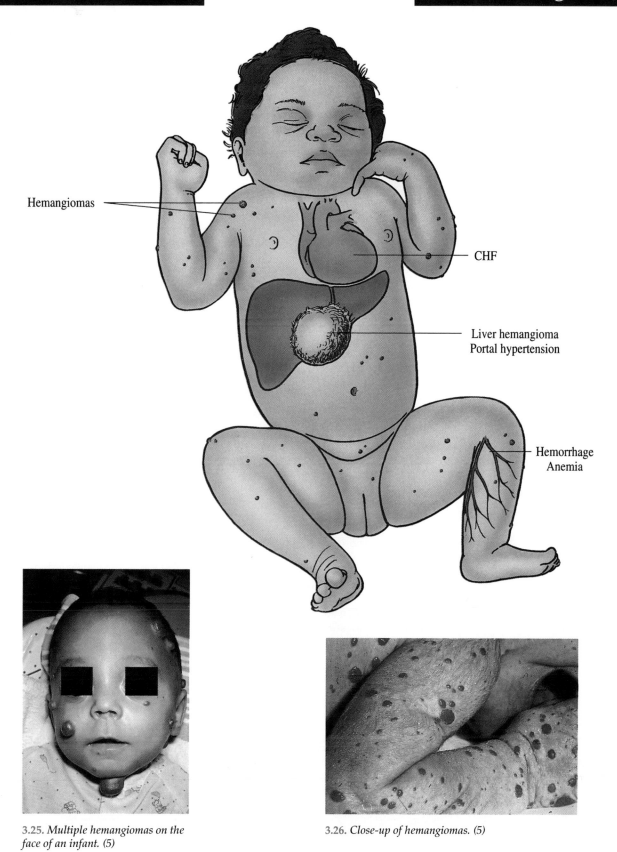

Hemangiomas

CHF

Liver hemangioma
Portal hypertension

Hemorrhage
Anemia

3.25. *Multiple hemangiomas on the face of an infant.* (5)

3.26. *Close-up of hemangiomas.* (5)

PHACE Syndrome

Synonym	**PHACE(S): P**osterior fossa brain malformations, large facial **H**emangioma, **A**rterial anomalies, **C**ardiac anomalies and aortic **c**oarctation, **E**ye abnormalities, and **S**ternal clefting and/or **S**upraumbilical raphe
Inheritance	Sporadic; x-linked dominant transmission with male lethality proposed given large predominance of female cases
Prenatal Diagnosis	First trimester ultrasound may pick up early intracranial structural defects
Incidence	Rare—may be underreported because of misdiagnosis as vascular malformation/Sturge-Weber syndrome; F > M
Age at Presentation	Birth to first few weeks of life
Pathogenesis	Unknown; may be secondary to a developmental error at 6 to 8 weeks' gestation caused by defects in morphoregulatory genes

Key Features

Skin
Large, facial, plaque-like **h**emangioma in a V_1 distribution alone or in combination with V_2 and V_3; unilateral left-sided most common, can be bilateral, more extensive lesions have greater CNS vascular/structural involvement; ulceration common **S**ternal cleft/pits, supraumbilical raphe

Central Nervous System
Posterior fossa malformations including Dandy-Walker malformation (most common), hypoplasia/agenesis of the cerebellum, cerebellar vermis, corpus callosum; anomalous branches/aneurysmal dilatation of the internal carotid arteries and cerebral **a**rteries with occlusion/stenosis/cerebral infarct; secondary seizures, developmental delay, contralateral hemiparesis, headache

Cardiac/Aorta
Coarctation of the aorta (most common), anomalies of the brachiocephalic arteries and aortic arch, patent ductus arteriosus, ventral septal defects, atrial septal defects, cor triatriatum, tricuspid and aortic atresia

Eye
Ipsilateral microphthalmos, optic atrophy, optic nerve hypoplasia, cataracts, increased retinal vascularity, strabismus, exophthalmos

Differential Diagnosis	Sturge-Weber syndrome (p. 100) Segmental hemangioma without extracutaneous findings Tufted angioma Kaposiform hemangioendothelioma
Laboratory Data	Cranial ultrasound, MRI, MRA Aortagraphy, echocardiogram
Management	Close follow-up with pediatric dermatologist, neurologist, cardiologist, and ophthalmologist
Prognosis	May have shortened life span depending on severity of extracutaneous findings

Clinical Pearls

The importance of PHACE is twofold. First, it should alert clinicians seeing infants with large, segmental facial hemangiomas to be aware of potential structural anomalies of the heart, eyes, CNS, and arterial vasculature. Second, knowledge about the timing of the associated anomalies suggests that the event(s) leading to PHACE occur very early in gestation, probably between 6 and 10 weeks. Thus, although hemangiomas are typically not visable at the time of birth, they truly represent a "birth defect" . . . Evaluation of infants at risk depends on clinical scenario . . . Careful cardiac, eye, and neurologic examinations should guide your referrals to pediatric specialists . . . MRI and MRA should be attempted on anyone at risk, however, given risk of general anesthesia in young children, these studies can be deferred/omitted if neurologic signs or symptoms are absent. *IF*

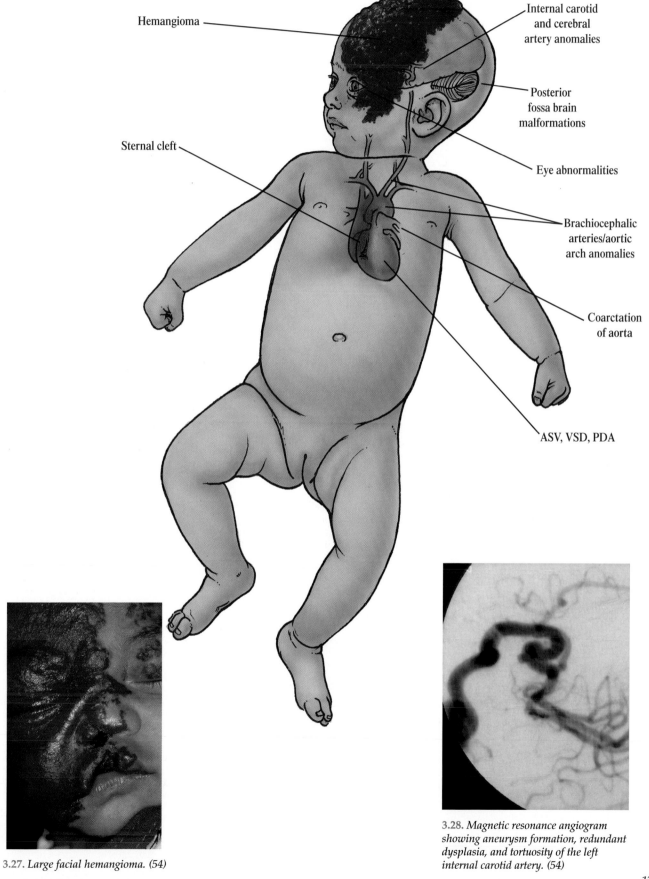

Hemangioma

Internal carotid
and cerebral
artery anomalies

Posterior
fossa brain
malformations

Sternal cleft

Eye abnormalities

Brachiocephalic
arteries/aortic
arch anomalies

Coarctation
of aorta

ASV, VSD, PDA

3.27. *Large facial hemangioma.* (54)

3.28. *Magnetic resonance angiogram
showing aneurysm formation, redundant
dysplasia, and tortuosity of the left
internal carotid artery.* (54)

Suggested Reading

Sturge-Weber Syndrome

Bains HS, Cirino AC, Tieho BH, et al. Photodynamic therapy using verteporfin for a diffuse choroidal hemangioma in Sturge-Weber syndrome. *Retina* 2004;24(l):152–1555.

Benedikt RA, Brown DC, Walker R, et al. Sturge-Weber syndrome: cranial MR imaging with Gd-DTPA. *Am J Neuroradiol* 1993;14:409–415.

Celebi S, Alagoz G, Aykan U. Ocular findings in Sturge-Weber syndrome. *Eur J Ophthalmol* 2000;10:239–243.

Comi AM, Hunt P, Vawter MP, Pardo CA, et al. Increased fibronectin expression in sturge-weber syndrome fibroblasts and brain tissue. *Pediatr Res* 2003;53:762–769.

Faller AS. The Sturge-Weber syndrome. *Dermatology* 1987;4:300–304.

Iwach AG, Hoskins HD Jr, Hetherington J Jr, et al. Analysis of surgical and medical management of glaucoma in Sturge-Weber syndrome. *Ophthalmology* 1990;97:904–909.

Kramer U, Kahana E, Shorer Z. et al. Outcome of infants with unilateral Sturge-Weber syndrome and early onset seizures. *Dev Med Child Neurol* 2000;42:756–759.

Lee JS, Asano E, Muzik O, et al. Sturge-Weber syndrome: correlation between clinical course and FDG PET findings. *Neurology* 2001;57:189–195.

Lin DD, Barker PB, Kraut MA, et al. Early characteristics of Sturge-Weber syndrome shown by perfusion MR imaging and proton MR spectroscopic imaging. *AJNR Am J Neuroradiol* 2003;24:1912–1915.

Mandal AK, Gupta N. Patients with Sturge-Weber syndrome. *Ophthalmology* 2004;111:606; author reply 606.

Marti-Bonmati L, Menor F, Mulas F. The Sturge-Weber syndrome: correlation between the clinical status and radiological CT and MRI findings. *Childs Nery Syst* 1993;9:07–109.

Michel S, Landthaler M, Hohenleutner U. Recurrence of port-wine stains after treatment with the flash-lamp pumped pulsed dye laser. *Br J Dermatol* 2000;143:1230–1234.

Pascual-Castroviejo I, Diaz-Gonzalez C, Garcia-Melian RM, et al. Sturge-Weber syndrome: study of 40 patients. *Pediatr Neurol* 1993;9:283–288.

Pinton F, Chiron C, Enjolras O, et al. Early single photon emission computed tomography in Sturge-Weber syndrome. *J Neurol Neurosurg Psychiatry* 1997;63:616–621.

Van der Horst C, Koster PH, de Borgie CA, et al. Effect of the timing of treatment of port-wine stains with the flash-lamp-pumped pulsed dye laser. *N Engl J Med* 1998;338:1028–1033.

Klippel-Trenaunay Syndrome

Aggarwal K, Jain VK, Gupta S, et al. Klippel-Trenaunay syndrome with a life-threatening thromboembolic event. *J Dermatol* 2003;30:236–240.

Enjolras O, Ciabrini D, Mazoyer E et al. Extensive pure venous malformations in the upper or lower limb, a review of 27 cases. *J Am Acad Dermatol* 1997;36: 219–225.

Gianlupi A, Harper R, Dwyre D, et al. Recurrent pulmonary embolism associated with Klippel—Trenaunay-Weber syndrome. *Chest* 1999;115: 1199–1201.

Gloviczki P, Stanson AW, Stickler GB, et al. Klippel-Trenaunay syndrome: the risks and benefits of vascular interventions. *Surgery* 1991;110:469–479.

Happle R. Lethal genes surviving by mosaicism: a possible explanation for sporadic birth defects involving the skin. *J Am Acad Dermatol* 1987;16: 899–906.

Levine C. The imaging of body asymmetry and hemihypertrophy. *Crit Rev Diagn Imaging* 1990;31:1–80.

Tian XL, Kadaba R, You SA, et al. Identification of an angiogenic factor that when mutated causes susceptibility to Klippel-Trenaunay syndrome. *Nature* 2004;427:640–645.

Viljoen D, Saxe N, Pearn J, et al. The cutaneous manifestations of the Klippel-Trenaunay-Weber syndrome. *Clin Exp Dermatol* 1987;12:12–17.

Vissers W, Van Steensel M, Steijlen P, et al. Klippel-Trenaunay syndrome and Sturge-Weber syndrome: variations on a theme? *Eur J Dermatol* 2003;13:238–241.

Ziyeh S, Spreer J, Rossler J, et al. Parkes Weber or Klippel-Trenaunay syndrome? Non-invasive diagnosis with MR projection angiography. *Eur Radiol* 2004 (*in press*).

Cobb Syndrome

Binkert CA, Kollias SS, Valavanis A. Spinal cord vascular disease: characterization with fast three-dimensional contrast-enhanced MR angiography. *Am J Neuroradiol* 1999;20:1785–1793.

Clinton TS, Cooke LM, Graham BS. Cobb syndrome associated with a verrucous (angiokeratomalike) vascular malformation. *Cutis* 2003;71:283–287.

Huffmann BC, Spetzger U, Reinges M, et al. Treatment strategies and results in spinal vascular malformations. *Neurol Med Chir (Tokyo)* 1998;38:231–237.

Jessen RT, Thompson S, Smith EB. Cobb syndrome. *Arch Dermatol* 1977;113: 1587–1590.

Kaito H, Kuwata T, Nohara T, et al. Cobb syndrome (cutaneomeningospinal angiomatosis). The first case reported in Japan [in Japanese]. *Nippon Naika Gakkai Zasshi* 1989;78:1758–1764.

Kaplan P, Hollenberg RD, Fraser FC. A spinal arteriovenous malformation with hereditary cutaneous hemangiomas. *Am J Dis Child* 1976;130:1329–1331.

Mercer RD, Rothner AD, Cook SA, et al. The Cobb syndrome: association with hereditary cutaneous hemangiomas. *Cleve Clin Q* 1978;45:237–240.

Rodesch G, Hurth M, Alvarez H, et al. Classification of spinal cord arteriovenous shunts: proposal for a reappraisal—the Bicetre experience with 155 consecutive patients treated between 1981 and 1999. *Neurosurgery* 2002;51:374–379; discussion 379–380.

Soeda A, Sakai N, Iihara K, et al. Cobb syndrome in an infant: treatment with endovascular embolization and corticosteroid therapy: case report. *Neurosurgery* 2003;52:711–715; discussion 714–715.

Proteus Syndrome

Biesecker LG, Happle R, Mulliken JB, et al. Proteus syndrome: diagnostic criteria, differential diagnosis, and patient evaluation. *Am J Med Genet* 1999;84:389.

Cohen MM Jr. Further diagnostic thoughts about the Elephant Man. *Am J Med Genet* 1988;29:777–782.

Cohen MM Jr. Proteus syndrome: clinical evidence for somatic mosaicism and selective review. *Am J Med Genet* 1993;47:645–652.

Cohen MM Jr. Understanding Proteus syndrome, unmasking the Elephant Man, and stemming elephant fever. *Neurofibromatosis* 1988;1: 260–280.

Cohen MM Jr, Turner JT, Biesecker LG. Proteus syndrome: misdiagnosis with PTEN mutations. *Am J Med Genet.* 2003;122A:323–324.

Cremin BJ, Viljoen DL, Wynchank S, Beighton P. The Proteus syndrome: the magnetic resonance and radiological features. *Pediatr Radiol* 1987;17: 486–488.

Hoeger PH, Martinez A, Maerker J, et al. Vascular anomalies in Proteus syndrome. *Clin Exp Dermatol* 2004;29:222–230.

Stricker S. Musculoskeletal manifestations of Proteus syndrome report of two cases with literature review. *J Pediatr Orthop* 1992;12:667–674.

Turner JT, Cohen MM, Biesecker LG. Natural history and complications in Proteus syndrome. *Am J Hum Genet* 2001;69:221.

Vaughn RY, Selinger AD, Howell CG, et al. Proteus syndrome: diagnosis and surgical management. *J Pediatr Surg* 1993;28:5–10.

Wiedemann HR, Burgio GR, Aldenhoff P, et al. The Proteus syndrome: partial gigantism of the hands and/or feet, nevi, hemihypertrophy, subcutaneous tumors, macrocephaly or other skull anomalies and possible accelerated growth and visceral affections. *Eur J Pediatr* 1983;140:5–12.

Zhou X, Hampel H, Thiele H, et al. Association of germline mutations in the PTEN tumor suppressor gene and Proteus and Proteus-like syndromes. *Lancet* 2001;358:210.

Beckwith-Wiedemann Syndrome

Alders M, Ryan A, Hodges M, et al. Disruption of a novel imprinted zinc-finger gene, ZNF215, in Beckwith-Wiedemann syndrome. *Am. J. Hum. Genet.* 2000;66:1473–1484.

Algar EM, Deeble GJ, Smith PJ. CDKN1C expression in Beckwith-Wiedemann syndrome patients with allele imbalance. *J Med Genet* 1999;36:524–531.

Beckwith JB. Children at increased risk for Wilms tumor: monitoring issues. *J Pediatr* 1998;132:377–379.

Beckwith JB. Macroglossia, omphalocele, adrenal cytomegaly, gigantism, and hyperplastic visceromegaly. *Birth Defects Orig Art Ser* 1969;V:188–196.

Emery LG, Shields M, Shah NR, et al. Neuroblastoma associated with Beckwith-Wiedemann syndrome. *Cancer* 1983;52:176–179.

Estabrooks LL, Lamb AN, Kirkmann H, et al. Beckwith-Wiedemann syndrome in twins with a duplication of chromosome (15q11.2–q13)mat. *Am J Hum Genet* 1989;14:A75.

Gerver WJM, Menheere PPCA, Schaap C, et al. The effects of a somatostatin analogue on the metabolism of an infant with Beckwith-Wiedemann syndrome and hyperinsulinaemia. *Eur J Pediatr* 1991;150:634–637.

Gicquel C, Gaston V, Mandelbaum J, et al. In vitro fertilization may increase the risk of Beckwith-Wiedemann syndrome related to the abnormal imprinting of the KCNQ1OT gene. (Letter) *Am J Hum Genet* 2003;72:1338–1341.

Goldman M, Shuman C, Weksberg R, et al. Hypercalciuria in Beckwith-Wiedemann syndrome. *J Pediatr* 2003;142:206–208.

Haas OA, Zoubek A, Grumayer ER, et al. Constitutional interstitial deletion of 11p11 and pericentric inversion of chromosome 9 in a patient with Wiedemann-Beckwith syndrome and hepatoblastoma. *Cancer Genet Cytogenet* 1986;23:95–104.

Hatada I, Ohashi H, Fukushima Y, et al. An imprinted gene p57KIP2 is mutated in Beckwith-Wiedemann syndrome. *Nat Genet* 1996;14:171–173.

Kubota T, Saitoh S, Matsumoto T, et al. Excess functional copy of allele at chromosomal region 11p15 may cause Wiedemann-Beckwith (EMG) syndrome. *Am J Med Genet* 1004;49:378–383.

Von Hippel-Lindau Syndrome

Chen F, Kishida T, Yao M, et al. Germline mutations in the von Hippel-Lindau disease tumor suppressor gene correlations with phenotype. *Hum Mutat* 1995;5:66–75.

Choyke PL, Filling-Katz MR, Shawler TH, et al. Von Hippel-Lindau disease: radiologic screening for visceral manifestations. *Radiology* 1990;174:815–820.

Hes F, Zewald R, Peeters T, et al. Genotype-phenotype correlations in families with deletions in the von Hippel-Lindau (VHL) gene. *Hum Genet* 2000;106:425–431.

Lamiell JM, Salazar FG, Hsia YE. Von Hippel-Lindau disease affecting 43 members of a single kindred. *Medicine* 1989;68:1–29.

Madhusudan S, Deplanque G, Braybrooke JP, et al. Antiangiogenic therapy for von Hippel-Lindau disease. *JAMA* 2004;291:943–944.

Maher ER, Bentley E, Yates JRW, et al. Mapping of the Von Hippel-Lindau disease locus to a small region of chromosome 3p by genetic linkage analysis. *Genomics* 1991;10:957–960.

Maher ER, Moore AT. Von Hippel-Lindau disease. *Br J Ophthalmol* 1992;76:743–745.

Richards FM, Crossey PA, Phipps ME, et al. Detailed mapping of germline deletions of the Von Hippel-Lindau disease tumour suppressor gene. *Hum Mol Genet* 1994;3:595–598.

Seizinger BR. Toward the isolation of the primary genetic defect in Von Hippel-Lindau disease. *Ann N Y Acad Sci* 1991;615:332–337.

Sgambati MT, Stolle C, Choyke PL, et al. Mosaicism in von Hippel-Lindau disease: lessons from kindreds with germline mutations identified in offspring with mosaic parents. *Am J Hum Genet* 2000;66:84–91.

Sharp WV, Platt RL. Familial pheochromocytoma: association with Von Hippel-Lindau's disease. *Angiology* 1971;22:141–146.

Shiao YH. The von Hippel-Lindau gene and protein in tumorigenesis and angiogenesis: a potential target for therapeutic designs. *Curr Med Chem* 2003;10:2461–2470.

Tse JY, Wong JH, Lo KW, et al. Molecular genetic analysis of the von Hippel-Lindau disease tumor suppressor gene in familial and sporadic cerebellar hemangioblastomas. *Am J Clin Pathol* 1997;107:459–466.

Van Velthoven V, Reinacher PC, Klisch J, et al. Treatment of intramedullary hemangioblastomas, with special attention to von Hippel-Lindau disease. *Neurosurgery* 2003;53:1306–1313; discussion 1313–1314.

Wait SD, Vortmeyer AO, Lonser RR, et al. Somatic mutations in VHL germline deletion kindred correlate with mild phenotype. *Ann Neurol* 2004;55:236–240.

Ataxia-Telangiectasia

Bridges BA, Arlett CF. Risk of breast cancer in ataxiatelangiectasia. [Letter]. *N Engl J Med* 1992;326:1357–1361.

Cabana MD, Crawford RO, Winkelstein JA, et al. Consequences of the delayed diagnosis of ataxia telangiectasia. *Pediatrics* 1998;102:98–100.

Gatti RA, Berkel I, Boder E, et al. Localization of an ataxia-telangiectasia gene to chromosom 11q22–23. *Nature* 1988;336:577–580.

Kahanna KK. Cancer risk and the ATM gene: a continuing debate. *J Natl Cancer Inst* 2000;92:795.

Kastan MB, Lim D. The many substrates and functions of ATM. *Mol Cell Biol* 2000;1:179.

Loeb DM, Lederman HM, Winkelstein JA. Lymphoid malignancy presenting sign of ataxia-telangiectasia. *J Pediatr Hematol Oncol* 2000;22:464–467.

Nowak-Wegrzyn A, Crawford TO, Winkelstein JA, et al. Immunodeficiency and infections in ataxia-telangiectasia. *J Pediatr* 2004;144:505–511.

Paller AS. Ataxia-telangiectasia. *Neurol Clin* 1987;5:447–449.

Savistky K, Bar-Shira A, Gilad S, et al. A single ataxia telangiectasia gene with a product similar to PI-3 kinase. *Science* 1995;268:1749.

Spacey SD, Gatti RA, Babb G. The molecular basis and clinical management of ataxia-telangiectasia: Can J Neurol Sci 2001;27:184–191.

Smith LL, Conerly SL. Ataxia-telangiectasia or Louis-Bar syndrome. *J Am Acad Dermatol* 1985;12:681–696.

Swift M, Morrell D, Massey RB, et al. Incidence of cancer in 161 families affected by ataxia-telangiectasia. *N Engl J Med* 1991;325:1831–1836.

Taylor AM, Byrd PJ, McConville CM, et al. Genetic and cellular features of ataxia-telangiectasia. *Int J Radiat Biol* 1994;65:65–70.

Taylor AM, Metcalfe JA, McConville C. Increased radiosensitivity and the basic defect in ataxia-telangiectasia. *Int J Radiat Biol* 1989;56:677–684.

Woods CG, Taylor AM. Ataxia-Telangiectasia in the British Isles: the clinical and laboratory features of 70 affected individuals. *Q J Med* 1992;82:169–179.

Hereditary Hemorrhagic Telangiectasia

Aassar OS, Friedman CM, White RI Jr. The natural history of epistaxis in hereditary hemorrhagic telangiectasia. *Laryngoscope* 1991;101:977–980.

Buchi KN. Vascular malformations of the gastrointestinal tract. *Surg Clin North Am* 1992;72:559–570.

Johnson DW, Berg JN, Baldwin MA, et al. Mutations in the activin receptor-like kinase 1 gene in hereditary haemorrhagic telangiectasia type 2. *Nat Genet* 1996;13:189.

Kanna B, Das B. Hemorrhagic pericardial effusion causing pericardial tamponade in hereditary hemorrhagic telangiectasia. *Am J Med Sci* 2004;327:149–151.

Li DY, Sorensen LK, Brooke BS, et al. Defective angiogenesis in mice lacking endoglin. *Science* 1999;284:1534.

Lischke R, Simonek J, Stolz A, et al. Bilateral pulmonary arteriovenous malformations in patient with Rendu-Osler-Weber disease. *Eur J Cardiothorac Surg* 2004,25:461.

McAllister KA, Grogg KM, Johnson DW, et al. Endoglin, a TGF-β binding protein of endothelial cells, is the gene for hereditary haemorrhagic telangiectasia type 1. *Nat Genet* 1994;8:345.

McDonald M, Papenberg K, Ghosh S, et al. (1993) Genetic linkage of hereditary hemorrhagic telangiectasia to markers on 9q. *Am J Hum Genet* 1993;53:A140.

Parnes LS, Heeneman H, Vinuela F. Percutaneous embolization for control of nasal blood circulation. *Laryngoscope* 1987;97:1312–1315.

Peery WH. Clinical spectrum of hereditary hemorrhagic telangiectasia (Osier-Weber-Rendu disease). *Am J Med* 1987;82:989–997.

Porteous MEM, Burn J, Proctor SJ. Hereditary haemorrhagictelangiectasia: a clinical analysis. *J Med Genet* 1992;29:527–530.

Press OW, Ramsey PG. Central nervous system infections associated with hereditary hemorrhagic telangiectasia. *Am J Med* 1984;77:86–92.

Remy J, Remy-Jardin M, Wattinne L, et al. Pulmonary arteriovenous malformations: evaluation with CT of the chest before and after treatment (see comments). *Radiology* 1992:182:809–816.

Shovlin CL, Guttmacher AE, Buscarini E, et al. Diagnostic criteria for hereditary hemorrhagic telangiectasia (Rendu-Oster-Weber syndrome). *Am J Med Genet* 2000;91:66.

Stankiewicz JA. Nasal endoscopy and control of epistaxis. *Curr Opin Otolaryngol Head Neck Surg* 2004;12:43–45.

Vincent P, Plauchu H, Hazan J, et al. (1995) A third locus for hereditary haemorrhagic telangiectasia map to chromosome 12. *Hum Mol Genet* 1995;4:945.

Cutis Marmorata Telangiectatica Congenita

Cohen PR, Zalar GL. Cutis marmorata telangiectatica congenita: cliniciopathologic characteristics and differential diagnosis. *Cutis* 1988;42:518–522.

Fujita M, Darmstadt GL, Dinulos JG. Cutis marmorata telangiectatica congenita with hemangiomatous histopathologic features. *J Am Med Dermatol* 2003;48:950–954.

Kanna B, Das B. Hemorrhagic pericardial effusion causing pericardial tamponade in hereditary hemorrhagic telangiectasia. *Am J Med Sci* 2004;327:149–151.

Lischke R, Simonek J, Stolz A, et al. Bilateral pulmonary arteriovenous malformations in patient with Rendu-Osler-Weber disease. *Eur J Cardiothorac Surg* 2004;25:461.

Lynch PJ. Cutis marmorata telangiectatica congenita associated with congenital glaucoma [letter; comment]. *J Am Acad Dermatol* 1991;22:857.

Pehr K, Moroz B. Cutis marmorata telangiectatica congenita: long-term follow-up, review of the literature, and report of a case in conjunction with congenital hypothyroidism. *Pediatr Dermatol* 1993;10:6–11.

Picascia DD, Esterly NB. Cutis marmorata telangiectatica congenita: report of 22 cases [see comments]. *J Am Acad Dermatol* 1989;20:1098–1104.

Requena LT, Sangueza OP: Cutaneous vascular anomalies: Hamartomas, malformations, and dilatation of preexisting vessels. *J Am Acad Dermatol* 1997;37:523.

Stankiewicz JA. Nasal endoscopy and control of epistaxis. *Curr Opin Otolaryngol Head Neck Surg* 2004;12:43–45.

Suarez SM, Grossman ME. Localized cutis marmorata telangiectatica congenita. *Pediatr Dermatol* 1991;8:329–331.

Weilepp AE, Eichenfield LF. Association of glaucoma with cutis marmorata telangiectatica congenita: a localized anatomic malformation. *J Am Acad Dermatol* 1996;35:276–278.

Maffucci Syndrome

Balcer LJ, Galetta SL, Cornblath WT et al. (1999) Neuro-ophthalmologic manifestations of Maffucciís syndrome and Ollieris disease. *J Neurophthalmol* 1999;19:62–66.

Collins PS, Han W, Williams LR, et al. Maffucciís syndrome (hemangiomatosis osteolytica): a report of four cases. *J Vasc Surg* 1992;16:364–371.

Kaplan RP, Wang JT, Amron DM, et al. Maffucciís syndrome: two case reports with a literature review. *J Am Acad Dermatol* 1993;29:894–899.

Sun TC, Swee RG, Shives TC, et al. Chondrosarcoma in Maffucciís syndrome. *J Bone Joint Surg Am* 1985;67:1214–1219.

Blue Rubber Bleb Nevus Syndrome

Beluffi G, Romano P, Matteotti C, et al. Jejunal intussusception in a 10-year-old boy with blue rubber bleb nevus syndrome. *Pediatr Radiol* 2004; (in press).

Buchi KN. Vascular malformations of the gastrointestinal tract. *Surg Clin North Am* 1992;72:559–570.

Gallo S, McClave S. Blue rubber bleb nevus syndrome: gastrointestinal involvement and its endoscopic presentation. *Gastrointest Endosc* 1992;38:72–26.

Goraya JS, Marwaha RK, Vatve M et al. Blue rubber bleb nevus syndrome. *Pediatr Hematol* 1998;15:261–264.

Kassarjian A, Fishman SJ, Fox VL, et al. Imaging characteristics of blue rubber bleb nevus syndrome. *AJR Am J Roentgenol* 2003;1:1041–1048.

Morris L, Lynch PM, Gleason WA Jr, et al. Blue rebber bleb nevus syndrome: laser photocoagulation of colonic hemangiomas in child with microcytic anemia. *Pediatr Dermatol* 1992;9:92–94.

Nahm WK, Moise S, Eichenfield LF, et al. Venous malformations in blue rubber bleb nevus syndrome: variable onset of presentation. *J Am Med Dermatol* 2004;50:101–106.

Oranje AP. Blue rubber bleb nevus syndrome. *Pediatr Dermatol* 1996;3:304–310.

Paules S, Baack B, Levisohn D. Tender Bluish papules on the trunk and extremities. Blue rubber-bleb nevus syndrome. *Arch Dermatol* 1993;129:1505–1506, 1508–1509.

Requena L, Sangueza OP. Cutaneous vascular anormalies: hamartomas, malformations, and dilatation of preexisting vessels. *J Am Acad Dermatol* 1997;37:523.

Kasabach-Merritt Syndrome

Alvarez-Mendoza A, Lourdes TS, Ridaura-Sanz C et al. Histopathology of vascular lesions found in Kasabach-Merritt syndrome: review based on 13 cases. *Pediatr Dev Pathol* 2000;3:556–560.

Drolet BA, Scott LA, Esterly NB, et al. Early surgical intervention in a patient with Kasabach-Merritt phenomenon. *J Pediatr* 2001;138:756–758.

Enjolras O, Muliken JB, Wassef M, et al. Residual lesions after Kasabach-Merritt phenomenon in 41 patients. *J Am Acad Dermatol* 2000;42:225–235.

Enjolras O, Riche MC, Merland JJ, et al. Management of alarming hemangiomas in infancy: a review of 25 cases [see comments]. *Pediatrics* 1990;85:491–498.

Enjolras O, Wassef M, Mazoyer E, et al. Infants with Kasabach-Merritt syndrome do not have "true" hemangiomas. *J Pediatr* 1997;130:631–640.

George M, Singhal V, Sharma V, et al. Successful surgical excision of a complex vascular lesion in an infant with Kasabach-Merritt syndrome. *Pediatr Dermatol* 2002;19:340–344.

Haisley-Roster CA, Enjolras O, Frieden IJ, et al. Kasabach-Merritt phenomenon: a retrospective study of treatment with vincristine. *J Pediatr Hematol Oncol* 2002;24:459–462.

Hall GW. Kasabach-Merritt syndrome: pathogensis and management. *Br J Haematol* 2001;112:851–862.

Hatley RM, Sabio H, Howell CG, et al. Successful retroperitoneum and Kasabach-Merritt syndrome with alpha-interferon. *J Pediatr Surg* 1993;28:1356–1357; discussion 1358–1359.

Lyons LL, North PE, MacMoune Lai F, et al. Kaposiform Hemangioendothelioma: a study of 33 cases emphasizing its pathologic, immunophenotypic, and biologic uniqueness from juvenile hemangioma. *Am J Surg Pathol* 2004;28:559–568.

Maceyko RF, Camisa C. Kasabach-Merritt syndrome. *Pediatr Dermatol* 1991;8:133–136.

Sarkar M, Muliken JB, Kozakewisch HP, et al. Thrombocytopenic coagulopathy (Kasabach-Merritt phenomenon) is associated with Kaposiform hemangioendothelioma and not with common infantile hemangioma. *Plast Reconstr Surg* 1997;100:1377–1386.

Shin HY, Ryu KH, Ahn HS. Stepwise multimodal approach in the treatment of Kasabach-Merritt syndrome. *Pediatr Int* 2000;42:620–624.

Diffuse Neonatal Hemangiomatosis

Blei F, Orlow SJ, Geronemus R. Multimodal management of diffuse neonatal hemangiomatosis. *J Am Acad Dermatol* 1997;37:1019–1021.

Ezekowitz RA, Muliken JB, Folkman J. Interferon alfa-2a therapy for life-threatening hemangiomas of infancy (see comments) *N Engl J Med* 1992;326:1456–1463 (published erratum appears in *N Engl J Med* 1994;330:300).

Fishman SJ, Muliken JB. Hemangiomas and vascular malformations of infancy and childhood. *Pediatric Clin North Am* 1993;40:1177–1200.

Gembruch U, Baschat AA, Gloeckner-Hoffinannlam K, et al. Prenatal diagnosis and management of fetuses with liver hemangiomata. *Ultrasound Obstet Gynecol* 2002;19:454–460.

Golitz LE, Rudikoff J, OíMeara OP. Diffuse neonatalhemangiomatosis. *Pediatr Dermatol* 1986;3:145–152.

Held JL, Haber RS, Silvers DN, et al. Benign neonatal hemangiomatosis: review and description of a patient with unusually persistent lesions. *Pediatr Dermatol* 1990;7:63–66.

Latifi HR, Siegel MJ. Diffuse neonatal hemangiomatosis: CT findings in an adult. *J Comput Assist Tomogr* 1992;16:971–973.

Rothe MJ, Rowse D, Grant-Kels JM. Benign neonatal hemangiomatosis with aggressive growth of cutaneous lesions. *Pediatr Dermatol* 1991;8:140–146.

Special symposia. The management of disseminated eruptive hemangiomata in infants. *Pediatr Dermatol* 1984;1:312.

Spiller JC, Sharma V, Woods GM, et al. Diffuse neonatal hemangiomatosis treated successfully with interferon alfa-2a. *J Am Acad Dermatol* 1992;27:102–104.

PHACE

Burrows PE, Robertson RL, Muliken JB, et al. Cerebral vasculopathy and neurologic sequelae in infants with cerviofacial hemangioma: report of eight patients. *Radiology* 1998;107:601–607.

Freiden IJ, Reese V, Cohen D. PHACE syndrome. The association of posterior fossa brain malformations, hemangiomas, arterial anomalies, coarctation of the aorta and cardiac defects, and eye abnormalities. *Arch Dermatol* 1996;132:317–311.

Metry DW, Dowd CF, Barkovich AJ, et al. The many faces of PHACE syndrome. *J Peidatr* 2001;139:117–123.

Slavotinek AM, Dubovsky E, Dietz HC, et al. Report of a child with aortic aneurysm, orofacial clefting, hemangioma, upper sternal defect, and marfanoid features: possible PHACE syndrome. *Am J Med Genet* 2002;110:283–288.

Chapter 4

Disorders of Connective Tissue

Clinical Pearls

Juoni Uitto, M.D., Ph.D. (JU), Ilona Frieden, M.D. (IF),
Kurt Hirschhorn, M.D. (KH), and Judith Willner, M.D. (JW)

Ehlers-Danlos Syndrome

Inheritance

Type
Classical (I and II):
autosomal dominant; gene locus 2q31, 9q34
Hypermobility (III):
autosomal dominant
Vascular (IV):
autosomal dominant; gene locus 2q31
Kyphoscoliosis (VI):
autosomal recessive; gene locus 1p36.3-p36.2
Arthrochalasia:
autosomal dominant (VIIA, VIIB); gene locus 7q22.1, 17q21-22
Dermatosparaxis (VIIC):
autosomal recessive ; gene locus 5q23
Other variants (V, VIII, X, XI)

Prenatal Diagnosis

Classical
Chorionic villus sampling (CVS)/amniocentesis-—deficient type V collagen in cultured cells
DNA mutation analysis
Vascular
CVS/amniocentesis—decreased type III collagen in cultured cells
DNA analysis
Kyphoscoliosis
Amniocentesis—decreased lysyl hydroxylase activity in cultured amniocytes
DNA analysis
Arthrochalasia/Dermatosparaxis
CVS/amniocentesis—deficient type I collagen in cultured cells

Incidence

Approximately 1:5,000; M=F, except X-linked (all male)
Classical
Approximately 80% of all Ehlers-Danlos syndrome (EDS)
Hypermobility
Approximately 10% of all EDS
Vascular
Approximately 4% of all EDS
All other types comprise remaining 6%

Age at Presentation

Birth to early childhood

Pathogenesis

Classical
Mutations in COL5A1 and COL5A2 chains in type V collagen account for about 50% of cases; deficiency in tenascin X in 3% of patients
Vascular
Mutations in COL3A1 results in abnormal synthesis, structure and secretion of type III collagen
Kyphoscoliosis
Mutation in procollagen lysyl 2-oxoglutarate 5 dioxygenase (*PLOD*) gene leads to deficient lysyl hydroxylase
Arthrochalasia
Mutations involving the amino terminal propeptide cleavage sites of COL1A1 (type A) or COL1A2 (type B) leads to defective conversion of procollagen to collagen type I
Dermatosparaxis
Recessive mutations in the type I collagen N-peptidase gene
Hypermobility
Unknown

Key Features

Classical (I, II)
  Skin
    Hyperextensible with "snap-back" elasticity, gaping wounds from minimal trauma, "cigarette-paper" scars, molluscoid pseudotumors, calcified subcutaneous nodules, varicose veins, ecchymoses
  Musculoskeletal
    Hypermobile joints with potential delay in ambulation, recurrent joint dislocations, pes planus, genu recurvatum, kyphoscoliosis, inguinal/umbilical hernias

Key Features
(continued)

Cardiovascular
Mitral valve prolapse

Craniofacial
Epicanthic folds, hypertelorism, blue sclerae, + Gorlin's sign (ability to touch nose with tongue tip)

Pregnancy
Prematurity caused by early rupture of fetal membranes in affected fetus; postpartum hemorrhage

Hypermobility (III)

Musculoskeletal
Severe joint laxity with delay in ambulation, recurrent dislocations, early-onset degenerative joint disease

Skin
Minimally affected with mild hyperextensiblity

Cardiovascular
Mitral valve prolapse

Vascular (IV)

Skin
Thin, translucent, fragile with easily seen venous network; inextensible, ecchymoses, varicose veins

Musculoskeletal
Minimal joint laxity (hands and feet)

Arterial
Aneurysm, dissection, rupture of large and medium-sized vessels; arteriovenous fistulas

Gastrointestinal
Colonic rupture, recurrent abdominal pain

Pregnancy
Uterine rupture, arterial rupture, tearing of vaginal tissues

Craniofacial
Acrogeric facies

Kyphoscoliosis (VI)

Skin
Hyperextensible, fragile, ecchymoses

Musculoskeletal
Newborn hypotonia, joint laxity, severe kyphoscoliosis

Eyes
Ruptured globe, retinal detachment, intraocular hemorrhage, keratoconus, blindness

Arthrochalasia (VIIA, B)

Skin
Mild hyperextensibility, fragility

Musculoskeletal
Congenital hip dislocation, severe joint hypermobility with dislocation of large and small joints, scoliosis, short stature

Dermatosparaxis (VIIC)

Skin
Severe fragility, laxity with sagging redundancy; easy bruisability, umbilical/inguinal hernias, premature rupture of fetal membranes; normal wound healing

Other Variants

Type VIII

Skin
Hyperextensible, fragile, ecchymoses; pretibial, yellow-brown, wrinkled scarring

Mouth
Severe periodontitis with resorption of alveolar bone and premature loss of permanent teeth

Type X

Skin
Mild hyperextensibility, petechiae, ecchymoses

Musculoskeletal
Joint laxity

Ehlers-Danlos Syndrome *(continued)*

Key Features
(continued)

Type XI
Musculoskeletal
Large joint (especially hips, shoulders, and patella) laxity with recurrent dislocations

Differential Diagnosis

Cutis laxa (p. 142)

Laboratory Data

Vascular
Skin biopsy—biochemical assay revealing decreased type III collagen in cultured fibroblasts
Two-dimensional echocardiography

Kyphoscoliosis
Skin biopsy: biochemical assay revealing reduced lysyl hydroxylase activity in cultured fibroblasts

Arthrochalasia/Dermatosparaxis
Electrophoresis reveals procollagen alpha1(I) or alpha 2(I) chains from cultured fibroblasts or collagen

Management

General
Referral to dermatologist, orthopedic surgeon
Skin protection from trauma
Advise surgeons regarding poor wound healing
Advise obstetrician regarding prematurity
Examine first-degree family members

Vascular
Referral to cardiologist/cardiovascular surgeon
Advise obstetrician regarding pregnancy avoidance/potential labor complications
Avoid arteriography
Avoid physical contact sports
Referral to gastroenterologist if symptomatic

Kyphoscoliosis
Referral to ophthalmologist
Oral ascorbic acid

Type VIII
Referral to dentist

Type X
Referral to hematologist

Prognosis

Normal life span except in vascular type with potential for premature death in second to third decade because of complications from arterial or colonic rupture or maternal death because of uterine or arterial rupture; kyphoscoliosis type may cause blindness

Clinical Pearls

This syndrome continues to be a challenge to practicing dermatologists. The wide spectrum of phenotypic manifestations blend at one end to the constitutive features in the general population and at the other end can be a cause of early demise. The molecular basis of all six major forms of EDS has now been deciphered, the mutations residing either in the genes encoding collagens, enzymes modifying the primary collagen translation products, or tenascin-X, another connective tissue protein.

The major type of EDS not to be missed is the vascular type (old EDS IV). They are at high risk for arterial and intestinal ruptures, and often unexpectedly, to uterine rupture during labor, with catastrophic consequences. As soon as you establish this diagnosis, get a cardiovascular evaluation, paying attention to the aortic root and possible aneurysms.

Another type not to miss is the kyphoscoliosis type (old EDS VI). In some cases one may be able to overcome the enzyme deficiency simply by supplementary ascorbic acid in the diet. In fact, some physicians advocate ascorbic acid for all EDS types.

The previous EDS IX has been excluded from EDS category and is known as the occipital horn syndrome (because of the characteristic bone protrusions at the base of the skull). It is allelic with Menkes syndrome.

General treatment of EDS is protection from trauma, use of shin guards when playing sports, avoid sharp edges of furniture at home. Loose jointedness, particularly affecting knees and hips, can result in early osteoarthrosis; a pediatric orthopedic consultation may be helpful. Mitral valve prolapse is exceedingly common among patients with EDS. *JU*

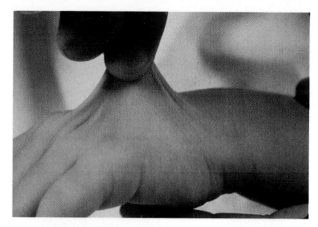

4.1. *Hyperextensible skin. (55)*

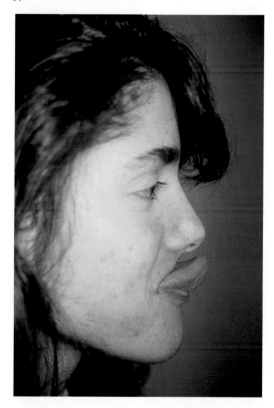

4.2. *Patient demonstrating a (+) Gorlin's sign. (5)*

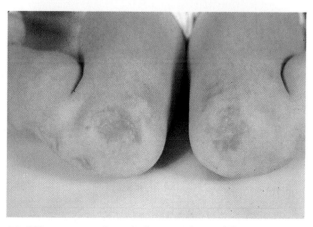

4.3. *"Cigarette paper" atypical scars on knees. (55)*

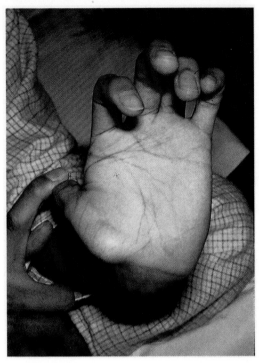

4.4. *Hypermobile joints.* (5)

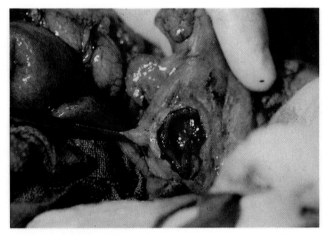

4.5. *Sigmoid perforation in a patient with vascular EDS.* (56)

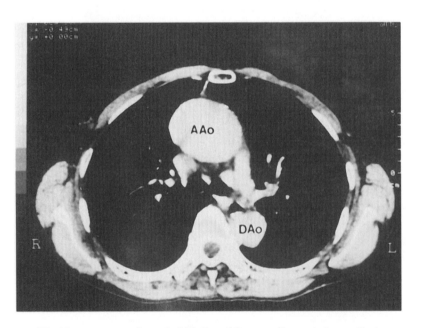

4.6. *CT with contrast reveals marked dilation of the ascending aorta in a patient with vascular EDS.* (57)

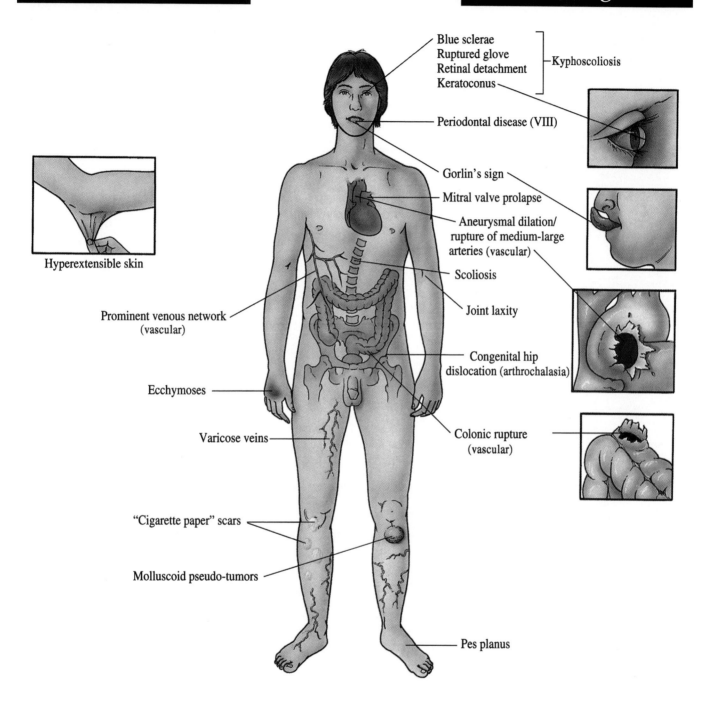

Blue sclerae
Ruptured glove
Retinal detachment
Keratoconus

Kyphoscoliosis

Periodontal disease (VIII)

Gorlin's sign

Mitral valve prolapse

Aneurysmal dilation/
rupture of medium-large
arteries (vascular)

Scoliosis

Joint laxity

Congenital hip
dislocation (arthrochalasia)

Colonic rupture
(vascular)

Hyperextensible skin

Prominent venous network
(vascular)

Ecchymoses

Varicose veins

"Cigarette paper" scars

Molluscoid pseudo-tumors

Pes planus

Marfan Syndrome

Inheritance	Autosomal dominant; mutation in fibrillin-1 on chromosome 15
Prenatal Diagnosis	DNA analysis
Incidence	1:10,000–20,000; M=F
Age at Presentation	Infancy if suspected by family history; usually second or third decade of life
Pathogenesis	Mutation in fibrillin gene, coding for a vital component of the microfibrillar system, results in a lack of fibrillin with concomitant defects in the ocular, cardiovascular, and musculoskeletal system
Key Features	**Musculoskeletal** Tall stature, lower body length longer than upper body length, arachnodactyly, dolichocephaly, pectus excavatum, high-arched palate, loose joints, poor muscle tone, kyphoscoliosis, pes planus, inguinal hernia **Eyes** Ectopia lentis (upward displacement in 75%) Myopia **Cardiovascular** Progressive aneurysmal dilatation of ascending aorta with secondary regurgitation, congestive heart failure (CHF), dissection and rupture Mitral valve prolapse **Skin (less common)** Striae distensae Elastosis perforans serpiginosa Decreased subcutaneous fat
Differential Diagnosis	Congenital contractural arachnodactyly Multiple endocrine neoplasia type IIb (p. 190) Homocystinuria (p. 332) Stickler syndrome
Laboratory Data	Echocardiagram Chest x-ray
Management	Referral to cardiologist/cardiac surgeon—surgical repair, β-blockers Referral to ophthalmologist Referral to orthopedic surgeon Estrogen therapy—prevent excessive tallness in females
Prognosis	Although the prognosis has improved dramatically with advanced cardiovascular surgical repair, patients may die prematurely from cardiac complications; marked variability in severity

Clinical Pearls

This systemic connective tissue disorder is caused by mutations in the fibrillin-1 gene. The phenotypic variability reflects the types of mutations and their consequences at the mRNA and protein levels. The major complications relate to cardiovascular findings, including aortic dilatation, dissection and aneurysms. The patients should be followed closely by cardiovascular surgeons. Lowering blood pressure and using beta-blockers is clearly helpful. The eye problems require regular follow-up by an ophthalmologist. *JU*

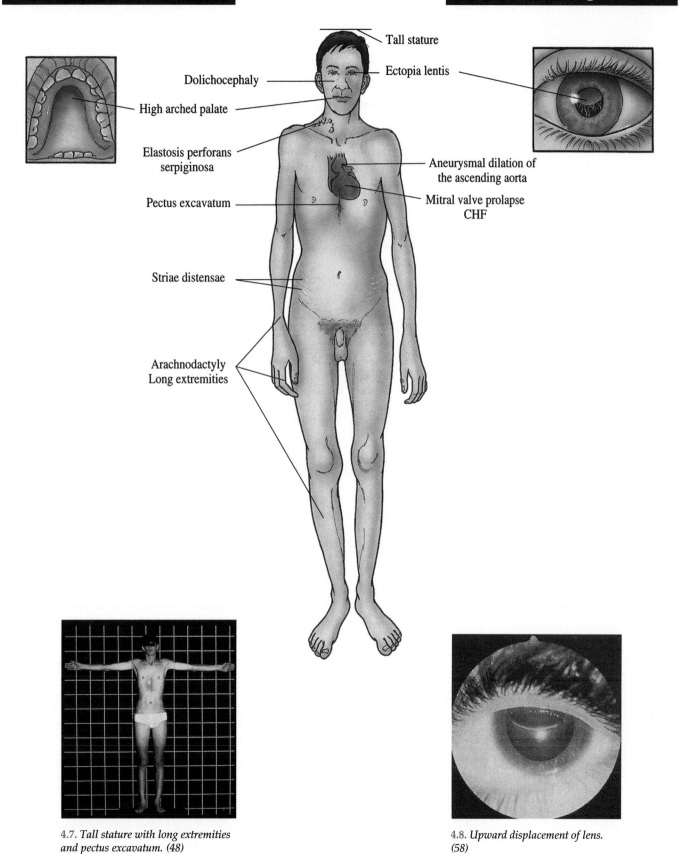

Tall stature

Ectopia lentis

Dolichocephaly

High arched palate

Elastosis perforans serpiginosa

Aneurysmal dilation of the ascending aorta

Pectus excavatum

Mitral valve prolapse CHF

Striae distensae

Arachnodactyly Long extremities

4.7. *Tall stature with long extremities and pectus excavatum.* (48)

4.8. *Upward displacement of lens.* (58)

Cutis Laxa

Synonym	Generalized elastolysis
Inheritance	Autosomal recessive (most common)-FBLN5 (fibulin 5) gene on 14q32; another locus on 5q23-31; autosomal dominant—elastin gene on 7q11 and FBLN5 on 14q32 (usually skin only); X-linked recessive—ATP7A on Xq12-13; acquired
Prenatal Diagnosis	DNA mutation analysis
Incidence	Rare
Age at Presentation	Birth to infancy
Pathogenesis	Heterogeneous mutations in fibulin 5 gene, elastin gene, or *ATP7A* gene (adenosine triphosphatase [ATPase] mutation that impairs copper transport necessary for lysyl oxidase activity and normal elastin production) contributes to variability in clinical severity

Key Features

Skin
Loose, redundant, pendulous skin folds with hound-dog facies, often generalized; inelastic, lacks recoil
Premature aged appearance

Oral
Vocal cord laxity causing deep, resonant voice

Lungs
Newborn—hypoplastic lungs
Emphysema (autosomal recessive)—may be complicated by tachypnea, pneumonitis, cor pulmonale

Gastrointestinal (autosomal recessive)
Esophageal, duodenal, rectal diverticulae

Genitourinary (autosomal recessive and x-linked)
Bladder diverticulae

Musculoskeletal (autosomal recessive and x-linked)
Inguinal, diaphragmatic, umbilical hernia, hip dislocation, occipital horn exostoses (x-linked)

Differential Diagnosis	Pseudoxanthoma elasticum (p. 144) EDS (p. 134) Granulomatous slack skin DeBarsy syndrome SCARF syndrome
Laboratory Data	Skin biopsy—decreased, fragmented elastic fibers visualized with Verhoeff-van Gieson stain Serum copper and ceruloplasmin levels Chest x-ray
Management	Referral to plastic surgeon Referral to pulmonologist, gastroenterologist, urologist, surgeon if symptomatic Sunscreen protection
Prognosis	Great variability in severity ranging from death in neonate if born with hypoplastic lungs to only skin involvement with normal life span if no pulmonary disease (majority with latter).

Clinical Pearls

The underlying pathology relates to perturbation in the elastic fiber network, and mutations have been demonstrated both in the elastin and fibulin-5 genes. The clinical spectrum spans from relatively mild skin involvement to extremely severe with skin problem associated with extracutaneous manifestations, including pulmonary emphysema, arterial aneurysms, and vesico-urinary diverticula. Therefore, careful systemic evaluation, especially in patients with congenital forms of cutis laxa, is in order. The inheritance can be either autosomal dominant or autosomal recessive. Acquired, late-onset cutis laxa is often associated with urticarial and/or inflammatory lesions and is sometimes a sequela of acute drug reaction, such as to penicillin. In the latter case, inflammatory cells that contain powerful elastases degrade elastin in the skin, resulting in paucity of elastic fibers. As a result, the entire skin shows progressive sagging, and because of relatively poor repair capacity, new elastic fibers are not formed in adult skin and the sagging is permanent. Solar elastosis tends to aggravate this condition, and sunscreen application should be stressed. Facelifts do provide improvement, but this may be only temporary. *JU*

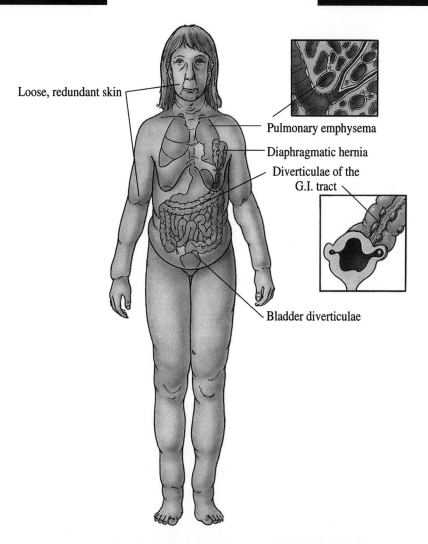

Loose, redundant skin

Pulmonary emphysema

Diaphragmatic hernia

Diverticulae of the
G.I. tract

Bladder diverticulae

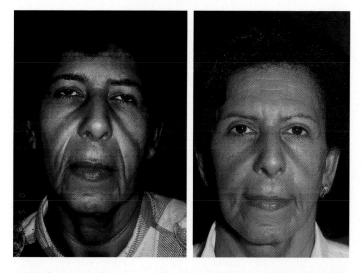

4.9. *Left: Twenty-three years-old patient with loose, pendulous skin folds.
Right: Same patient at 38 y.o. after 3 face-lifts, earlobe correction, and
resection of excess skin from the nasolabial folds and upper lip. (59)*

143

Pseudoxanthoma Elasticum

Inheritance
Autosomal recessive (most common); autosomal dominant; *ABCC6* (adenosine triphosphate [ATP]-binding cassette subfamily C member 6) transporter gene on 16p13

Prenatal Diagnosis
DNA mutation analysis if defect known

Incidence
Approximately 1:100,000; M=F

Age at Presentation
Childhood to second or third decade of life

Pathogenesis
Mutation in *ABCC6* transmembrane transporter gene that encodes a multidrug resistance protein; the correlation of this gene defect with the phenotype has not been elucidated

Key Features
Skin
Yellow papules coalescing to plaques overlying redundant, lax, soft skin folds on sides of neck, axillae, antecubital fossae, abdomen, groin, thighs
Mucous Membranes
Yellow papules on labial mucosa, soft palate, rectal and vaginal mucosa
Eyes
Angioid streaks (rupture in Bruch's membrane secondary to elastic fiber defect), macular degeneration, retinal hemorrhage causing blindness, retinal pigmentation alteration
Cardiovascular
Gastric artery hemorrhage (common) with epistaxis, hematemesis; claudication, decreased/absent peripheral pulses, hypertension, angina pectoris, myocardial infarction, cerebrovascular accidents, mitral valve prolapse
Obstetrics
Increased first trimester miscarraige, increased cardiovascular complications

Differential Diagnosis
Cutis laxa (p. 142)
Angioid streaks: Sickle cell anemia, Paget's disease of bone, hyperphosphatemia
EDS (p. 134)

Laboratory Data
Skin biopsy (affected, normal, or cicatricial skin)—Von Kossa stain (calcium), Verhoeff-van Gieson stain (curled elastin fibers)
Fundoscopy
X-ray of extremity or abdomen if symptomatic

Management   Complete physical examination and regular follow-up with primary care physician
Referral to dermatologist, ophthalmologist
Referral to gastroenterologist, cardiologist, neurologist if symptomatic
Referral to plastic surgeon—cosmetic correction
Advise obstetrician during pregnancy
Restriction of calcium intake (controversial)
Examination of first degree family members by dermatologist, ophthalmologist, cardiologist

Prognosis   Shortened life span secondary to cardiovascular complications

Clinical Pearls

This clinical entity can occasionally be a diagnostic problem, particularly because of delayed onset and considerable intrafamilial and interfamilial heterogeneity. Diagnosis can usually be confirmed by skin pathology, but recent identification of the mutated gene, *ABCC6*, provides a molecular tool to confirm the diagnosis. In cases without definitive cutaneous findings, but with angioid streaks and family history of pseudoxanthoma elasticum (PXE), mutation analysis can be used for presymptomatic diagnosis.

Patients need to be followed by ophthalmologists who may consider laser treatment of retinal hemorrhages. Avoidance of head trauma is important to prevent retinal bleeding. Although total blindness is extremely rare, some patients may become legally blind at a relatively early age. Plastic surgery may be helpful in improving the cosmetic appearance of skin. The major life-threatening problems are myocardial infarct and occasionally, massive gastrointestinal hemorrhages, particularly in families with predominant cardiovascular manifestations. Strongly advise patients against smoking, because it exacerbates intermittent claudication and other cardiovascular problems. Calcium intake is a controversial subject, as it has been suggested that high calcium intake during the childhood or early adolescence results in more severe phenotype. I do not recommend low-calcium diet for adults as it may accelerate development of osteoporosis, and balanced diet including modest amounts of dairy products should be fine for children as well.

Direct patients to the website of PXE International, a patient advocacy organization: www.pxe.org.   *JU*

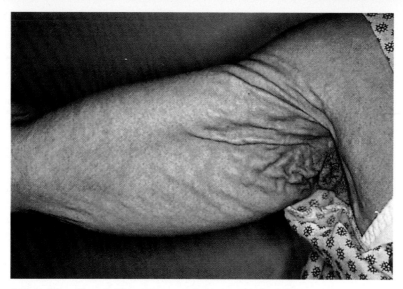

4.10. *Axilla with coalescing yellow papules over redundant skin.*

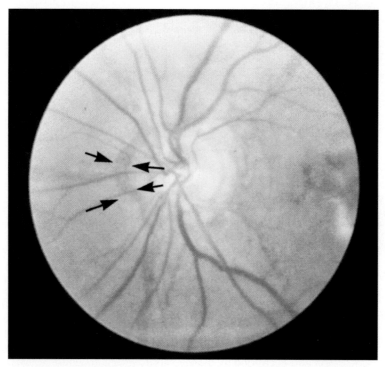

4.11. *Angioid streaks (arrows).*

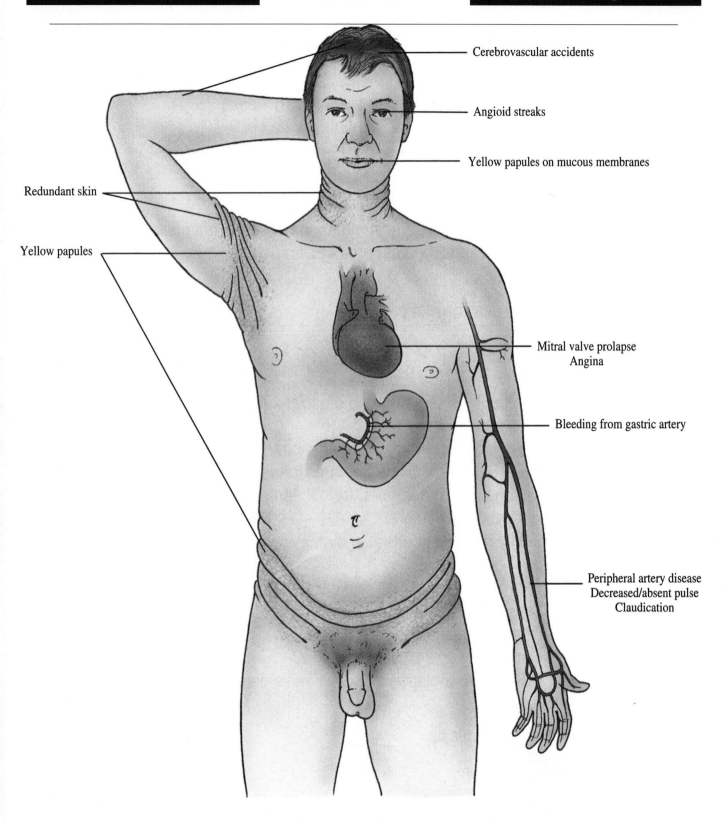

Cerebrovascular accidents

Angioid streaks

Yellow papules on mucous membranes

Redundant skin

Yellow papules

Mitral valve prolapse
Angina

Bleeding from gastric artery

Peripheral artery disease
Decreased/absent pulse
Claudication

Osteogenesis Imperfecta

Inheritance

Type I—autosomal dominant
Type II—autosomal dominant and recessive
Type III—autosomal dominant and recessive
Type IV—autosomal dominant
COL1A2 gene on 7q22 and COL1A1 gene on 17q22

Prenatal Diagnosis

Ultrasonography/in utero x-ray at 16 weeks
DNA analysis

Incidence

1:5–10,000—type I most common; M=F

Age at Presentation

Birth to adulthood depending on type

Pathogenesis

Heterogeneous genetic mutations in genes encoding type I collagen (α1 and α2 chains) provides for heterogeneous phenotype; mutation may alter amount of collagen produced (milder phenotype) or change the structure of type I collagen (mild-severe phenotype)

Key Features

Skin
   Thin, decreased elasticity; easy bruising (I, IV)
Eyes
   Blue sclerae (I, II, III [infant])
Ear-Nose-Throat
   Hearing loss secondary to otosclerosis
Musculoskeletal
   I (mild/moderate)—fractures, bowing of long bones, joints lax, kyphosis
   II (severe)—multiple fractures in utero; newborn with beaded ribs, crumpled humeri and femora; frontal, temporal bossing; limb avulsion during delivery, abducted thighs
   III—fractures in utero, at birth; progressive kyphoscoliosis, bowing with crippling deformities
   IV—fractures at birth and childhood with decreased frequency with age
Teeth
   Dentinogenesis imperfecta (I, IV)
Cardiac
   Mitral valve prolapse (I), aortic valve disease (I), autopsy reveals valvular disease (II)

Differential Diagnosis

Child abuse
Achondroplasia

Laboratory Data

Bone films
Echocardiography
Audiology examination

Management

Referral to orthopedist, psychiatrist, cardiologist, otolaryngologist, dentist if symptomatic
Intranasal calcitonin may reduce incidence of fractures
Bisphosphonate treatment

Prognosis

Variable with death in perinatal period (type II), increased mortality in third to fourth decade as a result of cardiorespiratory failure (type III), limb deformities after fractures, otherwise potential normal life span with limited morbidity

Clinical Pearls

Different mutations in type I collagen gene are responsible for varying severity of disease . . . Milder forms are often misdiagnosed as child abuse . . . However, osteogenesis imperfecta (OI) kids have thinner bones and fracture straight through, abused kids get spiral fractures . . . Blue sclerae should be looked for when evaluating for abuse . . . Can diagnose in utero with ultrasound . . . Looks like severe chondrodystrophies except you often see fractures . . . May need dentures as children . . . If teeth involved you usually have worse fractures . . . One of many dominant syndromes where you get an association with increased paternal age and a new mutation . . . Confirmation of prenatal and clinical diagnosis is available by collagen examination in cultured fibroblasts and by mutation screening.   *KH, JW*

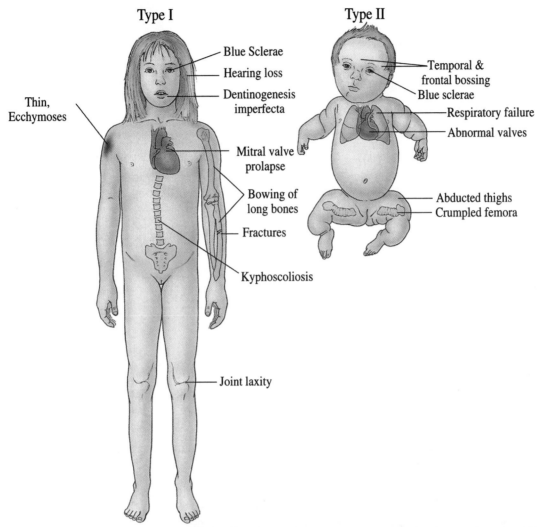

Type I

- Blue Sclerae
- Hearing loss
- Dentinogenesis imperfecta
- Thin, Ecchymoses
- Mitral valve prolapse
- Bowing of long bones
- Fractures
- Kyphoscoliosis
- Joint laxity

Type II

- Temporal & frontal bossing
- Blue sclerae
- Respiratory failure
- Abnormal valves
- Abducted thighs
- Crumpled femora

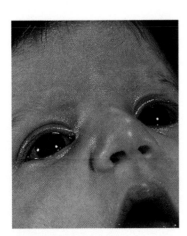

4.12. Blue sclerae. (60)

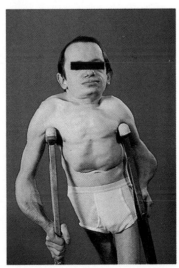

4.13. Severe bowing, kyphoscoliosis with crippling deformities. (60)

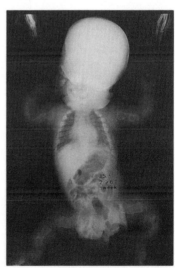

4.14. Crumpled humeri, femora with abducted thighs at one week of age. (60)

Buschke-Ollendorff Syndrome

Inheritance	Autosomal dominant; gene locus unknown
Prenatal Diagnosis	None
Incidence	Rare; likely underreported given asymptomatic and undiscovered lesions; M=F
Age at Presentation	Birth to adulthood
Pathogenesis	Increased elastic fiber content in skin; elastin mRNA levels in fibroblast cultures shown to be increased; unknown defect linking bone and skin

Key Features	**Skin**
	   Dermatofibrosis lenticularis disseminata
	      Skin-colored to yellow dermal papules with/without coalesced plaques often with symmetric distribution on trunk, buttocks, arms
	Bone
	   Osteopoikilosis
	      One- to 10-mm well-circumscribed round to oval opacities within carpal, tarsal bones and phalanges of the hands and feet, pelvis, and the epiphyses and metaphyses of long bones; asymptomatic x-ray finding

Differential Diagnosis	Tuberous sclerosis (p. 88) Pseudoxanthoma elasticum (p. 144) Familial cutaneous collagenoma
Laboratory Data	X-ray hands, feet, knees Skin biopsy with Verhoeff-van Gieson or orcein stain
Management	Advise patients of benignity—reassurance Examine first-degree family members
Prognosis	Normal life span; no adverse effects on health High penetrance, variable expression (patients may have bone and skin, bone only, skin only involvement in same family)

Clinical Pearls

The skin findings, i.e., multiple elastomas known as dermatofibrosis lenticularis disseminata, are primarily of cosmetic concern. The bone findings, i.e., osteopoikilosis reflecting ectopic calcification, are asymptomatic, and specifically, these patients are not prone to fractures. To confirm the diagnosis of this autosomal dominant syndrome in patients with multiple elastomas, x-rays of the hands and knees should pick up the bone lesions. It is important that the patients are aware that they have "spotty" bones so as to alert radiologists and thereby avoid misdiagnosis.   *JU*

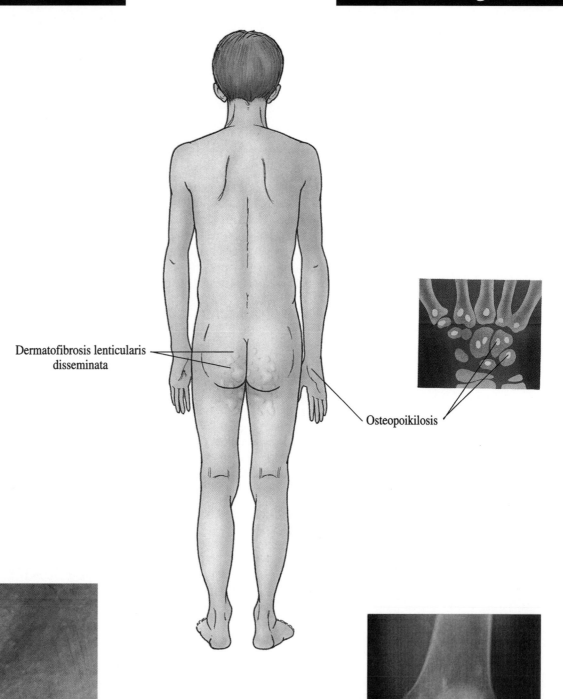

Dermatofibrosis lenticularis
disseminata

Osteopoikilosis

4.15. *Yellow dermal papules on the
trunk. (61)*

4.16. *Bone x-ray depicting multiple,
well-circumscribed oval-round
opacities. (62)*

Focal Dermal Hypoplasia

Synonym	Goltz syndrome
Inheritance	X-linked dominant; gene locus Xp22.31
Prenatal Diagnosis	DNA analysis available in future
Incidence	Over 200 cases reported; 90% female (lethal in male hemizygotes; however, 10% affected males might occur as a result of gametic half-chromatid mutations)
Age at Presentation	Birth
Pathogenesis	Unknown

Key Features

Skin
Asymmetric atrophic, hyperpigmented, or hypopigmented, telangiectatic linear streaks in Blaschko's lines on trunk, extremities
Soft red-yellow nodules (fat herniations) in Blaschko's lines
Ulcers at sites of congenital absence of skin that heal with atrophy (15%)
Papillomas on the lips, perineum, axilla, periumbilical area

Hair
Sparse, brittle; patchy alopecia in scalp or pubic area

Nails
Absent or dystrophic on fingers and toes

Eyes
Coloboma, strabismus, microphthalmia

Musculoskeletal
Syndactyly, polydactyly, oligodactyly with "lobster-claw" deformity; asymmetric trunk and limbs; **osteopathia striata** (vertical striations in metaphysis of long bones on x-ray)—greater than 80% of cases; short stature

Mouth
Hypodontia, oligodontia; small teeth with dysplastic enamel

Craniofacial
Small, rounded, asymmetric face; notched nasal alae, mandibular prognathism

Central Nervous System
Mild mental retardation (15%)

Differential Diagnosis	Incontinentia pigmenti (p. 72) Nevus lipomatosus superficialis Rothmund-Thomson syndrome (p. 238)
Laboratory Data	Skin biopsy X-ray long bones
Management	Referral to dermatologist, ophthalmologist, orthopedic surgeon upon diagnosis Referral to dentist with onset of oral disease Elicit family history/maternal history of spontaneous abortions, miscarriages, stillbirths
Prognosis	May be severely handicapped by skeletal deformities; cosmetic deformities from skin, ocular, and skeletal anomalies with psychosocial consequences; otherwise normal life span

Clinical Pearls

Usually noted at birth with skeletal abnormalities and skin lesions in linear distributions. The skeletal findings can be a useful marker for the disorder. Surgeons can help to surgically correct the anomalies.   *JU*

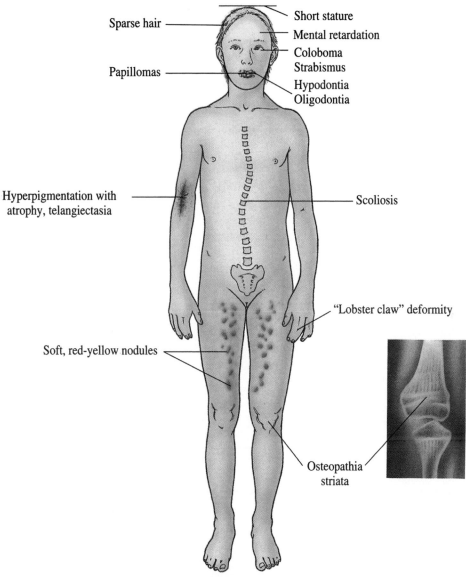

Sparse hair

Papillomas

Hyperpigmentation with
atrophy, telangiectasia

Soft, red-yellow nodules

Short stature

Mental retardation

Coloboma
Strabismus

Hypodontia
Oligodontia

Scoliosis

"Lobster claw" deformity

Osteopathia
striata

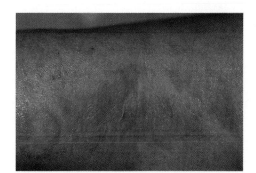

4.17. *Fat herniations presenting as soft red-yellow nodules in a linear distribution on the leg. (1)*

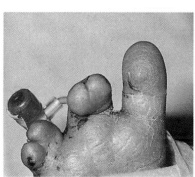

4.18. *Syndactyly on foot of child. (1)*

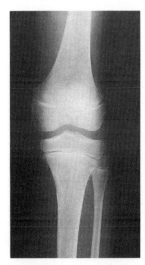

4.19. *Osteopathia striata. (63)*

Lipoid Proteinosis

Synonym	Urbach-Wiethe disease Hyalinosis cutis et mucosae
Inheritance	Autosomal recessive; extracellular matrix protein 1 (*ECM1*) gene on 1q21
Prenatal Diagnosis	DNA analysis in future
Incidence	Over 280 cases reported—increased in South Africa; M=F
Age at Presentation	Birth (hoarse cry) to first few years of life
Pathogenesis	Mutation in *ECM1* correlated with phenotype; unknown cause

Key Features

Skin
  Early
    Bullae with residual atrophic scarring on face, neck and extremities
  Late
    Yellow papules, nodules on face, neck, extremities with eyelid "string of pearls"
    Verrucous nodules of elbows, knees, and hands
Hair
  Patchy alopecia in scalp, beard, eyelashes
Mucous Membranes
  Infiltrative yellow papules and plaques on pharynx, lips, soft palate; with/without parotitis caused by stenotic parotid duct
Ear-Nose-Throat
  Hoarse cry because of vocal cord infiltration
  Large, wooden tongue
Central Nervous System
  Temporal and hippocampal calcification with/without seizures

Differential Diagnosis	Amyloidosis Erythropoietic protoporphyria (p. 224) Pseudoxanthoma elasticum (p. 144) Xanthomas
Laboratory Data	Skin biopsy (PAS (+) hyaline material) Brain magnetic resonance imaging (MRI)
Management	Retinoids, oral dimethylsulphoxide may be beneficial Referral to ear-nose-throat specialist—laser, surgical correction of vocal cords, tracheostomy Referral to dermatologist—diagnosis, dermabrasion, chemical peel Referral to neurologist if symptomatic
Prognosis	May progress to involve internal organs; however, chronic and benign course with normal life span; laryngeal involvement may lead to respiratory difficulties in childhood

Clinical Pearls

This is one of the few skin diseases where you can make the diagnosis without seeing the patient: classically hoarse cry in a newborn. This is followed later on by characteristic skin findings: pearly eyelid papules and verrucous lesions at the elbows; the elbows are occasionally misdiagnosed as psoriatic lesions. Get a neurologist and otolaryngologist involved in the treatment of these patients. The vocal cords can be lasered.

This condition is caused by mutations in the *ECM1* gene, which encodes a protein of unknown function. It is of interest that lichen sclerosus et atrophicus, another condition characterized by dermal hyalinization, is associated with antibodies to the ECM1 protein. *JU*

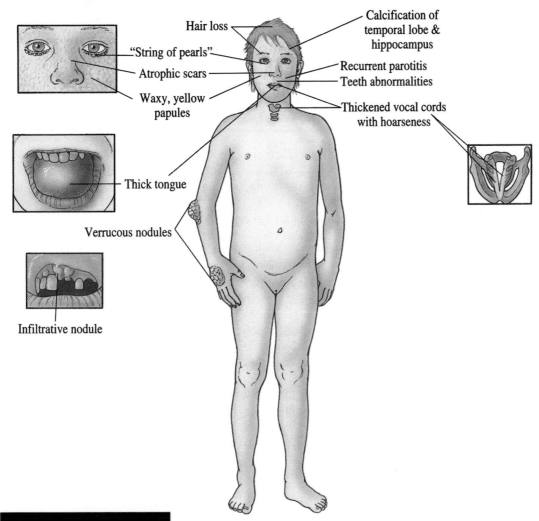

Hair loss

"String of pearls"

Atrophic scars

Waxy, yellow papules

Thick tongue

Verrucous nodules

Infiltrative nodule

Calcification of temporal lobe & hippocampus

Recurrent parotitis

Teeth abnormalities

Thickened vocal cords with hoarseness

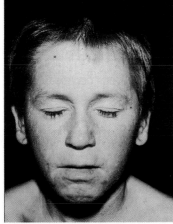

4.20. *Facial scarring, coalescing yellow infiltrative plaques with eyelid papules ("string of pearls"). (64)*

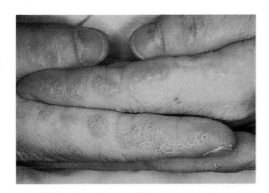

4.21. *Verrucous nodules in linear pattern on fingers. (1)*

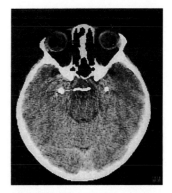

4.22. *CT brain scan shows symmetric calcifications just lateral to dorsum sellae. (64)*

Progeria

Synonym	Hutchinson-Gilford syndrome
Inheritance	Autosomal dominant; lamin A gene on 1q21
Prenatal Diagnosis	DNA analysis in the future
Incidence	Estimated 1:4–8,000,000; M:F=1.5:1
Age at Presentation	First to second year of life
Pathogenesis	Mutation in lamin A, a nuclear envelope protein, has been linked to phenotype

Key Features

Skin
Thin, atrophic, shiny in areas but wrinkled, dull in other areas; prominent scalp and thigh veins, loss of subcutaneous fat, mottled hyperpigmentation, sclerodermoid changes on lower trunk and thigh

Hair
Sparse to absent scalp hair, eyebrows, eyelashes; downy, fine hair may persist

Nails
Thin, dystrophic

Craniofacial
Large cranium relative to face, frontal and parietal bossing, thin beaked nose, small ears without lobules, micrognathia, prominent eyes

Musculoskeletal
Failure to thrive during second year of life; height at 10 years old approximately equal to that of a normal 3 year old; osteoporosis, prominent joints on extremities, shortened clavicle, coxa valga, muscular wasting

Cardiovascular
Premature, severe atherosclerosis with angina pectoris, cerebrovascular accidents, CHF, myocardial infarction

Mouth
Abnormal and delayed eruption of permanent teeth; high-pitched, squeaky voice

Psychosocial
Severe problems related to appearance, self-image

Differential Diagnosis	Cockayne syndrome (p. 242) Werner syndrome (p. 158) Hallerman-Streiff syndrome
Laboratory Data	Urinary hyaluronic acid increased
Management	Referral to cardiologist, orthopedic surgeon, rheumatologist, dermatologist, dentist
Prognosis	Premature death from atherosclerotic complication in second decade of life

Clinical Pearls

These patients appear normal at birth but start to develop characteristic facial features during the first or second year of life. Major problems relate to cardiovascular involvement, which causes premature demise usually in mid-teens. Scleroderma or scleroderma-like skin changes have been reported early on. This rare developmental disorder reflects de novo dominant mutations in the gene encoding lamin-a, a nuclear envelope protein. The families should be referred to patient advocacy group, Hutchinson-Gilford Progeria Syndrome Research Foundation: www.progeriaresearch.org. *JU*

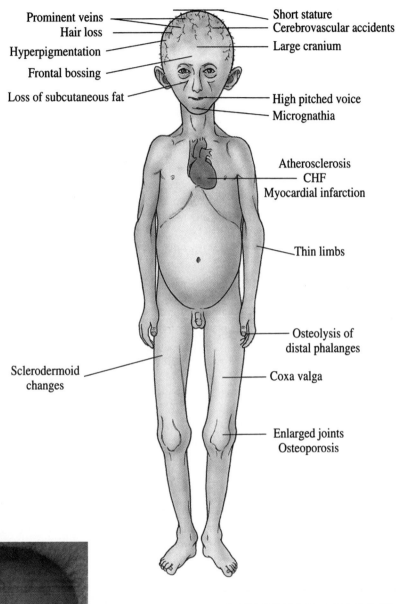

Prominent veins
Hair loss
Hyperpigmentation
Frontal bossing
Loss of subcutaneous fat

Short stature
Cerebrovascular accidents
Large cranium

High pitched voice
Micrognathia

Atherosclerosis
CHF
Myocardial infarction

Thin limbs

Osteolysis of
distal phalanges

Sclerodermoid
changes

Coxa valga

Enlarged joints
Osteoporosis

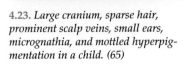

4.23. *Large cranium, sparse hair,
prominent scalp veins, small ears,
micrognathia, and mottled hyperpigmentation in a child. (65)*

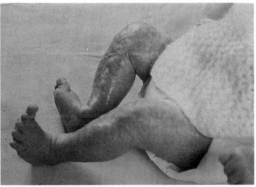

4.24. *Sclerodermoid changes on the legs of a baby with
progeria. (65)*

Werner Syndrome

Inheritance	Autosomal recessive; *RECQL2* gene (or *WRN* gene) on 8p12-p11
Prenatal Diagnosis	DNA analysis
Incidence	1–20:1,000,000; over 150 cases reported; M=F
Age at Presentation	Third to fourth decade of life
Pathogenesis	Mutation in *RECQL2*, a gene encoding a DNA helicase enzyme, leads to increased frequency of recombination with a predisposition toward accelerated aging and cancer

Key Features

Skin
Sclerodermoid changes increased acrally and facially with atrophy, mottled hyper-pigmentation, telangiectasias, soft-tissue calcifications, leg ulcerations; circum-scribed hyperkeratoses over bony prominences with ulceration; generalized loss of subcutaneous fat

Hair
Canities; progressive, premature hair loss

Craniofacial
Bird-like facies with beaked, pinched nose, taut circumoral skin, inelastic ears

Musculoskeletal
Short stature with growth arrest at puberty, muscular wasting, thin, spindly extremities, pes planus, osteoporosis, osteoarthritis

Eyes
Posterior, subcapsular cataracts

Ear-Nose-Throat
High-pitched, hoarse voice

Cardiovascular
Premature atherosclerosis with angina, myocardial infarction

Endocrine
Diabetes mellitus, hypogonadism

Neoplasm (10%)
Fibrosarcoma, osteosarcoma, cutaneous carcinoma, meningioma, adenocarcinoma

Differential Diagnosis	Progeria (p. 156) Rothmund-Thomson syndrome (p. 238) Scleroderma/CREST syndrome Myotonic dystrophy
Laboratory Data	Urinary hyaluronic acid increased; fasting serum glucose X-ray of extremities
Management	Referral to symptom-specific specialist: dermatologist, rheumatologist, ophthalmologist, cardiologist, endocrinologist, oncologist, orthopedic surgeon
Prognosis	Premature death from malignancy, myocardial infarction, or cerebrovascular accident by the fourth to sixth decade

Clinical Pearls

This systemic condition is characterized by premature degeneration of major organs, somewhat mimicking, but not precisely recapitulating accelerated chronologic aging. These patients often develop scleroderma-like skin changes, and their major skin problems relate to chronic ulcers that require meticulous care. This condition is caused by mutations in the *WRN* gene which encodes a DNA helicase. *JU*

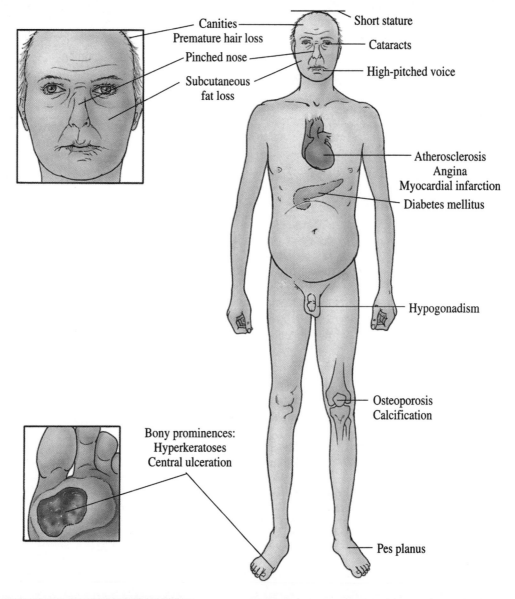

Canities —
Premature hair loss

Pinched nose —

Subcutaneous
fat loss

Short stature

Cataracts

High-pitched voice

Atherosclerosis
Angina
Myocardial infarction

Diabetes mellitus

Hypogonadism

Osteoporosis
Calcification

Bony prominences:
Hyperkeratoses
Central ulceration

Pes planus

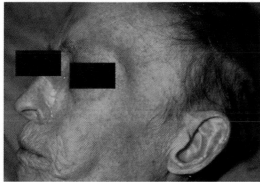

4.25. *Loss of subcutaneous fat on face with premature aged appearance. (5)*

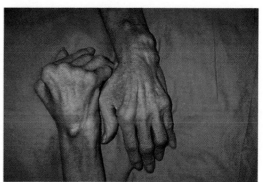

4.26. *Osteoarthritis, subcutaneous calcified nodules, and fat atrophy on hands. (5)*

Aplasia Cutis Congenita

Inheritance	Autosomal dominant (AD), recessive (AR), or sporadic dependent on subtype
Prenatal Diagnosis	Ultrasound
Incidence	Hundreds of case reports; M=F; group 1 most common
Age at Presentation	Birth
Pathogenesis	Depending on subtype, a genetic defect, trauma, teratogen, or infection causes a localized congenital absence of the epidermis, dermis, or subcutis with/without underlying bone (20% to 30%)
Key Features	

General

Aplasia cutis congenita (ACC)—0.5 to 10 cm solitary (70%) or multiple well-demarcated superficial erosions, deep ulcerations with thin membrane or atrophic scars with alopecia on scalp (80%) or any part of the body; heal with scar within weeks after birth; larger lesions usually the deepest with possible extension to dura and increased risk for meningitis, venous thrombosis, and sagittal sinus hemorrhage

Group 1 (AD or sporadic)

Scalp ACC without multiple anomalies

Group 2 (AD)

Scalp ACC (midline) with associated limb abnormalities

Associated Findings

Hypoplastic or absent phalanges, hands, lower extremities; cutis marmorata

Group 3 (sporadic)

Scalp ACC with associated epidermal or organoid nevi

Associated Findings

Epidermal, organoid nevi; corneal opacities, mental retardation, seizures

Group 4

ACC overlying embryologic malformations

Associated Findings

Meningomyeloceles, spinal dysraphia, omphalocoele, gastroschisis

Group 5 (sporadic)

ACC with associated fetus papyraceus or placental infarcts

Associated Findings

Multiple, symmetric, stellate, or linear ACC on trunk or extremities of surviving twin or triplet

Group 6

ACC associated with epidermolysis bullosa

Group 7 (AD or AR)

ACC localized to extremities without blistering

Group 8

ACC caused by teratogens or intrauterine infection

Associated Findings

Scalp ACC (methimazole); any area with varicella or herpes simplex

Group 9

ACC associated with malformation syndromes

Associated Findings

Trisomy 13, 4p-syndrome, ectodermal dysplasias, focal dermal hypoplasia, amniotic band syndrome, Opitz syndrome, Adams-Oliver syndrome, oculocerebrocutaneous syndrome, Johanson-Blizzard syndrome, Xp22 microdeletion syndrome, chromosome 16–18 defect

Aplasia Cutis Congenita *(continued)*

Differential Diagnosis

Trauma from fetal scalp monitor, forceps delivery
Nevus sebaceous
Localized scalp infection
Congenital dermoid cyst
Meningocele
Scarring alopecia
Heterotopic neural tissue
Herpes simplex virus

Laboratory Data

Skin biopsy (if diagnosis uncertain), viral culture
MRI (lumbosacral)
Cranial ultrasound screen beneath ACC in infants with open fontanelle

Management

Referral to dermatology—meticulous wound care to prevent secondary infection and further trauma
Referral to plastic surgery—assess need for skin/bone graft
Referral to symptom-specific specialist if significant associated findings

Prognosis

Most lesions heal within weeks to months leaving a hairless, smooth, yellowish atrophic scar; also dependent upon associated findings

Clinical Pearls

Isolated ACC of the scalp without associated findings is far and away the most common presentation . . . In my experience, 90% of these lesions occur on the scalp . . . Lesions specifically in the hair whorl are usually not associated with any other problems . . . The larger a lesion's diameter the deeper the defect and the increased likelihood of an underlying problem such as an arteriovenous malformation . . . Lesions > 5.0 cm in diameter tend not to heal secondarily . . . Always check for limb reduction abnormality . . . ACC that are sharply demarcated with increased hair growth at the periphery ("hair-collar sign") often represent heterotopic brain tissue . . . I do not biopsy routinely; if biopsy of scalp lesion is necessary to exclude other diagnoses, then imaging studies to rule out CNS connections should be performed prior to biopsy . . . Get skull x-ray if palpable bony defect exists . . . I generally do a cranial ultrasound on infants with scalp ACC to exclude underlying anomalies; if this reveals any abnormalities a confirmatory computed tomography or magnetic resonance scan is needed . . . Lumbosacral lesions should have an MRI scan . . . Obtain a history of oral medications, pregnancy problems . . . I like vaseline-impregnated gauze overlying polysporin to cover small lesions of ACC . . . The bottom line is that ACC is a finding, not a diagnosis . . . It's up to the M.D. to sort through the possible etiologies . . . The baby does not come with labels.   *IF*

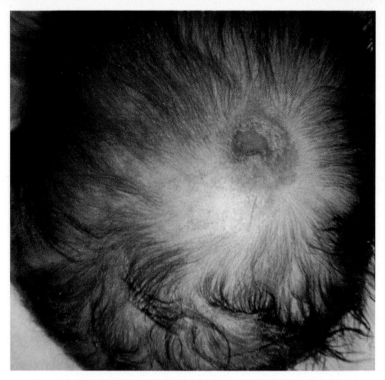

4.27. Solitary well-demarcated ulceration in patient with trisomy 13. (48)

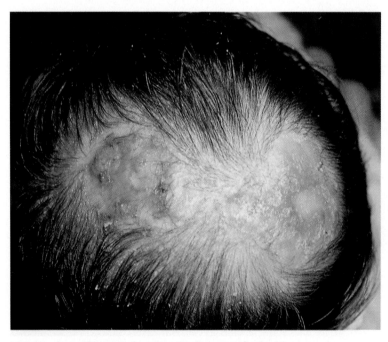

4.28. Two large "kissing" ulcerations healing secondarily. (1)

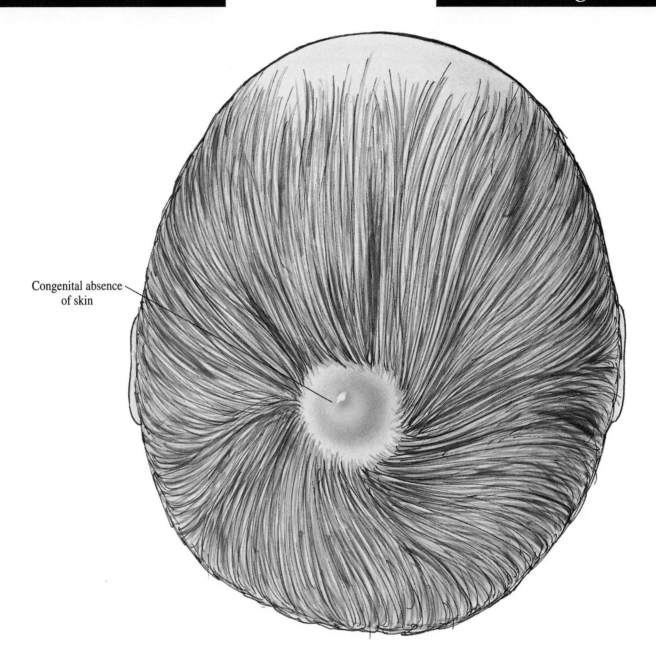

Congenital absence
of skin

Suggested Reading

Ehlers-Danlos Syndrome

Beighton P, De Paepe A, Steinmann B, et al. Ehlers-Danlos syndromes: revised nosology, Villefranche, 1997. *Am J Med Genet* 1998;77:31–37.

Byers PH. Inherited disorders of collagen gene structure and expression. *Am J Med Genet* 1989;34:72–80.

Cameron JA. Corneal abnormalities in Ehlers-Danlos syndrome type VI. *Cornea* 1993;12:54–59.

Cole WG, Chiodo AA, Lamande SR, et al. A base substitution at a splice site in the COL3A1 gene causes exon skipping and generates abnormal type III procollagen in a patient with Ehlers-Danlos syndrome type IV. *J Biol Chem* 1990;265:17070.

Colige A, Sicken AL, Li SW, et al. Human Ehlers-Danlos syndrome type VIIC and bovine dermatosparaxis are caused by mutations in the procollagen I N-proteinase gene. *Am J Hum Genet* 1999;65:308–317.

De Coster PJ, Malfait F, Martens LC, et al. Unusual oral findings in dermatosparaxis (Ehlers-Danlos syndrome type VIIC). *J Oral Pathol Med* 2003;32:568–570.

Dyne KM, Vitellaro-Zuccarello L, Bacchella L, et al. Ehlers-Danlos syndrome type VIII: biochemical, serological and immunocytochemical studies on dermis from a child with clinical signs of Ehlers-Danlos syndrome and a family history of premature loss of permanent teeth. *Br J Dermatol* 1993;128:458-463 (published erratum appears in *Br J Dermatol* 1993;129:226).

Fuchs JR, Fishman SJ. Management of spontaneous colonic perforation in ehlers-danlos syndrome type IV. *J Pediatr Surg* 2004;39:e1–3.

Germain DP, Herrera-Guzman Y. Vascular Ehlers-Danlos syndrome. *Ann Genet* 2004;47:1–9.

Gorlin RJ, Cohen MM Jr. Craniofacial manifestations of Ehlers-Danlos syndromes, cutis laxa syndromes, and cutis laxa-like syndromes. *Birth Defects* 1989;25:39–71.

Heikkinen J, Hautala T, Kivirikko KI, et al: Structure and expression of the human lysyl hydroxylase gene (PLOD): Introns 9 and 16 contain Alu sequences at the sites of recombination in Ehlers-Danlos syndrome type VI patients. *Genomics* 1994;24:464–471.

Kuivaniemi H, Peltonen L, Kivirikko KL. Type IX Ehlers-Danlos syndrome and Menkes syndrome: the decrease in lysyl oxidase protein. *Am J Hum Genet* 1985;37:798–808.

Leier CV, Call TD, Fulkerson PK, et al. The spectrum of cardiac defects in the Ehlers-Danlos syndrome, types I and III. *Ann Intern Med* 1980;92:171–178.

Levard G, Aigrain Y, Ferkadji L, et al. Urinary bladder diverticula and the Ehlers-Danlos syndrome in children. *J Pediatr Surg* 1989;24:1184–1186.

Lumley MA, Jordan M, Rubenstein R, et al. Psychosocial functioning in the Ehlers-Danlos syndrome. *Am J Med Genet* 1994;53:149–152.

Michalickovak K, Susic M, Willing MC, et al. Mutations of the alpha2(V) chain of type V collagen impair matrix assembly and produce Ehlers-Danlos syndrome type I. *Hum Mol Genet* 1998;7:249–255.

Nicholls AC, De Paepe A, Narcisi P, et al. LinkAge at a polymorphic marker for the type III collagen gene (COL2A1) to atypical autosomal dominant Ehlers-danlos syndrome type IV In a large Belgian pedigree. *Hum Genet* 1988;78:276–281.

Nuytinck L, Freund M, Lagae L, et al. Classical Ehlers-Danlos syndrome caused by a mutation in type I collagen. *Am J Hum Genet* 2000;66:1398–1402.

Owen SM, Durst RD. Ehlers-Danlos syndrome simulating child abuse. *Arch Dermatol* 1984;120:97–101.

Pepin M, Schwarze U, Superti-Furga A, et al. Clinical and genetic features of Ehlers-Danlos syndrome type IV, the vascular type. *N Engl J Med* 2000;342:673–680.

Pope FM, Narcisi P, Nicholls AC, et al. Clinical presentations of Ehlers-Danlos syndrome type VI. *Arch Dis Child* 1988;63:1016–1025.

Schievink WI. Cerebrovascular involvement in Ehlers Danlos syndrome. *Curr Treat Options Cardiovasc Med* 2004;6:231–236.

Serry C, Agomuoh OS, Goldin MD. Review of Ehlers-Danlos syndrome: successful repair of rupture and dissection of abdominal aorta. *J Cardiovasc Surg (Torino)* 1988;29:530–534.

Soucy P, Eidus L, Keeley F. Perforation of the colon in a 15-year old girl with Ehlers-Danlos syndrome type IV. *J Pediatr Surg* 1990;25:1180–1182.

Tiller GE, Cassidy SB, Wensel C, et al. Aortic root dilatation in Ehlers-Danlos syndrome types I, II and III. A report of five cases. *Clin Genet* 1998;53:460–465.

Uitto J, Ringpfeil F. Ehlers-danlos syndrome-molecular genetics beyond the collagens. *J Invest Dermatol* 2004;122:XII.

Wenstrup RJ, Florer JB, Willing MC, et al. COL5A1 haploinsufficiency is a common molecular mechanism underlying the classical form of EDS. *Am J Hum Genet* 2000;66:1766–1776.

Zweers MC, Van Vlijmen-Willems IM, Van Kuppevelt TH, et al. Deficiency of tenascin-x causes abnormalities in dermal elastic fiber morphology. *J Invest Dermatol* 2004;122:8135–1391.

Marfan Syndrome

Ades LC, Holman KJ, Brett MS, et al. Ectopia lentis phenotypes and the FBN1 gene. *Am J Med Genet*. 2004;126A:284–239.

Aoyama T, Francke U, Gasner C, et al. Fibrillin abnormalities and prognosis in Marfan syndrome and related disorders. *Am J Med Genet* 1995;58:169–176.

Biggin A, Holman K, Brett M, et al. Detection of thirty novel FBN1 mutations in patients with Marfan syndrome or a related fibrillinopathy. *Hum Mutat* 2004;23:99.

Carrel T, Beyeler L, Schnyder A, et al. Reoperations and late adverse outcome in Marfan patients following cardiovascular surgery. *Eur J Cardiothorac Surg* 2004;25:671–675.

Cohen PR, Schneiderman P. Clinical manifestations of the Marfan syndrome. *Int J Dermatol* 1989;28:291–299.

Dietz HC, Cutting GR, Pyeritz RE, et al. Marfan syndrome caused by a recurrent de novo missense mutation in the fibrillin gene. *Nature* 1991;352:337–339.

Francke U, Berg MA, Tynan K, et al. A Gly1127Ser mutation in an EGF-like domain of the fibrillin-1 gene is a risk factor for ascending aortic aneurysm and dissection. *Am J Hum Genet* 1995;56:1287–1296.

Gott VL, Pyeritz RE, Magovern GJ Jr, et al. Surgical treatment of aneurysms of the ascending aorta in the Marfan syndrome: results of composite-graft repair in 50 patients. *N Engl J Med* 1986;314:1070–1074.

Gray JR, Bridges AB, West RR, et al. Life expectancy in British Marfan syndrome populations. *Clin Genet* 1998;54:124–128.

Greco GM, Ambrosino L. Treatment of retinal detachment in Marfan syndrome. *Ann Ophthalmol* 1993;25:72–76.

Hwa J, Richards JG, Huang H, McKay D, et al. The natural history of aortic dilatation in Marfan syndrome. *Med J Aust* 1993;158:558–562.

Kainulainen K, Karttunen L, Puhakka L, et al. Mutations in the fibrillin gene responsible for dominant ectopia lentis and neonatal Marfan syndrome. *Nat Genet* 1994;6:64–69.

Kainulainen K, Pulkkinen L, Savolainen A, et al. Location on chromosome 15 of the gene defect causing Marfan syndrome. *N Engl J Med* 1990;323:935–939.

Prager RL, Deschner W, Kong B, et al. Early experience with homograft aortic root replacement for complex aortic pathology. *Surgery* 1993;114:794–798.

Pyeritz RE. The Marfan syndrome. *Annu Rev Med* 2000;51:481–510.

Pyeritz RE. Marfan syndrome: current and future clinical and genetic management of cardiovascular manifestations. *Semin Thorac Cardiovasc Surg* 1993;5:11–16.

Pyeritz RE, Francke U. The Second International Symposium on the Marfan Syndrome. *Am J Med Genet* 1993;47:127–135.

Rahman J, Rahman FZ, Rahman W, et al. Obstetric and gynecologic complications in women with Marfan syndrome. *J Reprod Med* 2003;48:723–728.

Rantamaki T, Kaitila I, Syvanen AC, et al. Recurrence of Marfan syndrome as a result of parental germ-line mosaicism for an FBN1 mutation. *Am J Human Genet* 1999;64:993–1001.

Robinson PN, Godfrey M. The molecular genetics of Marfan syndrome and related microfibrillopathies. *J Med Genet* 2000;37:9–25.

Shores J, Berger KR, Murphy EA, et al. Progression of aortic dilatation and the benefit of long-term beta-adrenergic blockade in Marfan syndrome. *N Engl J Med* 1994;330:1335–1341.

Simpson IA, de Belder MA, Treasure T, et al. Cardiovascular manifestations of Marfan's syndrome: improved evaluation by transoesophageal echocardiography. *Br Heart J* 1993;69:104–108.

Tagusari O, Ogino H, Kobayashi J, et al. Should the transverse aortic arch be replaced simultaneously with aortic root replacement for annuloaortic ectasia in Marfan syndrome? *J Thorac Cardiovasc Surg* 2004;127:1373–1380.

Tsipouras P, Devereux RB. Marfan syndrome: genetic basis and clinical manifestations. *Semin Dermatol* 1993;12:219–228.

Cutis Laxa

Banks ND, Redett RJ, Mofid MZ, et al. Cutis laxa: clinical experience and outcomes. *Plast Reconstr Surg* 2003;1I1:2434–2442; discussion 2443–244.

Dagenais SL, Adam AN, Innis JW, et al. A novel frameshift mutation in axon 23 of ATP7Am (MNK) results in occipital horn syndrome and not in Menkes disease. *Am J Hum Genet* 2001;69:420–427.

Fitzsimmons JS, Fitzsimmons EM, Guibert PR, et al. Variable clinical presentation of cutis laxa. *Clin Genet* 1985;28:284–285.

Gorlin RJ, Cohen MM Jr. Craniofacial manifestations of Ehlers-Danlos syndromes, cutis laxa syndromes, and cutis laxa-like syndromes. *Birth Defects Orig Artic Ser* 1989;25:39–71.

Khakoo A, Thomas R, Trompeter R, et al. Congenital cutis laxa and lysyl oxidase deficiency. *Clin Genet* 1997;51:109–114.

Koch SE, Williams ML. Acquired cutis laxa: case report and review of disorders of elastolysis. *Pediatr Dermatol* 1985;2:282–288.

Loeys B, Van Maldergem L, Mortier G, et al. Homozygosity for a missense mutation in fibulin (FBLNS) results in a severe form of curls laxa. *Hum Mol Genet* 2002;11:2113–2118.

Moller LB, Tumer Z, Lund L, et al. Similar splice-site mutations of the ATP7A gene lead to different phenotypes: classical Menkes disease or occipital horn syndrome. *Am J Hum Genet* 2000;66:1211–1220.

Nahas FX, Sterman S, Gemperli R, et al. The role of plastic surgery in congenital cutis laxa: a 10-year follow-up. *Plast Reconstr Surg* 1999;104:1174–1178.

Nanda A, Lionel J, Al-Tawari AA, et al. What syndrome is this? Autosomal recessive type II cutis laxa. *Pediatr Dermatol* 2004;21:167–170.

Tassabehji M, Metcalfe K, Hurst J, et al. Anelastln gene mutation producing abnormal tropoelastin and abnormal elastic fibers in a patient with autosomal dominant cutis laxa. *Hum Mol Genet* 1998;7:1921–1028.

Thomas WO, Moses MH, Craver RD, et al. Congenital cutis laxa: a case report and review of loose skin syndromes. *Ann Plast Surg* 1993;30:252–256.

Yanagisawa H, Davis EC, Starcher BC, et al. Fibulin-5 is an elastin-binding protein essential for elastic fiber development in vivo. *Nature* 2002;415:168.

Pseudoxanthoma Elasticum

Aralikatti AK, Lee MW, Lipton ME, et al. Visual loss due to cerebral infarcts in pseudoxanthoma elasticum. *Eye* 2002;16:785–786.

Bergen M, Plomp AS, Schuurman EJ, et al. Mutations in ABCC6 cause pseudoxanthoma elasticum. *Nat Genet* 2000;25:228–231.

Chassaing N, Martin L, Mazereeuw J, et al. Novel ABCC6 mutations in pseudoxanthoma elasticum. *J Invest Dermatol* 2004;122:608–613.

Christiano AM, Lebwohl MG, Boyd CD, et al. Workshop on pseudoxanthoma elasticum: molecular biology and pathology of the elastic fibers. Jefferson Medical College, Philadelphia, PA, June 10, 1992. *J Invest Dermatol* 1992;99:660–663.

Galadari H, Lebwohl M. Pseudoxanthoma elasticum: temporary treatment of chin folds and lines with injectable collagen. *J Am Acad Dermatol* 2003;49:S265–266.

Kazakis AM, Parish WR. Periumbilical perforating pseudoxanthoma elasticum. *J Am Acad Dermatol* 1988;19:384–388.

Le Saux O, Urban Z, Tschuch C, et al. Mutations in a gene encoding an ABC transporter cause pseudoxanthoma elasticum. *Nat Genet* 2000;25:223–227.

Lebwohl M, Halperin J, Phelps RG. Occult pseudoxanthoma elasticum in patients with premature cardiovascular disease. *N Engl J Med* 1993;329:1237–1239.

Lebwohl M, Lebwohl E, Bercovitch L. Prominent mental (chin) crease: a new sign of pseudoxanthoma elasticum. *J Am Acad Dermatol* 2003;48:620–622.

Lebwohl M, Neldner K, Pope FM, et al. Classification of pseudoxanthoma elasticum: report of a consensus conference. *J Am Acad Dermatol* 1994;30:103–107.

Lebwohl M, Phelps RG, Yannuzzi L, et al. Diagnosis of pseudoxanthoma elasticum by scar biopsy in patients without characteristic skin lesions. *N Engl J Med* 1987;317:347–350.

McCreedy CA, Zimmerman TJ, Webster SF. Management of upper gastrointestinal hemorrhage in patients with pseudoxanthoma elasticum. *Surgery* 1989;105:170–174.

Plomp AS, Hu X, de Jong PT, et al. Does autosomal dominant pseudoxanthoma elasticum exist? *Am J Med Genet* 2004;126A:403–412.

Ringpfeil F, Lebwohl MG, Christiano AM, et al. Pseudoxanthoma elasticum: mutations in the MRP6 gene encoding a transmembrane ATP-binding cassette (ABC) transporter. *Proc Natl Acad Sci USA* 2000;97:6001–6006.

Uitto J. Pseudoxanthoma elasticum—a connective tissue disease or a metabolic disorder at the genome/environment interface? *J Invest Dermatol* 2004;122:ix–x.

Uitto J, Pulkkinen L, Ringpfeil F. Molecular genetics of pseudoxanthoma elasticum: a metabolic disorder at the environment-genome interface? *Trends Mol Med* 2001;7:13–17.

Viljoen DL, Bloch C, Beighton P. Plastic surgery in pseudoxanthoma elasticum: experience in nine patients. *Plast Reconstr Surg* 1990;85:233–288.

Yap EY, Gleaton MS, Buettner H. Visual loss associated with pseudoxanthoma elasticum. *Retina* 1992;12:315–319.

Zachariah M, Thomas SB, Stokes IM. Pseudoaxanthoma elasticum and pregnancy. *J Obstet Gynaecol* 2003;23:433–434.

Osteogenesis Imperfecta

Ablon J. Personality and stereotype in osteogenesis imperfecta: behavioral phenotype or response to life's hard challenges? *Am J Med Genet* 2003;122A:201–214.

Arikoski P, Silverwood B, Tillmann V, et al. Intravenous pamidronate treatment in children with moderate to severe osteogenesis imperfecta: assessment of indices of dual-energy X-ray absorptiometry and bone metabolic markers during the first year of therapy. *Bone* 2004;34:539–546.

Badmanaban B, Sachithanandan A, MacGowan SW. Aortic valve replacement in osteogenesis imperfecta—technical and practical considerations for a successful outcome. *J Card Surg* 2003;18:554–556.

Binder H, Conway A, Hason S, et al. Comprehensive rehabilitation of the child with osteogenesis imperfecta. *Am J Genet* 1993;45:265–269.

Byers PH. Inherited disorders of collagen gene structure and expression. *Am J Med Genet* 1989;34:72–80.

Byers PH, Steiner RD. Osteogenesis imperfecta. *Annu Rev Med* 1992;43:269–282.

Chamberlain JR, Schwarze U, Wang PR, et al. Gene targeting in stem cells from individuals with osteogenesis imperfecta. *Science* 2004;303:1198–1201.

Cole DE. Psychosocial aspects of osteogenesis imperfecta: an update. *Am J Med Genet* 1993;45:207–211.

Cole WG. Orthopaedic treatment of osteogenesis imperfecta. *Ann NY Acad Sci* 1988;543:157–166.

Engelbert RH, Uiterwaal CS, Gerver WJ, et al. Osteogenesis imperfecta in childhood: impairment and disability, a prospective study with 4-year follow-up. *Arch Phys Med Rehabil* 2004;85:772–778.

Hanscom DA, Winter RB, Lutter L, et al. Osteogenesis imperfecta. Radiographic classification, natural history, and treatment of spinal deformities. *J Bone Joint Surg Am* 1992;74:598–616.

Hortop J, Tsipouras P, Hanley JA, et al. Cardiovascular involvement in osteogenesis imperfecta. *Circulation* 1986;73:54–61.

Lee CY, Ertel SK. Bone graft augmentation and dental implant treatment in a patient with osteogenesis imperfecta: review of the literature with a case report. *Implant Dent* 2003;12:291–295.

Lee YS, Low SL, Lim LA, et al. Cyclic pamidronate infusion improves bone mineralisation and reduces fracture incidence in osteogenesis imperfecta. *Eur J Pediatr* 2001;160:641–644.

Niyibizi C, Wang S, Mi Z, Robbins PD. Gene therapy approaches for osteogenesis imperfecta. *Gene Ther* 2004;11:408–416.

Paterson CR, Bums J, McAllion SJ. Osteogenesis imperfecta: the distinction from child abuse and the recognition of a variant form. *Am J Med Genet* 1993;45:187–192.

Rauch F, Glorieux FH. Osteogenesis imperfecta. *Lancet* 2004;363:1377–1385.

Sakkers R, Kok D, Engelbert R, et al. Skeletal effects and functional outcome with olpadronate in children with osteogenesis imperfecta: a 2-year randomised placebo-controlled study. *Lancet* 2004;363:1427–1431.

Saldanha KA, Saleh M, Bell MJ, et al. Limb lengthening and correction of deformity in the lower limbs of children with osteogenesis imperfecta. *J Bone Joint Surg Br* 2004;86:259–265.

Schafer IA, Stein J, Hyland JC, et al. Gene symbol: COL1A1. Disease: osteogenesis imperfecta type 1. *Hum Genet* 2004;114:404.

Shapiro JR, McCarty EF, Ressiter K, et al. The effect of intravenous pamidronate on bone mineral density, bone histomorphometry, and parameters of bone turnover in adults with type IA osteogenesis imperfecta. *Calcif Tissue Int* 2003;72:103–112.

Sykes B, Ogilvie D, Wordsworth P, et al. Consistent linkAge at dominantly inherited osteogenesis imperfecta to the type I collagen loci: COLIA and COL1A2. *Am J Hum Genet* 1990;46:293–307.

Thompson EM. Non-invasive prenatal diagnosis of osteogenesis imperfecta. *Am J Med Genet* 1993;45:201–206.

Willing MC, Pruchno CJ, Byers PH. Molecular heterogeneity in osteogenesis imperfects type I. *Am J Med Genet* 1993;45:223–227.

Zacharin M, Bateman J. Pamidronate treatment of osteogenesis imperfecta—lack of correlation between clinical severity, age at onset of treatment, predicted collagen mutation and treatment response. *J Pediatr Endocrinol Metab* 2002;15:163–174.

Buschke-Ollendorff Syndrome

Ehrig T, Cockerell CJ. Buschke-Ollendorff syndrome: report of a case and interpretation of the clinical phenotype as a type 2 segmental manifestation of an autosomal dominant skin disease. *J Am Med Dermatol* 2003;49:1163–1166.

Giro MG, Duvic M, Smith LT, et al. Buschke-Ollendorff syndrome associated with elevated elastin production by affected skin fibroblasts in culture. *J Invest Dermatol* 1992;99:129–137.

Kim GH, Dy LC, Caldemeyer KS, et al. Buschke-Ollendorff syndrome. *J Am Acad Dermatol* 2003;48:600–601.

Milewicz DM, Urban Z, Boyd C. Genetic disorders of the elastic fiber system. *Matrix Biol J* 2000;19:471–480.

Roberts NM, Langtry JA, Branfoot AC, et al. Case report: osteopoikilosis and the Buschke-Ollendorff syndrome. *Br J Radiol* 1993;66:468–470.

Thieberg MD, Stone MS, Siegfried EC. What syndrome is this? Buschke-Ollendorff syndrome. *Pediatr Dermatol* 1993;10:85–87.

Walpole IR, Manners PJ. Clinical considerations in Buschke-Ollendorff syndrome. *Clin Genet* 1990;37:59–63.

Woodrow SL, Pope FM, Handfield-Jones SE. The Buschke-Ollendorff syndrome presenting as familial elastic tissue naevi. *Br J Dermatol* 2001;144:890–893.

Focal Dermal Hypoplasia

Alster TS, Wilson F. Focal dermal hypoplapia (Goltzi syndrome). Treatment of cutaneous lesions with the 585-nm flashlamp-pumped pulsed dye laser. *Arch Dermatol* 1995;131:143–144.

Bellosta M, Tresprolli D, Ghiselli E, et al. Focal dermal hypoplasia: report of a family with 7 affected women in 3 generations. *Eur J Dermatol* 1996;6:499.

Boothroyd AE, Hall CM. The radiological features of Goltz syndrome: focal dermal hypoplasia. A report of two cases. *Skeletal Radiol* 1988;17:505–508.

Goltz RW. Focal dermal hypoplasia syndrome. An update (editorial; comment). *Arch Dermatol* 1992;128:1108–1111.

Goltz RW, Henderson RR, Hitch JM, et al. Focal dermal hypoplasia syndrome: a review of the literature and report of two cases. *Arch Dermatol* 1970;101:1–11.

Han XY, Wu SS, Conway DH, et al. Truncus arteriosus and other lethal internal anomalies in Goltz syndrome. *Am J Med Genet* 2000;90:45–48.

Kilmer SL, Grix AW Jr, Isseroff RR. Focal dermal hypoplasia: four cases with widely varying presentations. *J Am Acad Dermatol* 1993;28:839–843.

Landa N, Oleaga JM, Raton JA, et al. Focal dermal hypoplasia (Goltz syndrome): an adult case with multisystemic involvement. *J Am Acad Dermatol* 1993;28:86–89.

Larregue M, Duterque M. Striated osteopathy in focal dermal hypoplasia. *Arch Dermatol* 1975;111:1365–1366.

Ogunbiyi AO, Adewole IO, Ogunleye O, et al. Focal dermal hypoplasia: a case report and review of literature. *West Afr J Med* 2003;22:346–349.

Pujol RM, Casanova JM, Perez M, et al. Focal dermal hypoplasia (Goltz syndrome): report of two cases with minor cutaneous and extracutaneous manifestations. *Pediatr Dermatol* 1992;9:112–116.

Stephen LX, Behardien N, Beighton P. Focal dermal hypoplasia: management of complex dental features. *J Clin Pediatr Dent* 2001;25:259–261.

Lipoid Proteinosis

Chan I. The role of extracellular matrix protein 1 in human skin. *Clin Exp Dermatol* 2004;29(1):52–56.

Hamada T, Wessagowit V, South AP, et al. Extracellular matrix protein 1 gene (ECM1) mutations in lipoid proteinosis and genotype-phenotype correlation. *J Invest Dermatol* 2003;120:345–350.

Konstantinov K, Kabakchiev P, Karchev T, et al. Lipoid proteinosis. *J Am Acad Dermatol* 1992;27:293–297.

Moy LS, Moy RL, Matsuoka LY, et al. Lipoid proteinosis: ultrastructural and biochemical studies. *J Am Acad Dermatol* 1987;16:1193–1201.

Pierard GE, Van Cauwenberge D, Buda J, et al. A clinicopathologic study of six cases of lipoid proteinosis. *Am J Dermatopathol* 1988;10:300–305.

Rosenthal G, Lifshitz T, Monos T, et al. Carbon dioxide laser treatment for lipoid proteinosis (Urbach-Wiethe syndrome) involving the eyelids. *Br J Opthalmol* 1997;81:252.

Savage MM, Crockett DM, McCabe BF. Lipoid proteinosis of the larynx: a cause of voice change in the infant and young child. *Int J Pediatr Otorhinolaryngol* 1988;15:33–38.

Sharma V, Kashyap S, Betharia SM, et al. Lipoid proteinosis: a rare disorder with pathognomonic lid lesions. *Clin Experiment Ophthalmol* 2004;32:110–112.

Urbach E, Wiethe C. Lipoidosis cutis at mucosae. *Virchow Arch Pathol Mater* 1929;273:285–319.

Wong CK, Lin CS. Remarkable response of lipoid proteinosis to oral dimethyl sulphoxide. *Br J Dermatol* 1988;119:541–544.

Progeria

Badame AJ. Progeria. *Arch Dermatol* 1989;125:540–544.

Bridger JM, Kill IR. Aging of Hutchinson-Gilford progeria syndrome fibroblasts is characterised by hyperproliferation and increased apoptosis. *Exp Gerontol* 2004;39:717–724.

Cao H, Hegele RA. LMNA is mutated in Hutchinson-Gilford progeria (MIM 176670) but not in Wiedemann-Rautenstrauch progeroid syndrome (MIM 264090). *J Hum Genet* 2003;45:271–274.

Csoka AB, Cao H, Sammak PJ, et al. Novel lamin A/C gene (LMNA) mutations in atypical progeroid syndromes. *J Med Genet* 2004;41:304–308.

De Sandre-Giovannoli A, Bernard R, Cau P, et al. Lamin a truncation in Hutchinson-Gilford progeria. *Science* 2003;300:2055.

Eriksson M, Brown WT, Gordon LB, et al. Recurrent de novo point mutations in lamin A cause Hutchinson-Gilford progeria syndrome. *Nature* 2003;423:293–298.

Fernandez-Palazzi F, McLaren AT, Slowie DF. Report on a case of Hutchinson-Golford progeria, with special reference to orthopedic problems. *Eur J Pediatr Surg* 1992;2:378–382.

Fossel M. The progerias. *J Anti Aging Med* 2003;6:123–138.

Gillar PJ, Kaye CI, McCourt JW. Progressive early dermatologic changes in Hutchinson-Gifford progeria syndrome. *Pediatr Dermatol* 1991;8:199–206.

Hall JW, Denneny JC. Audiologic and otolaryngologic findings inprogeria: case report. *J Am Acad Audiol* 1993;4:116–121.

Hamada T, McLean WH, Ramsay M, et al. Lipoid proteinosis maps to 1q21. and is caused by mutations in the extracellular matrix protein 1 gene. *Hum Mol Genet* 2002;11:833–840.

Hamada T, Wessagowit V, South AP, et al. Extracellular matrix protein I gene (ECMI) mutations in lipoid proteinosis and genotype-phenotype correlation. *J Invest Dermatol* 2003;120:345–350.

Navarro C, Fachal C, Rodriguez C, et al. Lipoid proteinosis: a biochemical and ultrastructural investigation of two new cases. *Br J Dermatol* 1999;141:326–340.

Vastag B. Cause of progeria's premature aging found: expected to provide insight into normal aging process. *JAMA* 2003;289:2481–2482.

Werner Syndrome

Anderson NE, Haas LF. Neurological complications of Werner's syndrome. *J Neurol* 2003;250:1174–1178.

Bohr VA. Werner syndrome and its protein: clinical, cellular and molecular advances. *Mech Aging Dev* 2003;124:1073–1082.

Chen L, Lee L, Kudlow BA, et al. LMNA mutations in atypical Werner's syndrome. *Lancet* 2003;362:440–445.

Cohen JI, Arnett EN, Kolodny AL, et al. Cardiovascular features of the Werner syndrome. *Am J Cardiol* 1987;59:493–495.

Gray MD, Shen JC, Kamath-Loeb AS, et al. The Werner syndrome protein is a DNA helicase. *Nat Genet* 1997;17:100–103.

Fry M. The Werner syndrome helicase-nuclease—one protein, many mysteries. *Sci Aging Knowledge Environ* 2002;2002:re2.

Furuichi Y. Premature aging and predisposition to cancers caused by mutations in RecQ family helicases. *Ann NY Acad Sci* 2001;928:121–131.

Hickson ID. RecQ helicases: caretakers of the genome. *Nat Rev Cancer* 2003;3:169–178.

Monnat RJ Jr, Saintigny Y. Werner syndrome protein—unwinding function to explain disease. *Sci Aging Knowledge Environ* 2004;2004:re3.

Swanson G, Saintigny Y, Emond MJ, et al. The Werner syndrome protein has separable recombination and survival functions. *DNA Repair (Amst)* 2004;3:475–482.

Wang W, Seki M, Narita Y, et al. Functional relation among RecQ family helicases RecQL1, RecQL5, and ELM in cell growth and sister chromatid exchange formation. *Mol Cell Biol* 2003;23:3527–3535.

Yeong EK, Yang CC. Chronic leg ulcers in Werner's syndrome. *Br J Plast Surg* 2004;57:86–88.

Yu CE, Oshima J, Wijsman EM, et al. Mutations in the consensus helicase domains of the Werner syndrome gene. Werner's Syndrome Collaborative Group. *Am J Hum Genet* 1997;60:330–341.

Aplasia Cutis Congenita

Argenta LC, Dingman RO. Total reconstruction of aplasia cutis congenita involving scalp, skull and dura. *Plast Reconstr Surg* 1986;77:650–653.

Al-Sawan RMZ, Soni AL, AI-Kobrosly AM, et al. Truncal aplasia cutis congenita associated with ileal atresia and mesenteric defect. *Pediatr Dermatol* 1999;16:498–509.

Blunt K, Quan V, Carr D, et al. Aplasia cutis congenita: a clinical review and associated defects. *Neonatal Netw* 1992;11:17–27.

Evers ME, Steijlen PM, Hamel BC. Aplasia cutis congenita and associated disorders: an update. *Clin Genet* 1995;47:295–301.

Frieden IJ. Aplasia cutis congenita: a clinical review and proposal for classification. *J Am Acad Dermatol* 1986;14:646–660.

Itin P, Pletscher M. Familial aplasia cutis congenita of the scalp without other defects in 6 members of three successive generations. *Dermatologica* 1988;177:123–125.

Kim CS, Tatum SA, Rocziewicz G. (2001) Scalp aplasia cutis congenita presenting with sagittal sinus hemorrhage. *Arch Otolaryngol Head Neck Surv* 2001;127:71–74.

Lestringant G, al Towairky A. Three siblings with extensive aplasia cutis congenita of the scalp and underlying bone defect: autosomal recessive inheritance [letter]. *Int J Dermatol* 1989;28:278–279.

Sybert VP. Aplasia cutis congenita: a report of 12 new families and review of the literature. *Pediatr Dermatol* 1985;3:1–14.

Simman R, Priebe CJ, Simon M. Reconstruction of aplasia cutis congenita of the trunk in a newborn infant using acellular allogenic dermal graft and cultured epithelial autografts. *Ann Plast Surg* 2000;44:451–454.

Chapter 5

Disorders With Malignant Potential

Clinical Pearls

Lawrence Eichenfield, M.D. (LE)

Basal Cell Nevus Syndrome

Synonym	Nevoid basal cell carcinoma syndrome Gorlin syndrome
Inheritance	Autosomal dominant; *PTCH1* (*PATCHED1*) gene on 9q22–31
Prenatal Diagnosis	DNA mutation analysis
Incidence	Approximately 1:60,000; M=F
Age at Presentation	Birth (bossing, skeletal anomalies); childhood (jaw cysts, basal cell carcinoma)
Pathogenesis	Mutations in *PTCH1*, a tumor suppressor gene encoding the sonic hedgehog transmembrane receptor protein; receptor interacts with signaling proteins important for controlling cell fate, patterning, and growth

Key Features

Skin
Basal cell carcinomas (BCCs)—multiple, skin-colored to tan, dome-shaped papules on face, neck, trunk
Palmoplantar pits—2- to 3-mm erythematous pits, rarely develop into BCCs; milium, epidermoid cysts

Musculoskeletal
Jaw cysts (odontogenic keratocysts)—secondary pain, swelling, drainage, increased in molar and premolar areas in maxilla, usually multiple, lining with malignant potential
Frontal bossing, bifid ribs, vertebral fusion, kyphoscoliosis

Central Nervous System
Calcification of falx cerebri, agenesis of corpus callosum, medulloblastoma, mental retardation (less common)

Eyes
Hypertelorism, congenital blindness, cataracts, colobomas, strabismus

Genitourinary
Ovarian fibromas, fibrosarcoma

Differential Diagnosis
Bazex syndrome
Unilateral linear nevoid basal cell carcinomas
Melanocytic nevi
Rombo syndrome
Xeroderma pigmentosa (XP) (p. 174)

Laboratory Data
Skin biopsy
Skeletal surveys of skull, maxilla, mandible, ribs, vertebrae

Management

Referral to dentist/oral surgeon
Referral to dermatologist/Moh's surgeon—surgical excision, electrodesiccation and curettage with/without general anesthesia, topical 5-fluorouracil, imiquimod; frequent cutaneous examinations
Oral retinoids—suppression of new BCCs
Avoid radiotherapy/x-rays—induces new BCCs
Sun avoidance, broad-spectrum sunscreen, protective clothing
Referral to orthopedist, neurologist, ophthalmologist

Prognosis

Normal life span if BCCs treated early on and no other malignancies develop; close surveillance with physician throughout life; disfiguring scars may create psychosocial problems

Clinical Pearls

The syndrome is caused by gene defects that regulate growth and differentiation; mutations in the *PTCH* gene impair the PTCH protein inhibition of SMOOTHENED (SMO), a transmembrane protein. SMOs active signaling contributes to tumor formation . . . Clues to the diagnosis in early life include a family history, frontal bossing, and hypertelorism . . . Cleft lip and palate may be associated . . . BCCs begin in early childhood, and are often small, banal appearing monomorphic, brown, smooth dome shaped papules, very acrochordon-like, and not looking like typical adult BCC's at all . . . Learning difficulties are common . . . A pediatric dentist should be part of the care team . . . Photoprotection is important, and should include sun-protective garments, hats, and broad-spectrum sunscreens . . . X-rays and radiotherapy should be avoided . . . Consider topical imiquimod as a treatment option . . . *LE*

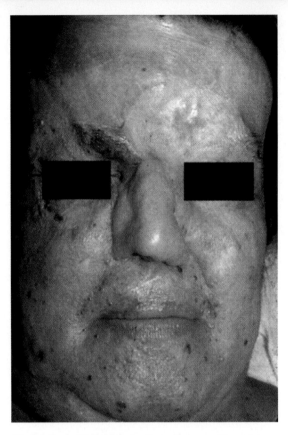

5.1. Pigmented facial basal cell carcinomas with post-surgical scars and glabellar graft. (5)

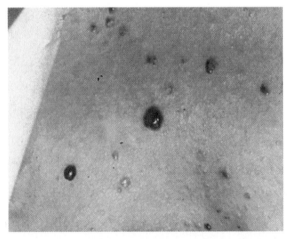

5.2. Multiple tan-brown basal cell carcinomas on patient's back. (5)

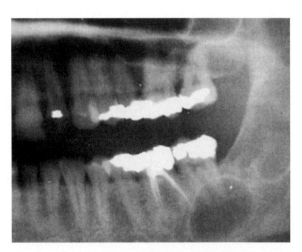

5.3. Large jaw cysts in maxilla and mandible. (5)

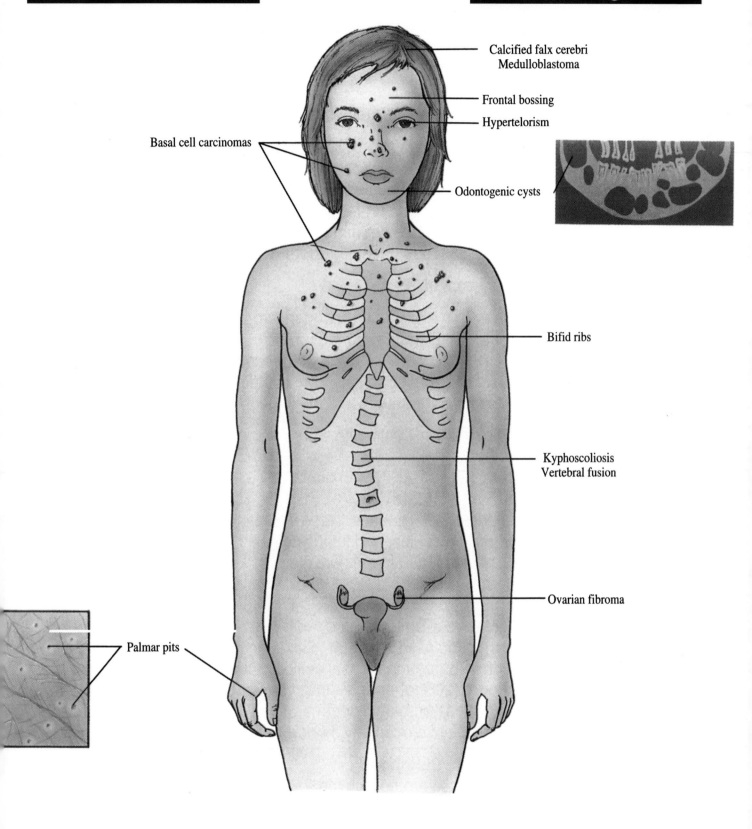

Calcified falx cerebri
Medulloblastoma

Frontal bossing

Hypertelorism

Basal cell carcinomas

Odontogenic cysts

Bifid ribs

Kyphoscoliosis
Vertebral fusion

Ovarian fibroma

Palmar pits

Xeroderma Pigmentosum

Inheritance

Autosomal recessive
XPA gene encodes DNA damage binding protein 1 (*DDB1*) gene on 9q22
XPB gene encodes excision-repair cross-complementing 3 (*ERCC3*) gene on 2q21
XPC gene encodes endonuclease on 3p25
XPD gene encodes ERCC2 on 19q13
XPE gene encodes DDB2 on 11p12
XPF gene encodes ERCC4 on 16p13
XPG gene encodes endonuclease on 13q33
XPV (Variant) gene encodes polymerase η on 6p21

Prenatal Diagnosis

DNA analysis
UDS (unscheduled DNA synthesis) assay on cultured amniotic fluid cells

Incidence

1:1,000,000 in the United States; 1:40,000 in Japan; M=F
XPA, C, and V comprise 75% of all patients
XPA—most common form in Japan, over 90% with identical single base substitution mutation; skin with mild–severe neurologic manifestations
XPB—rare in the United States; skin and neurologic; association with Cockayne syndrome, trichothiodystrophy
XPC—most common form in the United States, rare in Japan; skin without neurologic manifestations
XPD—moderate frequency; association with trichothiodystrophy and XP-Cockayne complex, skin and neurologic manifestations
XPE—rare; mild skin without neurologic manifestations
XPF—moderate rare; most seen in Japan; skin without neurologic manifestations
XPG—extremely rare; association with Cockayne, skin with Cockayne-like neurologic manifestations
XPV—approximately 30% of all cases; United States, Europe, Japan; mild–severe skin without neurologic manifestations

Age of Presentation

First few years of life

Pathogenesis

Mutations in genes encoding DNA repair enzymes (DNA helicase, endonuclease, or DNA damage-binding protein) leads to defective DNA excision repair upon exposure to ultraviolet radiation; defective postreplication repair in XPV group
Complementation groups (total of 8), based on correction of reduced post-UV UDS after fusion of skin fibroblasts from two different patients, have distinct clinical characteristics, frequency and distribution

Key Features

Skin (severity may vary with different complementation groups)
  Infancy
   Acute sun sensitivity with sunburn-like reaction (erythema, inflammation, bullae)
  First Years of Life
   Childhood/adolescence (listed in order of appearance)—pigmented macules, achromic macules, and telangiectasias in photodistribution; dry, scaly, atrophic, with narrowing of mouth and nares; actinic keratoses, keratoacanthomas; 1,000-fold increased risk for basal cell carcinoma, squamous cell carcinoma, malignant melanoma

Eyes

Progressive symptomatology with photophobia, conjunctivitis, telangiectasia and pigmentation of lid and conjunctiva; ectropion, corneal vascularization, opacification; benign lid papillomas; BCC, malignant melanoma

Neurologic (20% of cases—most in XPA and XPD)

Progressive neurologic degeneration with mental retardation, sensorineural deafness; with/without microcephaly, hyporeflexia, spasticity, ataxia

Differential Diagnosis

Infancy/Early Childhood

Erythropoietic protoporphyria (p. 224)

Congenital erythropoietic porphyria (p. 226)

Bloom syndrome (p. 234)

Cockayne syndrome (p. 242)

Hartnup disease (p. 250)

Rothmund-Thomson syndrome (p. 238)

Laboratory Data

DNA analysis

UDS assay from cultured skin fibroblasts

Management

Referral to dermatologist—sun avoidance/limit outdoor activity to early morning, late afternoon and night; photoprotect with physical block sunscreen, long-sleeve, long pants, frogskin clothing, wide-brimmed hat, UV-blocking glasses with side shields, long hair styles

Dermatologic cancer screening every 3 months with weekly examination by informed parent

Removal of cutaneous neoplasms, cryotherapy, 5-fluorouracil, imiquimod

Isotretinoin—prevention of new skin cancers

Referral to ophthalmologist—corneal protection with methylcellulose drops, soft contact lens; corneal transplantation, regular cancer screening

Referral to neurologist if symptomatic

Referral to XP support group

Prognosis

Early diagnosis with UV protection and close malignancy surveillance will prevent skin cancers; otherwise premature death at early age; UV exposure prior to diagnosis and protection may induce neoplasm; neurologic symptoms are progressive and unaffected by UV protection; severe psychosocial impact

Clinical Pearls

XP is caused by gene mutations responsible for the repair of UV-induced DNA damage, which involves recognition of damaged DNA, unwinding of the DNA by helicase, and incision and removal of injured DNA strands by endonucleases; each step has mutations associated with one or several complementation groups . . . Photosensitivity in infants can show up as crying on sun exposure . . . Families shouldn't make their life adjustments alone; the XP support group and website www.xps.org, is invaluable in keeping "state of the art" with XP care . . . Sunprotective garments or UV suits, window tinting, and UV meters are important parts of care, along with constant broad-spectrum sunscreen, to be worn inside and out . . . Children may be tutored at home, although we have been able to accommodate classrooms with UV filters and set-up special programs . . . Consider developmental delay, and refer early for evaluation and management . . . Vigilant cancer screening is crucial, and serial photography is very useful to track changing skin lesions . . . "Camp Sundown" is a must—it is a camp dedicated to sun-sensitive children and their families . . . *LE*

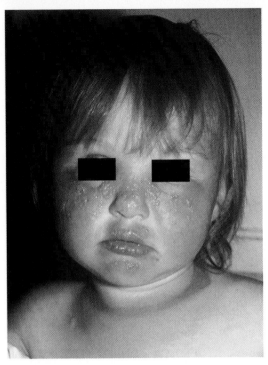

5.4. *Photodistributed bullae, erythema, and inflammation in girl with XP. Note sharp cut-off of eruption on exposed neck. (66)*

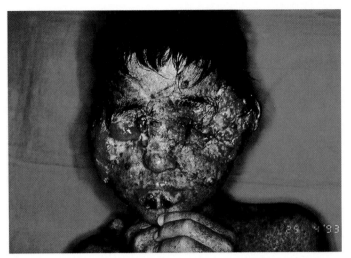

5.5. *Destructive cutaneous carcinomas and squamous cell carcinoma of the tongue in this unfortunate terminal boy. (20)*

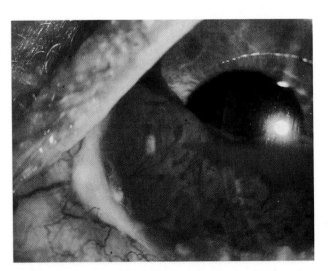

5.6. *Iris melanoma and blood obliterate the anterior chamber of the eye. (67)*

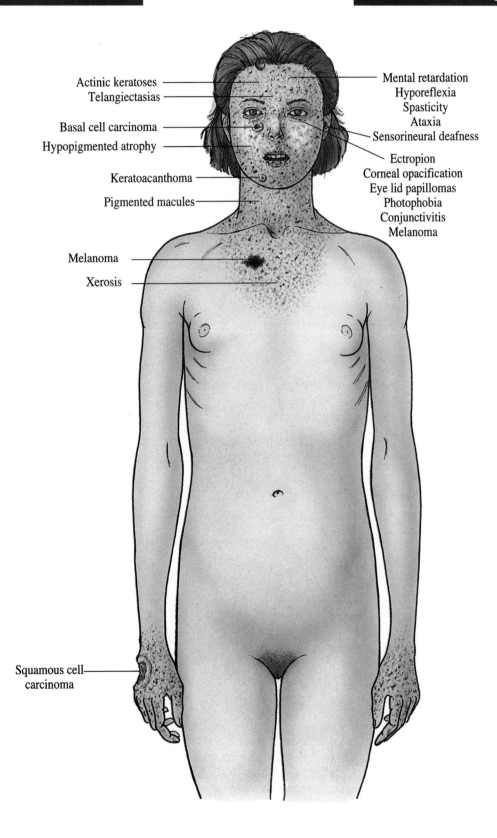

Actinic keratoses
Telangiectasias
Basal cell carcinoma
Hypopigmented atrophy
Keratoacanthoma
Pigmented macules
Melanoma
Xerosis
Squamous cell carcinoma

Mental retardation
Hyporeflexia
Spasticity
Ataxia
Sensorineural deafness
Ectropion
Corneal opacification
Eye lid papillomas
Photophobia
Conjunctivitis
Melanoma

Muir-Torre Syndrome

Synonym

Torre syndrome
Torre-Muir syndrome

Inheritance

Autosomal dominant; *MSH1* and *MSH2* genes on 3p21 and 2p22–21, respectively

Prenatal Diagnosis

DNA analysis

Incidence

At least 65 cases reported; M=F

Age of Presentation

Fifth to sixth decade of life (internal malignancies usually precede cutaneous lesions)

Pathogenesis

Mutations in *MSH2* (most common) and *MSH1*, DNA mismatch repair genes, produces phenotype; syndrome is linked to the Lynch II cancer family syndrome

Key Features

Skin
Multiple sebaceous tumors: adenomas (most common), carcinomas, hyperplasias, epitheliomas, basal cell carcinoma with sebaceous differentiation
Keratoacanthomas
Neoplasms
Adenocarcinoma of the colon (most common), other gastrointestinal tract, genitourinary tract, lung, breast, and hematologic malignancies described

Differential Diagnosis

Cowden syndrome (p. 188)
Gardner syndrome (p. 184)

Laboratory Data

Skin biopsy
Endoscopy/gastrointestinal x-ray

Management

Close follow-up by internist screening for malignancy
Referral to dermatologist
Referral to gastroenterologist

Prognosis

Malignancies usually low-grade with good prognosis; may have normal life span with close surveillance and early detection of malignancy

Clinical Pearls

Ophthalmic sebaceous tumors may be a presenting sign . . . Sebaceous adenoma or carcinoma should prompt a trip to an internist for a screening evaluation, looking for visceral malignancies . . . Sebaceous hyperplasia and sebaceous epitheliomas arising witin nevus sebaceous of Jadassohn are not part of the syndrome . . . The associated visceral malignancies may be indolent, and detection can lead to prolonged survival . . . Both hereditary nonpolyposis colorectal cancer and Muir-Torre syndrome are caused by inherited DNA mismatch repair defect . . . Mutations in the *MSH2* gene located on 2p are commonly implicated, while mutations in the MSH1 gene located on 3p, can also cause the syndrome . . . *LE*

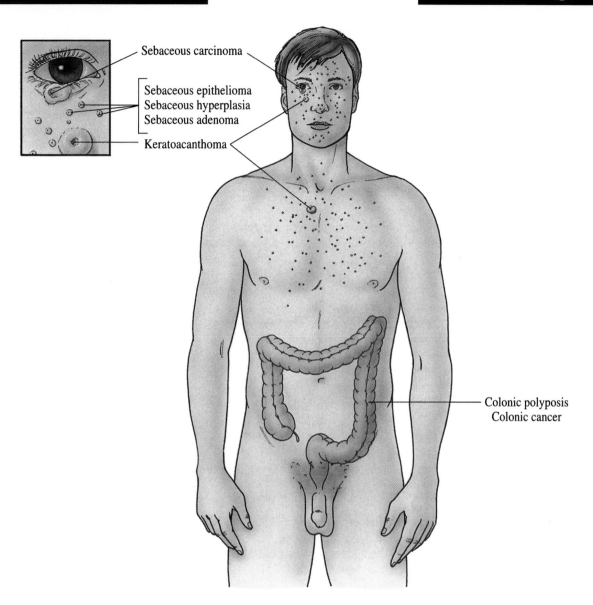

Sebaceous carcinoma

Sebaceous epithelioma
Sebaceous hyperplasia
Sebaceous adenoma

Keratoacanthoma

Colonic polyposis
Colonic cancer

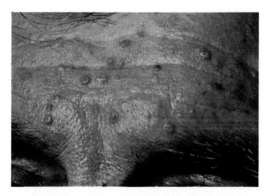

5.7. *Multiple sebaceous hyperplasia and sebaceous adenomas on patient's forehead.* (68)

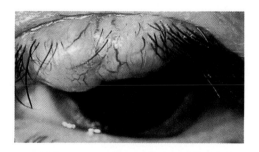

5.8. *Sebaceous carcinoma of upper eyelid.* (69)

Dyskeratosis Congenita

Synonym	Zinsser-Engman-Cole syndrome
Inheritance	X-linked recessive (most common); dyskerin (*DKC1*) gene on Xq28; autosomal dominant and recessive patterns have been described; telomerase RNA component (*TERC*) gene on 3q21–q28 in autosomal dominant cases
Prenatal Diagnosis	DNA analysis
Incidence	Over 100 cases reported; M:F=10:1
Age at Presentation	First decade of life (cutaneous, nail, mucosal changes)
Pathogenesis	Mutation in the *DKC1* gene encoding the dyskerin protein has untoward effects on RNA nucleolar function and RNA telomerase activity with subsequent problems in cell proliferation in blood and epithelium; *TERC* gene mutations responsible for the RNA component of telomerase, has been implicated in autosomal dominant cases
Key Features	**Skin** Reticulated gray-brown hyperpigmentation on neck, face, trunk, upper thighs; atrophy, hypopigmentation, and telangiectasias within pigmentation Palmoplantar hyperkeratosis, hyperhidrosis, friction bullae, acrocyanosis **Hair** Thinning alopecia on scalp, eyebrows, eyelashes **Nails** Dystrophic with longitudinal ridges, pterygium; atrophic, or absent **Mouth** Premalignant leukoplakia of the tongue, buccal mucosa, pharynx; dental caries with early loss of teeth **Mucous Membranes** Premalignant leukoplakia of any mucosal surface **Hematologic** Fanconi's type pancytopenia with secondary infection, hemorrhage **Eyes** Blepharitis, conjunctivitis, lacrimal duct obstruction with epiphora, ectropion **Central Nervous System** Mild to moderate mental retardation (50%)
Differential Diagnosis	Fanconi syndrome Pachyonychia congenita (p. 294) Rothmund-Thomson syndrome (p. 238) Chronic graft vs. host disease

Dyskeratosis Congenita *(continued)*

Laboratory Data
Mucosal biopsy
Bone marrow biopsy
DNA analysis

Management
Referral to hematologist/oncologist—bone marrow transplantation, transfusions, oral retinoids
Referral to dermatologist, otolaryngologist, gastroenterologist, ophthalmologist
Counsel against excessive sun exposure, smoking

Prognosis
Death usually in 20s to 30s secondary to malignancy (usually squamous cell carcinoma), gastrointestinal hemorrhage, or opportunistic infection

Clinical Pearls

Dyskeratosis congenita is caused by inherited defects in the telomerase complex . . . Autosomal dominant dyskeratosis congenita is associated with mutations in the RNA component of telomerase, *hTERC*, while X-linked dyskeratosis congenita is caused by mutations in the gene encoding dyskerin, a protein implicated in both telomerase function and ribosomal RNA processing . . . X-linked dyskeratosis congenita is clearly the most common . . . X-linked recessive and autosomal recessive cases have a high incidence of nail dystrophy, skin changes and leukoplakia, with earlier presentation (median is approximately 15 years) . . . Autosomal dominant cases are usually milder, and may present later (median age at diagnosis, 28 years) . . . Some patients may be thought to have twenty-nail dystrophy; pigmentary and mucosal changes are sufficient to make the differentiation . . . Bone marrow dysfunction can be the first manifestation . . . Mucosal surfaces should be followed carefully with liberal biopsies of any worrisome changes . . . Hematopoietic stem cell transplantation is the standard treatment of bone marrow complications; nonmyeloablative conditioning regimens may be more successful.   *LE*

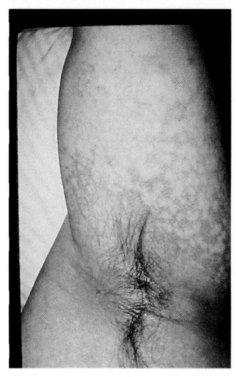

5.9. *Poikilodermatous changes in the axilla extending on to arm. (1)*

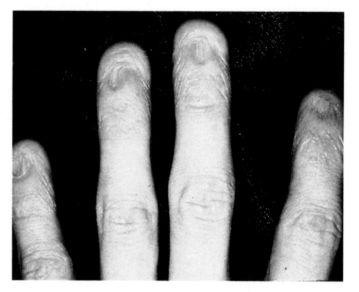

5.10. *Dystrophic and absent nails. (1)*

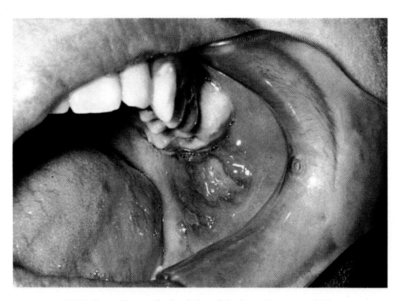

5.11. *Premalignant leukoplakia of the buccal mucosa. (70)*

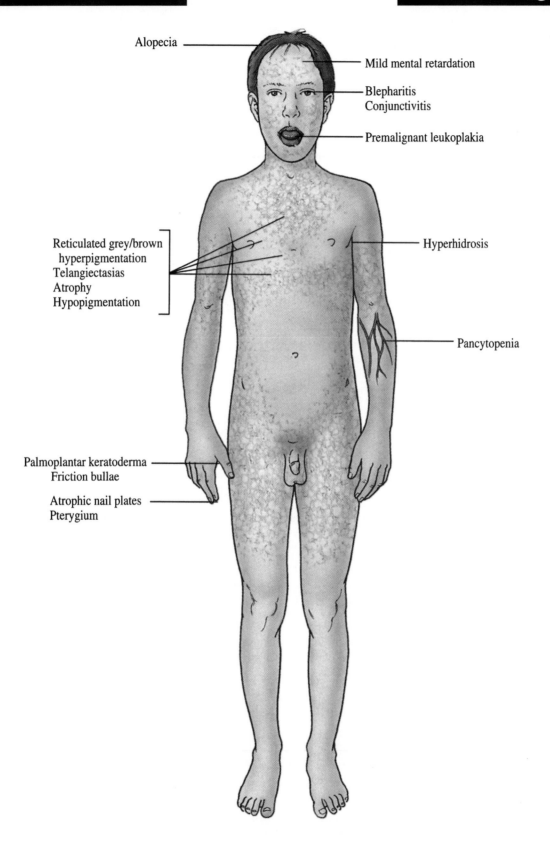

Alopecia

Mild mental retardation

Blepharitis
Conjunctivitis

Premalignant leukoplakia

Hyperhidrosis

Reticulated grey/brown
hyperpigmentation
Telangiectasias
Atrophy
Hypopigmentation

Pancytopenia

Palmoplantar keratoderma
Friction bullae

Atrophic nail plates
Pterygium

Gardner Syndrome

Inheritance   Autosomal dominant; adenomatous polyposis coli (*APC*) gene on 5q21–22

Prenatal Diagnosis   DNA analysis

Incidence   Approximately 1:14,000; M=F

Age at Presentation   Infancy to early childhood (bone, skin lesions); second to fourth decade (gastrointestinal lesions)

Pathogenesis   Mutations in *APC*, a tumor suppressor gene that regulates B-catenin, an adherens junction protein controlling cell growth and early embryonic axis formation, promotes tumor formation; high dietary fat may play a role in patients with the genetic defect

Key Features

Skin
   Epidermoid cysts—increased on head and neck; may have unusual location on toe, scalp, shin
   Fibromas
Musculoskeletal
   Osteomas—maxilla, mandible, other skull bones; small, multiple
Gastrointestinal
   Polyposis with high predisposition to malignant adenocarcinoma; most common in colon/rectum
   Desmoid tumors—postabdominal surgery; uteral or intestinal obstruction
Eyes
   Congenital hypertrophy of retinal pigment epithelium (CHRPE)—congenital marker for diagnosis
Teeth
   Odontomas, supernumerary teeth

Differential Diagnosis   Epidermoid cysts
Familial polyposis coli
Turcot syndrome

Laboratory Data   Colonoscopy/biopsy of polyp
Endoscopy
Radiologic evaluation of upper and lower gastrointestinal tract
Skull films/skeletal survey
DNA analysis

Management   Referral to gastroenterologist—semiannual evaluation of gastrointestinal tract, high-fiber diet
Referral to surgeon—prophylactic colectomy
Referral to ophthalmologist, dentist
Referral to dermatologist—excision of cysts
Examination of family members

Prognosis   If total colectomy performed early, prior to metastases, then normal life span

Clinical Pearls

Gardner syndrome is caused by mutations in the adenomatous polyposis of the colon gene (*APC*) . . . CHRPE is very useful marker for the disease . . . Children at risk as a result of family history may be followed early with eye examinations, stool guaics, and sigmoidoscopy . . . Annual sigmoidoscopy is advised beginning at age 12 years, and total colectomy may be needed . . . Nonsteroidal anti-inflammatory drugs (NSAIDs) and cyclooxygenase-2 inhibitors have been used to try to decrease polyps or colorectal cancer, but I would check new studies to see if these medications are really considered useful. . . . When a patient presents with multiple epidermoid cysts, it should prompt eliciting a family history of polyps and/or colonic cancer . . . Gastroenterology, general surgery, oral surgery, radiology, ophthalmology, endocrinology and neurology are all appropriate specialties to assist with care.   *LE*

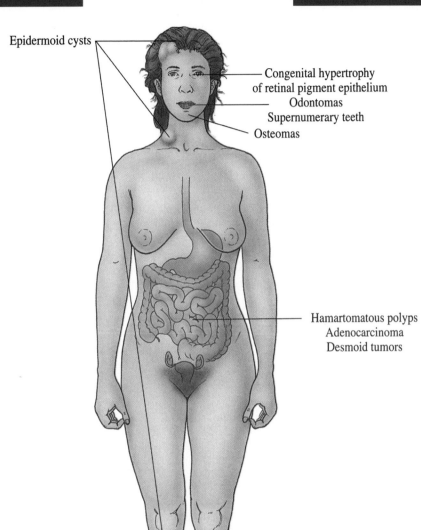

Epidermoid cysts

Congenital hypertrophy
of retinal pigment epithelium
Odontomas
Supernumerary teeth
Osteomas

Hamartomatous polyps
Adenocarcinoma
Desmoid tumors

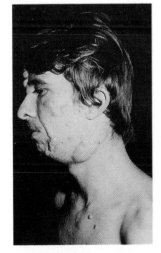

5.12. Multiple epidermoid cysts of the face. (71)

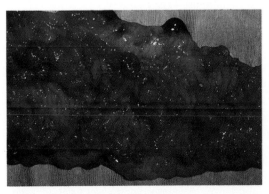

5.13. Gross surgical specimen demonstrating multiple polyps of the colon. (72)

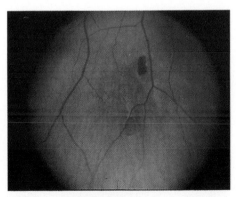

5.14. Fundoscopic exam demonstrates CHRPE. (73)

Peutz-Jeghers Syndrome

Synonym	Periorificial lentiginosis
Inheritance	Autosomal dominant; serine/threonine kinase 11 (*STK11*) gene on 19p13 Spontaneous mutation (approximately 40%)
Prenatal Diagnosis	DNA analysis
Incidence	Over 500 cases reported; M=F
Age at Presentation	Birth to first few years of life (pigmented macules); first to third decade of life (polyps)
Pathogenesis	Mutations in *STK11*, a tumor suppressor gene encoding STK protein involved in catalyzing addition of serine and threonine, may affect cell cycle progression
Key Features	**Skin** Pigmented macules—0.2 to 7 mm, brown to black in color, variation in shape on periorificial skin, lips, buccal mucosa, digits, nails, palms, soles, any mucosal surface; all except buccal mucosal lesions may fade with time **Gastrointestinal** Hamartomatous polyps—small intestine > large intestine, secondary abdominal pain, gastrointestinal bleeding, anemia, intussusception, obstruction; adenocarcinoma may develop within polyps **Neoplasm** Increased frequency of ovarian, breast, and pancreatic carcinoma
Differential Diagnosis	LEOPARD syndrome (p. 76) Carney complex (p. 78) Laugier-Hunziker syndrome Cronkhite-Canada syndrome Addison's disease Gardner syndrome (p. 184)
Laboratory Data	Bowel x-rays, gastroscopy/colonoscopy screening every 1 to 2 years, polyp biopsy Stool guaiac Mammography
Management	Referral to gastroenterologist/surgeon—removal of symptomatic polyps and those larger than 1.5 cm via endoscopic perioperative panpolypectomy; screening every 2 years if asymptomatic Referral to obstetrician/gynecologist—regular pelvic/breast examinations/screening Referral to dermatologist—laser surgery
Prognosis	Normal life span if malignancy detected early

Clinical Pearls

The disorder is caused by mutations in the serine/threonine kinase *STK11* gene . . . The pigmented macules on the lips are very amenable to treatment with ruby or Alexandrite lasers . . . We coordinate laser treatment with endoscopy, utilizing the sedation/anesthesia to make the laser "painless" . . . Endoscopy should be routine, with removal of polyps to minimize bowel wall invasion . . . For history buffs, Keller et al. (*Familial Cancer* 2002;1:181–185) reviews the history of Peutz-Jeghers syndrome, including biographic information about Jan Peutz and Harold Jeghers.   *LE*

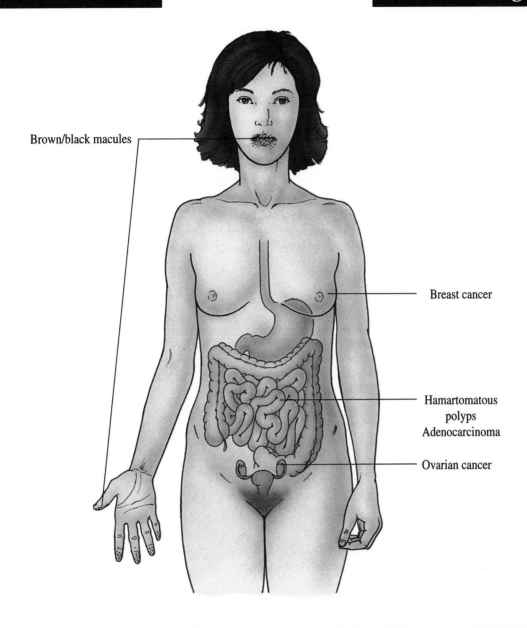

Brown/black macules

Breast cancer

Hamartomatous
polyps
Adenocarcinoma

Ovarian cancer

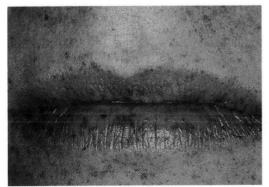

5.15. *Perioral brown macules. (74)*

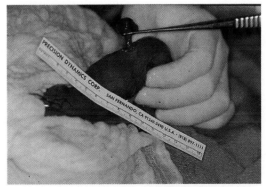

5.16. *Resection of hamartomatous polyp via perioperative endoscopy. (74)*

187

Cowden Syndrome

Synonym	Multiple hamartoma syndrome
Inheritance	Autosomal dominant; phosphatase and tensin homologue deleted on chromosome ten (*PTEN*) gene on 10q23
Prenatal Diagnosis	DNA analysis
Incidence	1:300,000; M:F=1:2
Age at Presentation	Usually second to third decade of life; range from 4 to 75 years
Pathogenesis	Mutations in *PTEN*, a tumor suppressor gene that encodes a tyrosine phosphatase protein necessary to remove phosphate from proteins and regulate their activation, leads to cell proliferation in epidermis, gastrointestinal and oral mucosa, thyroid, and breast tissue; also implicated in Banayan-Riley-Ruvalcaba and Proteus

Key Features

Skin
  Facial tricholemmomas—tan-yellow verrucous papules
  Oral papillomas-"cobblestone" appearance on lips, gingival, labial, and buccal mucosa, oropharynx
  Acral keratotic papules—dorsal hands, wrists
  Palmoplantar translucent punctate keratoses
  Lipomas, angiomas (rare)
Breasts
  Fibrocystic disease, virginal hypertrophy, fibroadenomas, adenocarcinoma, gynecomastia (males)
Thyroid
  Goiter, adenomas, thyroglossal duct cysts, follicular adenocarcinoma
Gastrointestinal
  Hamartomatous polyps—throughout gastrointestinal tract but increased in colon, usually benign
Genitourinary
  Ovarian cysts, menstrual irregularities
Craniofacial/Skeletal
  Adenoid facies, high-arched palate, craniomegaly, kyphoscoliosis

Differential Diagnosis	Lipoid proteinosis (p. 154) Muir-Torre syndrome (p. 178) Multiple endocrine neoplasia IIb (p. 190) Tuberous sclerosis (p. 88)
Laboratory Data	Mammography Thyroid scan Thyroid function tests, complete blood count (CBC), urinalysis, stool guaiac
Management	Referral to obstetrician/gynecologist—periodic breast examinations, mammography, prophylactic bilateral mastectomy, pelvic examinations Referral to endocrinologist, gastroenterologist Referral to dermatologist—surgery, retinoids for cosmesis
Prognosis	If carcinoma detected early on, may have normal life span

Clinical Pearls

PTEN mutations are responsible for Cowden syndrome . . . There is overlap with Bannayan-Riley-Ruvalcaba syndrome, and cancer surveillance is appropriate for patients with both syndromes . . . Patients usually present in their 30s or 40s, while breast disease in women may be seen in their 20s . . . Breast cancer has been reported in males as well . . . Laser vaporization of trichilemmomas may be useful for cosmetic improvement . . . The most important intervention is excellent screening for malignancies by an internist . . . *LE*

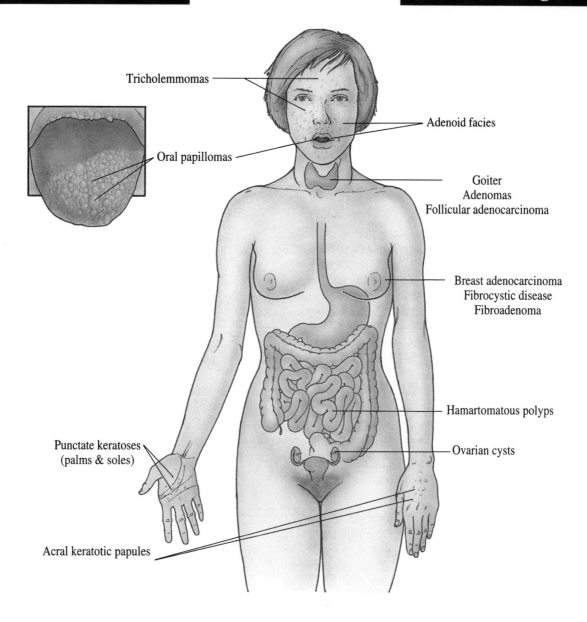

Tricholemmomas

Oral papillomas

Adenoid facies

Goiter
Adenomas
Follicular adenocarcinoma

Breast adenocarcinoma
Fibrocystic disease
Fibroadenoma

Hamartomatous polyps

Punctate keratoses
(palms & soles)

Ovarian cysts

Acral keratotic papules

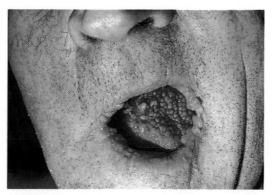

5.17. Multiple oral papillomas providing a "cobble-stone" appearance. (75)

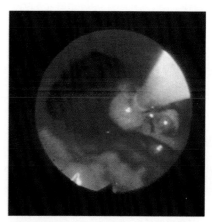

5.18. Smooth hamartomatous polyps in colon. (76)

Multiple Endocrine Neoplasia Type IIb

Synonym
Multiple endocrine neoplasia (MEN) type III
Multiple mucosal neuroma syndrome

Inheritance
Autosomal dominant; *RET* proto-oncogene on 10q11.2
Sporadic mutation in 50%

Prenatal Diagnosis
DNA analysis

Incidence
Rare; approximately 150 cases reported; M=F

Age at Presentation
Birth to first few years of life (mucosal lesions may precede internal malignancies by a decade)

Pathogenesis
Mutation in *RET* proto-oncogene encoding a tyrosine kinase receptor in neural-crest derived tissue, promotes neoplasia

Key Features
Mucocutaneous
Mucosal neuromas on tongue and lips; may involve buccal, palatal, gingival, nasal, and laryngeal mucosa
Thickened "blubbery" lips
Endocrine
Medullary carcinoma of the thyroid
Pheochromocytoma
Musculoskeletal
Marfanoid habitus (see Marfan syndrome, p. 140)
Eyes
Conjunctival neuromas; upper eyelids thickened and everted; thickened white medullated nerve fibers in cornea
Gastrointestinal
Ganglioneuromatosis with secondary megacolon, diarrhea, constipation

Differential Diagnosis
MEN IIA-Sipple syndrome
Neurofibromatosis I (p. 82)
Marfan syndrome (p. 140)

Laboratory Data
Serum/urine calcitonin level
Urine catecholamine level
Thyroid scan/thyroid function tests
Abdominal CT/Ultrasound
Barium enema

Management
Referral to endocrinologist/surgeon—thyroidectomy, removal of pheochromocytoma
Referral to gastroenterologist, ophthalmologist, dermatologist
Examine family members

Prognosis
If thyroid carcinoma detected early on, may have normal life span; otherwise, often fatal by 20 to 30 years of age

Clinical Pearls

Both MEN IIB and IIA are caused by mutations in the *RET* proto-oncogene . . . Thick, full lips can be noticed first, and pedunculated neuromas can occur on the tongue and eyelids as well . . . Diagnosis is often made in early teenage years . . . Neuromas are not usually bothersome . . . Medullary thyroid carcinoma can occur very early in life, and some experts recommend treatment even in the first 6 months of life!   *LE*

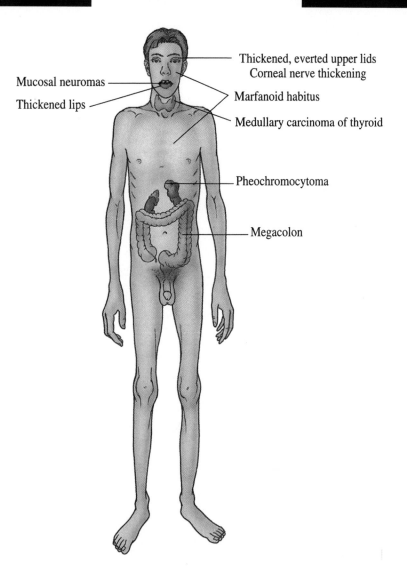

Thickened, everted upper lids
Corneal nerve thickening

Mucosal neuromas

Thickened lips

Marfanoid habitus

Medullary carcinoma of thyroid

Pheochromocytoma

Megacolon

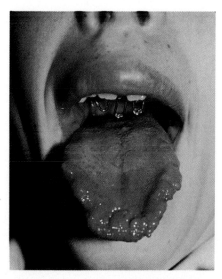

5.19. *Coalescing mucosal neuromas of the tongue. (77)*

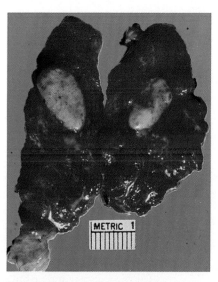

5.20. *Cross-section of thyroid gland revealing white nodules representing bilateral medullary thyroid carcinoma. (78)*

Birt-Hogg-Dube Syndrome

Synonym	Fibrofolliculomas with trichodiscomas, and acrochordons
Inheritance	Autosomal dominant; *BHD* gene encoding folliculin on 17p11
Prenatal Diagnosis	DNA mutation analysis
Incidence	Unknown; most likely underdiagnosed
Age at Presentation	Often greater than 25 years of age
Pathogenesis	Protein-truncating mutations in folliculin contribute to phenotype and may help understand the role this kidney cancer gene plays in skin, lung and kidney development

Key Features	**Skin**
	   Fibrofolliculomas, trichodiscomas, and acrochordons (may be one lesion, namely fibrofolliculomas)
	Kidney
	   Renal cell carcinoma, (often bilateral)
	Lung
	   Recurrent spontaneous pneumothoraces, lung cysts, bullous emphysema

Differential Diagnosis	Cowden syndrome Tuberous sclerosis Brooke-Spiegler syndrome Rombo syndrome Basaloid follicular hamartoma syndrome
Laboratory Data	Skin biopsy Abdominal computed tomography (CT) scan, renal ultrasound periodic screening Chest x-ray
Management	Referral to nephrology, pulmonology after thorough history, physical examination and diagnosis confirmed by dermatologist Screen all first-degree relatives for kidney and lung manifestations
Prognosis	If renal cell cancer detected early and pulmonary sequelae not debilitating, then good prognosis

Clinical Pearls

Birt-Hogg-Dube is a syndrome caused by mutations in the gene encoding folliculin . . . The three tumors initially associated with this syndrome—fibrofolliculoma, trichodiscoma, and acrochordon—are all apparently variations of fibrofolliculomas . . . Multiple firm papules, 2 to 4 mm, on the face, neck, and/or trunk, with or without soft pedunculated achrocordon-like lesions should raise clinical suspicion . . . Lesions usually occur after age 25 . . . Specific history should be elicited including pulmonary disease (including recurrent spontaneous pneumothorax, lung cysts, and/or bullous emphysema) and renal malignancy . . . *BHDS* is autosomal dominant, so screening abdominal CT and renal ultrasound should be done for patients and at-risk relatives . . . *LE*

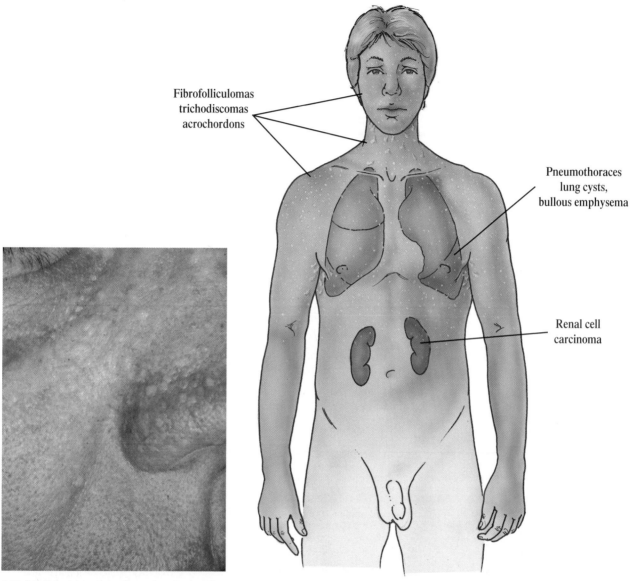

Fibrofolliculomas
trichodiscomas
acrochordons

Pneumothoraces
lung cysts,
bullous emphysema

Renal cell
carcinoma

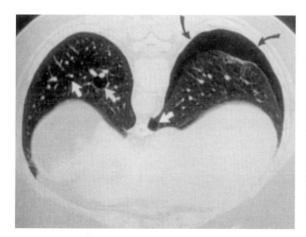

5.21. Mutiple dome-shaped papules representing fibrofolliculomas on the nose and cheek. (79)

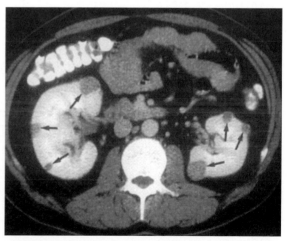

5.22. Left. Transverse CT scan demonstating pneumothorax (black arrows) and several pulmonary cysts (white arrows). Right Transverse abdominal CT revealing solid chromophobe renal cancers (arrows). (80)

Basal Cell Nevus Syndrome

Barr RJ, Headley JL, Jensen JL, et al. Cutaneous keratocysts of nevoid basal cell carcinoma syndrome. *J Am Acad Dermatol* 1986;14:572–576.

Boutet N, Bignon YJ, Drouin-Garraud V, et al. Spectrum of PTCH1 mutations in French patients with Gorlin syndrome. *J Invest Dermatol* 2003;121:478–481.

Doctoroff A, Oberlender SA, Purcell SM. Full-face carbon dioxide laser resurfacing in the management of a patient with the nevoid basal cell carcinoma syndrome. *Dermatol Surg* 2003;29:1236–1240.

Evans DG, Famdon PA, Burnell LD, et al. The incidence of Gorlin syndrome in 173 consecutive cases of medulloblastoma. *Br J Cancer* 1991;64:959–961.

Evans DG, Ladusans EJ, Rimmer S, et al. Complications of the naevoid basal cell carcinoma syndrome: results of a population based study. *J Med Genet* 1993;30:460–464.

Frentz G, Munch-Petersen B, Wulf HC, et al. The nevoid basal cell carcinoma syndrome: sensitivity to ultraviolet and x-ray irradiation. *J Am Acad Dermatol* 1987;17:637–643.

Gailani MR, Bale SJ, Leffell DJ, et al. Developmental defects in Gorlin syndrome related to a putative tumor suppressor gene on chromosome 9. *Cell* 1992;69:111–117.

Goldberg LH, Hsu SH, Alcatay J. Effectiveness of isotretinoin in preventing the appearance of basal cell carcinomas in basal cell nevus syndrome. *J Am Acad Dermatol* 1989;21:144–145.

Goldstein AM, Bale SJ, Peck GL, et al. Sun exposure and basal cell carcinomas in the nevoid basal cell carcinoma syndrome. *J Am Med Dermatol* 1993;29:34–41.

Gorlin RF. Nevoid basal cell carcinoma syndrome. *Medicine* 1987;66:98–113.

Gorlin RJ. Nevoid basal cell carcinoma (Gorlin) syndrome: unanswered issues. *J Lab Clin Med* 1999;134:551–552.

Gorlin RJ, Goltz RW. Multiple nevoid basal cell epithelioma, jaw cysts and bifid rib: a syndrome. *N Engl J Med* 1960;262:908–912.

Hasenpusch-Theil K, Bataille V, Laehdetie J, et al. Gorlin syndrome: identification of 4 novel germ-line mutations of the human patched (PTCH) gene. Mutations in brief no. 137. Online. *Hum Mutat* 1998;11:480.

Johnson AD, Hebert AA, Esterly NB. Nevoid basal cell carcinoma syndrome: bilateral ovarian fibromas in a 3 1/2 year old girl. *J Am Acad Dermatol* 1986;14:371–374.

Kagy MK, Amonette R. The use of imiquimod 5% cream for the treatment of superficial basal cell carcinomas in a basal cell nevus syndrome patient. *Dermatol Surg* 2000;26:577, 2000.

Kimonis VE, Goldstein AM, Pastakia B, et al. Clinical manifestations in 105 persons with nevoid basal cell carcinoma syndrome. *Am J Med Genet* 1997;69:299–308.

Lacombe D, Chateil JF, Fontan D, et al. Medulloblastoma in the nevoid basal cell carcinoma syndrome: case reports and review of the literature. *Genet Couns* 1990;1:273–277.

Lam CW, Leung CY, Lee KC, et al. Novel mutations in the PATCHED gene in basal cell nevus syndrome. *Mol Genet Metab* 2002;76:57–61.

Ottinger LW, Vickery AL Jr. Case records of the Massachusetts General Hospital (Case 10–1986). *N Engl J Med* 1986;314:700–706.

Palacios E, Serou M, Restrepo S, et al. Odontogenic keratocysts in nevoid basal cell carcinoma (Gorlin's) syndrome CT and MRI evaluation. *Ear Nose Throat J* 2004;83:40–42.

Reis A, Kuster W, Linn G, et al. Localisation of gene for the naevold basal cell carcinoma syndrome [letter]. *Lancet* 1992;339:617.

Sanchez-Conejo-Mir J, Camacho F. Nevoid basal cell carcinoma syndrome: combined etretinate and surgical treatment. *J Dermatol Surg Oncol* 1989;15:868–871.

Stone D, Hynes M, Armanini M, et al. The tumour-suppressor gene patched encodes a candidate receptor for Sonic hedgehog. *Nature* 1996;384:129–134.

Vogt A, Chuang PT, Hebert J, et al. Immunoprevention of basal cell carcinomas with recombinant hedgehog-interacting Protein. *J Exp Med* 2004;199:753–761.

Wicking C, Gillies S, Smyth I, et al. De novo mutations of the Patched gene in nevoid basal cell carcinoma syndrome help to define the clinical phenotype. *Am J Med Genet* 1997;73:304–307.

Zedan W, Robinson PA, Markham AF, et al. Expression of the Sonic Hedgehog receptor "PATCHED" in basal cell carcinomas and odontogenic keratocysts. *J Pathol* 2001;194:473–477.

Xeroderma Pigmentosum

Bernard F, Asselineau D, Vioux C, et al. Clues to epidermal cancer proneness revealed by reconstruction of DNA repair-deficient xeroderma pigmentosum skin in vitro. *Proc Natl Acad USA* 2001;98:7817–7822.

Cleaver JE, Thompson LH, Richardson AS, et al. A summary of mutations in the UV sensitive disorders: xeroderma pigmentosum, Cockayne syndrome, and trichothiodystrophy. *Hum Mutat* 1999;14:9–22.

Friedberg EC. The discovery that xeroderma pigmentosum (XP) results from defective nucleotide excision repair. *DNA Repair (Amst)* 2004;3:183–195.

Friedberg EC. Xeroderma pigmentosum,

Cockayne's syndrome, helicases, and DNA repair: what's the relationship? *Cell* 1992;71:887–889.

Gaspari AA, Fleisher TA, Kraemer KH. Impaired interferon production and natural killer cell activation in patients with the skin cancer-prone disorder, xeroderma pigmentosum. *J Clin Invest* 1993;92:1135–1142.

Johnson RT, Squires S. The XPD complementation group. Insights into xeroderma pigmentosum, Cockayne's syndrome and trichothiodystrophy. *Mutat Res* 1992;273:97–118.

Kraemer KH, DiGiovanna JJ, Moshell AN, et al. Prevention of skin cancer in xeroderma pigmentosum with the use of oral isotretinoin. *N Engl J Med* 1988;318:1633–1637.

Kraemer KH, DiGiovanna JJ, Peck GL. Chemoprevention of skin cancer in xeroderma pigmentosum. *J Dermatol* 1992;19:715–718.

Kraemer KH, Lee MM, Scotto J. Xeroderma pigmentosum. Cutaneous, ocular, and neurologic abnormalities in 830 published cases. *Arch Dermatol* 1987;123:241–250.

Kraemer KH, Seetharam S, Seidman MM, et al. Defective DNA repair in humans: clinical and molecular studies of xeroderma pigmentosum. *Basic Life Sci* 1990;53:95–104.

Kraemer KH, Slor H. Xeroderma pigmentosum. *Clin Dermatol* 1985;3:33–69.

Lehmann AR. The xeroderma pigmentosum group D (XPD) gene: one gene, two functions, three diseases. *Genes Dev* 2001;15:15–23.

Magnaldo T. Xeroderma pigmentosum: from genetics to hopes and realities of cutaneous gene therapy. *Expert Opin Biol Ther* 2004;4:169–179.

Nagore E, Sevila A, Sanmartin O, et al. Excellent response of basal cell carcinomas and pigmentary changes in xeroderma pigmentosum to imiquimod 5% cream. *Br J Dermatol* 2003;149:858–861.

Rapin I, Lindenbaum Y Dickson DW, et al. Cockayne syndrome and xeroderma pigmentosum. *Neurology* 2000;55:1442–1449.

Stefanini M, Lagomarsini P, Arlett CF, et al. Xeroderma pigmentosum (complementation group D) mutation is present In patients affected by trichothiodystrophy with photosensitivity. *Hum Genet* 1986;74:107–112.

Shiomi N, Kito S, Oyama M, et al. Identification of the XPG region that causes the onset of Cockayne syndrom by using Xpg mutant mice generated by the cDNA-mediated knock-in method. *Mol Cell Biol* 2004;24:3712–3719.

Zafeiriou DI, Thorel F, Andreou A, et al. Xeroderma pigmentosum group G with severe neurological involvement and features of Cockayne syndrome in infancy. *Pediatr Res* 2001;49:407–412.

Muir-Torre Syndrome

Finan MC, Ray MK. Gastrointestinal polyposis syndromes. *Dermatol Clin* 1989;7:419–434.

Fusaro RM, Lemon SJ, Lynch HT. Muir-Torre syndrome and defective DNA mismatch repair genes. *J Am Acad Dermatol* 1996;35:493–494.

Hall NR, Murday VA, Chapman P, et al. Genetic linkage in Muir-Torre syndrome to the same chromosomal region as cancer family syndrome. *Eur J Cancer* 1994;30A:180–182.

Harrington CR, Egbert BM, Swetter SM. Extraocular sebaceous carcinoma in a patient with muir-torre syndrome. *Dermatol Surg* 2004;30:817–819.

Honchei R, Hailing KC, Schaid DJ, et al. Microsatellite instability in Muir-Torre syndrome. *Cancer Res* 1994;54:1159–1163.

Jakobiec FA, Zimmerman LE, La Plana F, at al. Unusual eyelid tumors with sebaceous differentation in the Muir-Torre syndrome. Rapid clinical regrowth and frank squamous transformation after biopsy. *Ophthalmology* 1988;95: 1543–1548.

Kruse R, Ruzicka T. DNA mismatch repair and the significance of a sebaceous skin tumor for visceral cancer prevention. *Trends Mol Med* 2004;10:136–141.

Lynch HT, Fusaro RM. The Muir-Torre syndrome in kindreds with hereditary nonpolyposis colorectal cancer (Lynch syndrome): a classic obligation in preventive medicine. *J Am Acad Dermatol* 1999;41:797–799.

Mathiak M, Rutten A, Mangold E, et al. Loss of DNA mismatch repair proteins in skin tumors from patients with Muir-Torre syndrome and MSH2 or MLH1 germline mutations: establishment of immunohistochemical analysis as a screening test. *Am J Surg Pathol* 2002;26:338–343.

Rishi K, Font RL. Sebaceous gland tumors of the eyelids and conjunctiva in the Muir-Torre syndrome: a clinicopathologic study of five cases and literature review. *Ophthal Plast Reconstr Surg* 2004;20:31–36.

Rothenberg J, Lambert WC, Vail JT Jr, et al. The Muir-Torre (Torre's) syndrome: the significance of a solitary sebaceous tumor. *J Am Acad Derm* 1990;23:638–640.

Schwartz RA, Goldberg DJ, Mahmood F, et al. The Muir-Torre syndrome: a disease of sebaceous and colonic neoplasms. *Dermatologica* 1989;178:23–28.

Schwartz RA, Torre DP. The Muir-Torre syndrome: a 25 year retrospect. *J Am Acad Dermatol* 1995;33:90–104

Spielvogel RL, DeVillez RL, Roberts LC. Oral isotretinoin therapy for familial Muir-Torre syndrome. *J Am Acad Dermatol* 1985;12:475–480.

Dyskeratosis Congenita

Amgrimsson R, Dokal I, Luzzatto L, et al. Dyskeratosis congenita: three additional families show linkage to a locus In Xg28. *J Med Genet* 1993;30:818–619.

Connor JM, Gatherer D, Gray FC, et al. Assignment of the gene for dyskeratosis congenita to Xq28. *Hum Genet* 1966;72:348–351.

Connor JM, Teague RH. Dyskeratosis congenita: report of a large kindred. *Br J Dermatol* 1981;105:321–325

Dokal I, Vulliamy T. Dyskeratosis congenita: its link to telomerase and aplastic anaemia. *Blood Rev* 2003;17:217–225.

Drachtman RA, Alter BP. Dyskeratosis congenita: clinical and genetic heterogeneity. Report of a new case and review of the literature. *Am J Pediatr Hematol Oncol* 1992;14:297–304.

Hassock S, Vetrie D, Giannelli F. Mapping and characterization of the X-linked dyskeratosis congenita (DKC) gene. *Genomics* 1999;55:21–27.

Heiss NS, Megarbane A, Klauck SM, et al. One novel and two recurrent missense DKC1 mutations in patients with dyskeratosis congenita (DKC). *Genet Couns* 2001;12:129–136.

Knight SW, Heiss NS, Vulliany TJ, et al. X-linked dyskeratosis congenita is predominantly: caused by missense mutations in the DKC1 gene. *Am J Hum Genet* 1999;65:50–58.

Knight SW, Vulliamy TJ, Morgan B, et al. Identification of novel DKC1 mutations in patients with dyskeratosis congenita: implications for pathophysiology and diagnosis. *Hum Genet* 2001;108:299–303.

Mallory SB. What syndrome is this characteristic of? Dyskeratosis congenita. *Pediatr Dermatol* 1991;8:81–83.

Marrone A, Mason PJ. Dyskeratosis congenita. *Cell Mol Life Sci* 2003;60:507–517.

Mason PJ. Stem cells, telomerase and dyskeratosis congenita. *Bioessays* 2003;25:126–133.

Mitchell JR, Wood E, Collins K. A telomerase component is defective in the human disease dyskeratosis congenita. *Nature* 1999;402:551–555.

Phillips RJ, Judge M, Webb D, et al. Dyskeratosis congenita: delay in diagnosis and successful treatment of pancytopenia by bone marrow transplantation. *Br J Dermatol* 1992;127:278–280.

Pytterman C, Safadi R, Ziotogori J, et al. Treatment of the hematological manifestations of dyskeratosis congenita. *Ann Hematol* 1993;66:209–212.

Steier W, Van Voolen GA, Setmanowitz VJ. Dyskeratosis congenita: relationship to Fanconi's anemia. *Blood* 1972;39:510–521.

Theimer CA, Finger LD, Trantirek L, et al. Mutations linked to dyskeratosis congenita cause changes in the structural equilibrium in telomerase RNA. *Proc Natl Acad Sci USA* 2003;100:449–454.

Youssoufian H, Gharibyan V, Qatanani M. Analysis of epitope-tagged forms of the dyskeratosis congenital protein (dyskerin): identification of a nuclear localization signal. *Blood Cells Mol Dis* 1999;25:305–309.

Gardner Syndrome

Burt RW, Bishop DT, Lynch HT, et al. Risk and surveillance of Individuals with heritable factors for colorectal cancer. WHO Collaborating Centre for the Prevention of Colorectal Cancer. *Bull WHO* 1990;68:655–665.

Davies DR, Armstrong JG, Thakker N, et al. Severe Gardner syndrome in families with mutations restricted to a specific region of the APC gene. *Am J Hum Genet* 1995;57:1151–1158.

Einstein DM, Tagliabue JR, Desai RK. Abdominal desmoids: CT findings in 25 patients. *Am J Roentgenol* 1991;157:275–279.

Halata MS, Miller J, Stone RK, et al. Gardner syndrome. Early presentation with a desmoid tumor. Discovery of multiple colonic polyps. *Clin Pediatr* 1989;28:538–540.

Harped RK, Buck JL, Olmsted WW, et al. Extracolonic manifestations of the familial adenomatous polyposis syndrome. *Am J Roentgenol* 1991;156:481–485.

Lyons LA, Lewis RA, Strong LC, et al. A genetic study of Gardner syndrome and congenital hypertrophy of the retinal pigment epithelium. *Am J Hum Genet* 1988;42:290–296.

Nakamura Y, Lathrop M, Lepper M. Localization of the genetic defect in familial adenomatous polyposis within a small region of chromosome 5. *Am J Hum Genet* 1988;43:638–644.

Nilbert M, Fernebro J, Kristoffersson U. Novel germline APC mutations in Swedish patients with familial adenomatous polyposis and Gardner syndrome. *Scand J Gastroenterol* 2000;35:1200–1203.

Parks ET, Caldemeyer KS, Mirowski GW. Gardner syndrome. *J Am Acad Dermatol.* 2001;45:940–942.

Patel SR, Evans HL, Benjamin RS. Combination chemotherapy in adult desmoid tumors. *Cancer* 1993;72:3244–3247.

Traboulsi El, Krush AJ, Gardner EJ, et al. Prevalence and importance of pigmented ocular fundus lesions in Gardner's syndrome. *N Engl J Med* 1987;316:661–667.

Tsao H. Update on familial cancer syndromes and the skin. *J Am Med Dermatol* 200042:939–969; quiz 970–972.

Peutz-Jeghers Syndrome

Ballhausen WG, Gunther K. Genetic screening for Peutz-Jeghers syndrome. *Expert Rev Mol Diagn* 2003;3:471–479.

Benedict LM, Cohen B. Treatment of Peutz-Jeghers lentigines with the carbon dioxide laser. *J Dermatol Surg Oncol* 1991;17:954–955.

Boardman LA, Couch FJ, Burgart U, et al. Genetic heterogeneity in Peutz-Jeghers syndrome. *Hum Mutat* 2000;16:23–30.

Buck JL, Harned RK, Lichtenstein JE, Sobin LH. Peutz-Jeghers syndrome. *Radiographics* 1992;12:365–378.

Daniel ES, Ludwig SL, Lewin KJ, et al. The Cronkhite-Canada syndrome: an analysis of clinical and pathologic features and therapy in 55 patients. *Medicine* 1982;61:293–309.

Edwards DP, Khosraviani K, Stafferton R, et al. Long-term results of polyp clearance by intraoperative enteroscopy in the Peutz-Jeghers syndrome. *Dis Colon Rectum* 2003;46:48–50.

Foley TR, McGarrity TJ, Abt AB. Peutz-Jeghers syndrome: a clinicopathologic survey of the 'Harrisburg Family' with a 49-year follow-up. *Gastroenterology* 1988;95:1535–1540.

Giardiello FM, Brensinger JD, Tersmette AC, et al. Very high risk of cancer in familial Peutz-Jeghers syndrome. *Gastroenterology* 2000;119:1447–1453.

Kato S, Takeyama J, Tanita Y, et al. Ruby later therapy for labial lentigines in Peutz-Jeghers syndrome. *Eur J Pediatr* 1998;157:622–624.

Keller JJ, Offerhaus GJ, Giardiello FM, et al. Jan Peutz, Harold Jeghers and a remarkable combination of polyposis and pigmentation of the skin and mucous membranes. *Fam Cancer* 2001;1:181–185.

Koch SE, LeBoit PE, Odom RB. Laugier-Hunziker syndrome. *J Am Acad Dermatol* 1987;16:431–434.

Konishi F, Wyse NE, Muto T, et al. Peutz-Jeghers polyposis associated with carcinoma of the digestive organs. Report of three cases and review of the literature. *Dis Colon Rectum* 1987;30:790–799.

Kurugoglu S, Aksoy H, Kantarci F, et al. Radiological work-up in Peutz-Jeghers syndrome. *Pediatr Radiol* 2003;33:766–771.

Lim W, Hearle N, Shah B, et al. Further observations on LKBI/STK11 status and cancer risk in Peutz-Jeghe syndrome. *Br J Cancer* 2003;89:308–313.

McGarrity TJ, Kulin HE, Zaino RJ. Peutz-Jeghers syndrome. *Am J Gastroenterol* 2000;95:596–604.

McGrath DR, Spigelman AD. Preventive measures in Peutz-Jeghers syndrome. *Fam Cancer* 2001;1:121–125.

Meur NL, Martin C, Saugier-Veber P, et al. Complete germline deletion of the STK11 gene in a family with Peutz-Jeghers syndrome. *Eur J Hum Genet* 2004;12:415–418.

Nakagawa H, Koyama K, Tanaka T, et al. Localization of the gene responsible for Peutz-Jeghers syndrome within a 6-cM region of chromosomes 19p13.3. *Hum Genet* 1998;102:203–206.

O'Neill JF, James WD. Inherited patterned lentiginosis in blacks. *Arch Dermatol* 1989;125:1231–1235.

Parsi MA, Burke CA. Utility of capsule endoscopy in Peutz-Jeghers syndrome. *Gastrointest Enclose Clin North Am* 2004;14:159–167.

Seenath MM, Scott MJ, Morris AI, et al. Combined surgical and endoscopic clearance of small bowel polyps in Peutz Jeghers syndrome. *J R Soc Med* 2003;96:505–506.

Shaw RJ, Kosmatka M, Bardeesy N, et al. The tumor suppressor LKB1 kinase directly activates AMP-activated kinase and regulates apoptosis in response to energy stress. *Proc Natl Acad Sci USA* 2004;101:3329–3335.

Sudduth RH, Bute BG, Schoelkopf L, et al. Small bowel obstruction in a patient with Peutz-Jeghers syndrome: the role of intraoperative endoscopy. *Gastrointest Endosc* 1992;36:69–72.

Cowden Syndrome

Bardenstein DS, McLean IW, Nerney J, et al. Cowden's disease. *Ophthalmology* 1988;95:1038–1041.

Barax CN, Lebwohl M, Phelps RG. Multiple hamartoma syndrome. *J Am Acad Dermatol* 1987;17:342–346.

Braunstein BL, Pfau RG. Facial and acral wartlike papules. Multiple hamartoma syndrome or Cowden's disease. *Arch Dermatol* 1986;122:821, 824–825.

Chen YM, Ott DJ, Wu WC, et al. Cowden's disease: a case report and literature review. *Gastrointest Radiol* 1987;12:325–329.

DiCristofano A, Pesce B, Cordon Cardo C, et al. Pten is essential for embryonic development and tumour suppression. *Nat Genet* 1998;19:348–355.

Eng C. Will the real Cowden syndrome please stand up: revised diagnostic criteria. *J Med Genet* 2000;37:828–830.

Fackenthal JD, Marsh DJ, Richardson AL, et al. Male breast cancer in Cowden syndrome patients with germline PTEN mutations. *J Med Genet* 2001;38:159–164.

Mills GB, Lu Y, Fang X, et al. The role of genetic abnormalities of PTEN and the phosphatidylinositol, 3-kinase pathway in breast and ovarian tumorigenesis, prognosis, and therapy. *Semin Oncol* 2001;28:125–141.

Reifenberger J, Rauch L, Beckmann MW, et al. Cowden's disease: clinical and molecular genetic findings in a patient with a novel PTEN germline mutation. *Br J Dermatol* 2003;148:1040–1046.

Starink TM, van der Veen JP, Arwert F, et al. The Cowden syndrome: a clinical and genetic study in 21 patients. *Clin Genet* 1986;29:222–233.

Taylor AJ, Dodds WJ, Stewart ET. Alimentary tract lesions in Cowden's disease. *Br J Radiol* 1989;62:890–892.

Tsou HC, Ping XL, Xie XX, et al. The genetic basis of Cowden's syndrome: three novel mutations in PTEN/MMAC1/TEP1. *Hum Genet* 1998;102:467–473.

Walton BJ, Morain WD, Baughman RD, et al. Cowden's disease: a further indication for prophylactic mastectomy. *Surgery* 1986;99:82–86.

Williard W, Bergen P, Bol R, et al. Cowden's disease. A case report with analyses at the molecular level. *Cancer* 1992;69:2969–2974.

Zambrano E, Holm I, Glickman J, et al. Abnormal distribution and hyperplasia of thyroid c-cells in PTEN-associated tumor syndromes. *Endocr Pathol* 2004;15:55–64.

Multiple Endocrine Neoplasia Type IIB

Decker RA, Toyama Wm, O'Neal LW, et al. Evaluation of children with multiple endocrine neoplasia type lib following thyroidectomy. *J Pediatr Surg* 1990;25:939–943.

Eng C, Smith DP, Mulligan LM, et al. Point mutation within the tyrosine kinase domain of the RET proto-oncogene in multiple endocrine neoplasia type 2B and related sporadic tumours. *Hum Mol Genet* 1994;3:237–241.

Hofstra RMW, Landsvater RM, Ceccherini I, et al. A mutation In the RET proto-ongogene associated with multiple endocrine neoplasia type 2B and sporadic medullary thyroid carcinoma. *Nature* 1994;367:375–376.

Ichihara M, Murakumo Y, Takahashi M. RET and neuroendocrine tumors. *Cancer Lett* 2004;204:197–211.

Kaplan M, Love OR, Mole SE, et al. Genetic linkage studies map the multiple endocrine neoplasia type 2 loci to a small interval on chromosome 10q11.2. *Hum Mol Genet* 1993;2:241–246.

Kinoshita S, Tanaka F, Ohashi Y, et al. Incidence of prominent corneal nerves in multiple endocrine neoplasia type 2A. *Am J Ophthalmol* 1991;111:307–311.

Kirk JF, Flowers FP, Ramos-Caro FA, et al. Multiple endocrine neoplasia type III: case report and review. *Pediatr Dermatol* 1991;8:124–128.

Sanso GE, Domene HM, Garcia R, et al. Very early detection of RET proto-oncogene mutation is crucial for preventive thyroidectomy in multiple endocrine neoplasia type 2 children: presence of C-cell malignant disease in asymptomatic carriers. *Cancer* 2002;94:323–330.

Sizemore GW, Carney JA, Gharib H, et al. Multiple endocrine neoplasia type 2B: eighteen-year follow-up of a four-generation family. *Henry Ford Hosp Med J* 1992;40:236–244.

Stratakis CA. Clinical genetics of multiple endocrine neoplasias, Carney complex and related syndromes. *J Endocrinol Invest* 201;24:370–383.

Telander RL, Zimmerman D, Sizemore GW, et al. Medullary carcinoma in children. Results of early detection and surgery. *Arch Surg* 1989;124:841–843.

Torre M, Martucciello G, Ceccherini I, et al. Diagnostic and therapeutic approach to multiple endocrine neoplasia type 28 in pediatric patients. *Pediatr Surg Int* 2002;18:378–383.

Vasen HF, van der Feltz M, Raue F, et al. The natural course of multiple endocrine neoplasia type lib. A study of 18 cases. *Arch Intern Med* 1992;152:1250–1252.

Yip L, Cote GJ, Shapiro SE, et al. Multiple endocrine neoplasia type 2: evaluation of the genotype-phenotype relationship. *Arch Surg* 2003;138:409–416; discussion 416.

Birt-Hogg-Dube

da Silva NF, Gentle D, Hesson LB, et al. Analysis of the Birt-Hogg-Dube (BHD) tumour suppressor gene in sporadic renal cell carcinoma and colorectal cancer. *J Med Genet* 2003;40:820–824.

Jacob CI, Dover JS. Birt-Hogg-Dube syndrome: treatment of cutaneous manifestations with laser skin resurfacing. *Arch Dermatol* 2001;37:98–99.

Khoo SK, Giraud S, Kahnoski K, et al. Clinical and genetic studies of Birt-Hogg-Dube syndrome [published erratum appears in *J Med Genet* 2003;40:150]. *J Med Genet* 2002;39:906–912.

Lindor NM, Hand J, Burch PA, et al. Birt-Hogg-Dube syndrome: an autosomal dominant disorder with predisposition to cancers of the kidney, fibrofolliculomas, and focal cutaneous mucinosis. *Int J Dermatol* 2001;40:653–656.

Nickerson ML, Warren MB, Toro JR, et al. Mutations in a novel gene lead to kidney tumors, lung wall defects, and benign tumors of the hair follicle in patients with the Birt-Hogg-Dube syndrome. *Cancer Cell* 2002;2:157–164.

Okimoto K, Sakurai J, Kobayashi T, et al. A germ-line insertion in the Birt-Hogg-Dube (BHD) gene gives rise to the Nihon rat model of inherited renal cancer. *Proc Natl Acad Sci USA* 2004;101:2023–2027.

Roth JS, Rabinowitz AD, Benson M, et al. Bilateral renal cell carcinoma in the Birt-Hogg-Dube syndrome. *J Am Acad Dermatol* 1993;29:1055–1056.

Toro JR, Shevchenko YO, Compton JG, et al. Exclusion of PTEN, CTNNB1, and PTCH as candidate genes for Birt-Hogg-Dube syndrome. *J Med Genet* 2002;39:E10.

Vincent A, Farley M, Chan E, et al. Birt-Hogg-Dube syndrome: a review of the literature and the differential diagnosis of firm facial papules. *J Am Acad Dermatol* 2003;49:698–705.

Zbar B, Alvord WG, Glenn G, et al. Risk of renal and colonic neoplasms and spontaneous pneumothorax in the Birt-Hogg-Dube syndrome. *Cancer Epidemiol Biomarkers Prev* 2002;11:393–400.

Chapter 6

Epidermolysis Bullosa

Juoni Uitto, M.D., Ph.D. (JU)

Clinical
Pearls

Epidermolysis Bullosa Simplex

Inheritance Autosomal dominant; very few autosomal recessive kindreds; keratin 5 and 14 genes on 12q and 17q, respectively

Prenatal Diagnosis DNA analysis

Incidence Approximately 10 to 30 cases per million live births; M=F

Age at Presentation **Weber-Cockayne**—first to third decade
Generalized (Koebner)—birth to early infancy
Dowling-Meara—birth to first month of life

Pathogenesis Mutations in keratin 5 and 14 genes produces a weakened basalar cytoskeleton (keratin intermediate filaments) and mechanical fragility with resultant intraepidermal bullae after trauma; plectin gene mutations affect hemidesmosomal protein and play a role in EB with muscular dystrophy and Ogna variant

Key Features **Weber-Cockayne**
Skin
  Palmoplantar bullae, callouses, hyperhidrosis; with/without pain, superinfection; worsening in summer months, warm temperatures
Generalized (Koebner)
Skin
  Generalized bullae with/without superinfection; worsening in summer months, warm temperatures
Mouth
  Mucosal erosions (mild)
Dowling-Meara
Skin
  Widespread bullae with "herpetiform" grouping of lesions—may have marked severity with increased morbidity, mortality in infancy; nonscarring, postinflammatory hyperpigmentation, milia; palmoplantar keratoderma with age
Nails
  Dystrophy with shedding
Mucous Membranes
  May have blistering, erosions in oral cavity (with/without secondary hoarseness) and esophagus

Differential Diagnosis **Weber-Cockayne**
  Pachyonychia congenita (p. 294)
  Tinea pedis
  Dyshidrotic eczema
  Congenital syphilis
Generalized (Koebner) and Dowling-Meara
  Neonatal herpes simplex virus (HSV)
  Bacterial sepsis
  Incontinentia pigmenti (p. 72)
  Congenital syphilis
  Bullous impetigo
  Linear IgA disease

Epidermolysis Bullosa Simplex *(continued)*

Laboratory Data

Skin biopsy for light microscopy (intraepidermal bullae), electron microscopy (clumped tonofilaments in Dowling-Meara) and immunomapping with monoclonal antibodies (see Junctional and Dystrophic EB, p. 204; 208)
Viral and bacterial cultures
DNA analysis with blood, buccal swabs

Management

Referral to dermatologist—diagnosis, trauma avoidance, wound care with whirlpool, modified Dakin's solution, topical mupirocin, topical corticosteroids, cool environment with well-ventilated leather shoes; Dowling-Meara patients may improve with increased temperature
Referral to podiatry—silicone, plastizoate orthotics; thin, white cotton socks to decrease friction and sweat
Admit to neonatal intensive care unite (NICU) if severe blistering in neonate—monitor fluids, electrolytes, sepsis

Prognosis

Debilitating with normal life span; all types tend to blister less with aging
Dowling-Meara—significant morbidity, mortality in first few months of life

Clinical Pearls

EB is a group of mechano-bullous disorders with one unifying diagnostic feature: fragility of skin. The severity of skin involvement and association of extracutaneous findings produces a broad spectrum of clinical manifestations. This clinical complexity, compounded with a plethora of eponyms, has resulted in the identification of as many as 30 different subtypes (Lamprecht IA, Gedde-Dahl T. Epidermolysis Bullosa. In: Rimoin, Connor M, Pyeritz RE, et al. *Principles and Practice of Medical Genetics*, 4th edition. New York: Churchill Livingstone, 2002.). More recently, molecularly based classification recognizes four major categories (simplex, hemidesmosomal, junctional, and dystrophic), and distinct mutations in 10 different genes expressed at the cutaneous basement membrane zone have been identified. The level of expression of the mutated genes along the basement membrane zone and in extracutaneous tissues, the types and combinations of mutations, their positions along the mutated genes, and their consequences at the mRNA and protein levels, when superimposed on individuals' genetic background, explain the tremendous phenotypic variability in this group of diseases. Precise classification of individual cases requires determination of the level of tissue separation by diagnostic immunoepitope mapping and/or transmission electron microscopy. Routine light microscropy may be helpful in identification of the simplex forms, but is often not diagnostic for the junctional and dystrophic subtypes. *JU*

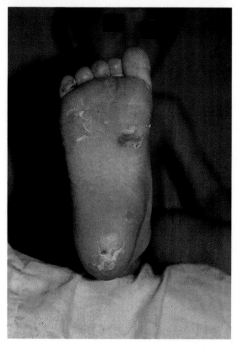

6.1. *Bullae, callous, and erosions at points of friction on plantar surface of patient with Weber-Cockayne. (81)*

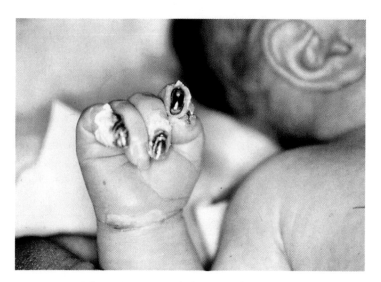

6.2. *Severe nail dystrophy prior to shedding in infant with Dowling-Meara. (82)*

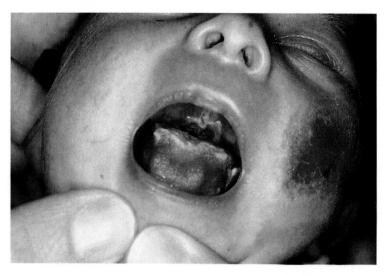

6.3. *Same patient (Fig. 6.2) with oral mucosa bullae and erosions. (82)*

Dowling-Meara

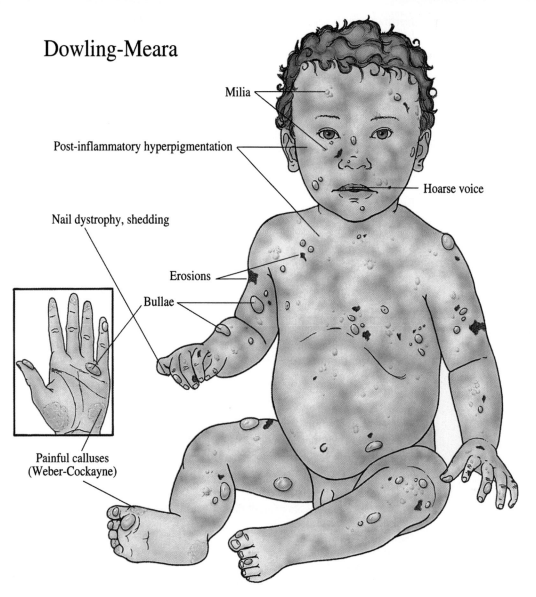

Milia

Post-inflammatory hyperpigmentation

Hoarse voice

Nail dystrophy, shedding

Erosions

Bullae

Painful calluses
(Weber-Cockayne)

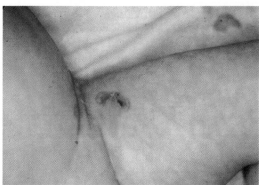

6.4. *Herpetiform bullae on thigh of same infant (Figs. 6.2,6.3). (82)*

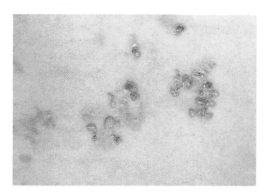

6.5. *Close-up of grouped bullae in a patient with Dowling-Meara. (83)*

Junctional Epidermolysis Bullosa (JEB)

Inheritance

Herlitz variant—autosomal recessive; *LAMA3*, *LAMB3* (80% of mutations), and *LAMC2* genes encoding laminin 5 polypeptide chains on 1q32
Non-Herlitz variant—autosomal recessive; laminin 5 and *COL17A1* on 1q32 and 10q24, respectively (other mutations identified)
JEB-pyloric atresia—autosomal recessive; *ITGA6* (integrin α6) and *ITGB4* (integrin β4) genes on chromosome 2 and 17q11, respectively

Prenatal Diagnosis

DNA analysis if mutation in family known; preimplantation determination of genotype at eight-cell stage

Incidence

Approximately 2 to 3 cases per million live births; M=F

Age at Presentation

Birth

Pathogenesis

Heterogeneous gene mutations encoding proteins at the dermal-epidermal junction are responsible for phenotype; basal cell adhesion to the basement membrane is altered resulting in a split within the lamina lucida
Herlitz—*LAMA3*, *LAMB3*, *LAMC2* gene mutations coding for the polypeptide chains within laminin 5 responsible for anchoring filament development in the lamina lucida
Non-Herlitz—laminin 5 and *COL17A1* (BP180–180 kDa bullous pemphigoid antigen) gene mutations, the latter encoding type 17 collagen (hemidesmosome protein in the lamina lucida)
JEB with pyloric atresia—*ITGB4* and *ITGA6* mutations encoding α6, β4 integrin, a hemidesmosome transmembrane protein complex

Key Features

Herlitz Variant
Skin
  Generalized bullae without scarring, milia—mild atrophy with healing; nonhealing granulation tissue periorally, scalp, neck, upper trunk, nail folds, buttocks, pinnae of the ears
Nails
  Absent (shed)
Ear-Nose-Throat
  Dysplastic teeth with enamel defects, oral erosions, laryngeal involvement with hoarseness, croup, edema
Hematologic
  Multifactorial anemia
Musculoskeletal
  Growth retardation secondary to malnutrition
Non-Herlitz Variant
Skin
  Bullae increased on extremities, heal with atrophic scarring; worse in warm environment
Nails
  Dystrophy
Hair
  Scarring alopecia
  Otherwise similar to Herlitz without granulation tissue, anemia, growth retardation and poor prognosis (see Prognosis)
Junctional EBS-Pyloric Atresia
  Skin/mucosa
    Severe congenital blistering, mucosal erosions
  Gastrointestinal
    Pyloric atresia
  Genitourinary
    Hydronephrosis, renail failure secondary to stricture development

Junctional Epidermolysis Bullosa (JEB) *(continued)*

Differential Diagnosis   Other forms of EB (p. 204; 208)
Epidermolytic hyperkeratosis (p.6)
Neonatal HSV
Bullous impetigo
Staphylococcal scalded skin syndrome
Toxic epidermal necrolysis

Laboratory Data   Bacterial, viral cultures
Skin biopsy for light, electron microscopy, immunofluoresence, cell culture
DNA analysis with blood, buccal swabs

Management

Herlitz Variant
See EBS (p. 206), tissue-engineered skin grafts, nutritional support, iron supplementation, referral to ophthalmologist; protein and/or gene therapy in the future

Non-Herlitz Variant
See EBS

JEB-Pyloric Atresia
Referral to surgeon/urologist-surgical release of GI/GU strictures, dilatation and gastrostomy

Prognosis   **Herlitz variant**—usually fatal by 3 to 4 years of age secondary to profound hypoproteinemia, anemia, and infection
Non-Herlitz variant—normal life span; bullae may improve with age
JEB-pyloric atresia—usually fatal early on

Clinical Pearls (continued from EBS)

Before the biopsy, it is helpful to induce small mini-blisters by lightly rotating a pencil eraser at the site of the biopsy. Alternatively, a biopsy could be taken from the outer edge of a blister; never biopsy center of the blister, as the dermis and epidermis become separated and lost, and secondary changes complicate the diagnosis. Molecular diagnostics can be used to confirm the assignment of the patient to a subcategory, but mutation analysis by itself cannot be performed without prior knowledge of the candidate gene/proteins through ultrastructural and immunologic analysis. The impact of molecular genetics is most evident in terms of prenatal diagnosis that is readily available for all major subtypes by DNA-based analysis from chorionic villus sample as early as the tenth week of gestation. The mutation analysis is also helpful in deciphering the mode of inheritance in instances where there is no previous family history of EB and thereby assisting in accurate genetic counseling regarding the recurrence risk. Specifically, molecular diagnostics of type VII collagen mutations can distinguish between *de novo* dominant dystrophic EB and mild recessive (mitis) EB. Similarly, mutation analysis of keratin 5 and 14 genes can distinguish between *de novo* dominant and relatively rare autosomal recessive forms of EBS. Some families may also be interested in preimplantation genetic diagnosis that, when performed in the context of *in vitro* fertilization, makes the diagnosis before the pregnancy starts and therefore avoids the ethical issues related to termination of pregnancy.   *JU*

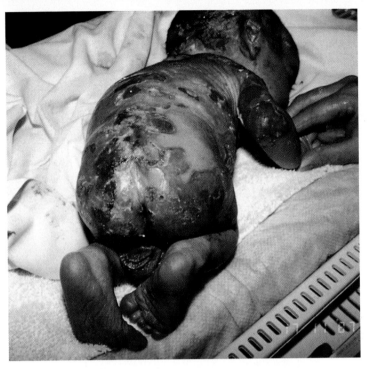

6.6. *Generalized bullae and erosions with nonhealing granulation tissue. (20)*

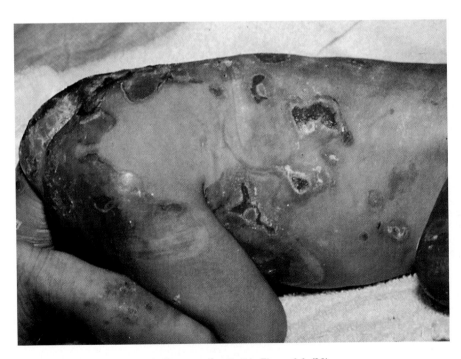

6.7. *Close-up of patient in Figure 6.6. (20)*

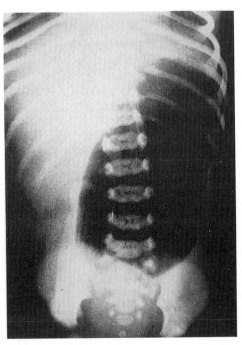

6.8. *Abdominal x-ray reveals huge stomach bubble secondary to pyloric atresia. (84)*

Herlitz
Variant

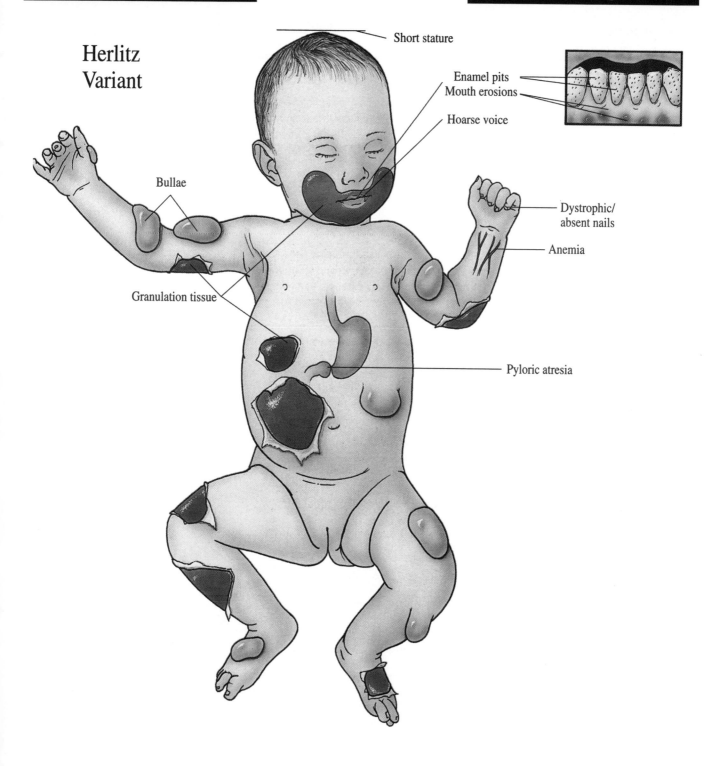

Short stature

Enamel pits
Mouth erosions

Hoarse voice

Bullae

Dystrophic/
absent nails

Anemia

Granulation tissue

Pyloric atresia

Dystrophic Epidermolysis Bullosa

Inheritance

Dominant dystrophic epidermolysis bullosa (DDEB)—autosomal dominant; *COL7A1* gene on 3p21
Recessive dystrophic epidermolysis bullosa (RDEB)—autosomal recessive; *COL7A1* gene on 3p21

Prenatal Diagnosis

DNA analysis
Chorionic villus sampling/amniocentesis analysis of fetal cells

Incidence

Approximately 2.5 cases per million live births in the United States. (DDEB more common than RDEB); M=F

Age at Presentation

DDEB—birth to early infancy
RDEB—birth

Pathogenesis

Mutations in the *COL7A1* gene responsible for type VII collagen formation, the main structural protein in anchoring fibrils, disrupts the integrity of the dermal-epidermal junction; structurally defective and reduced numbers of anchoring fibrils contribute to phenotype
RDEB-Hallopeau-Siemens subtype—more severe phenotype secondary to premature termination codon mutations causing lack of anchoring fibrils
RDEB–non-Hallopeau-Siemens subtype—less severe phenotype secondary to missence or frameshift mutations in COL7A1 producing defective anchoring fibrils
DDEB—less severe phenotype secondary to glycine substitutions that impact upon the triple helix assembly of type 7 collagen

Key Features

DDEB
Skin
Bullae can be localized to extremities or widespread; healing with/without milia, scar; mild oral disease; with/without albopapuloid lesions—hypopigmented scar-like papules increased on trunk
Nails
Dystrophic to absent
RDEB (Hallopeau-Siemens)
Skin
Generalized bullae with erosions healing with atrophic scarring, hyper/hypopig-mentation, milia; squamous cell carcinoma may occur within scars
Nails
Marked dystrophy with loss
Musculoskeletal
Digital fusions and "mitten" deformities of hands and feet secondary to repeated episodes of blistering and scarring; flexural contractures of knees, elbows, wrists; short stature secondary to malnutrition
Mucous Membranes
Oral/pharyngeal/laryngeal erosions with scarring, pain on eating, hoarse voice; esophageal erosions with strictures/stenosis; anal erosions with pain on defeca-tion/fecal impaction; conjunctival/corneal erosions with conjunctivitis/keratitis, scarring/visual loss (less common); genitourinary scarring
Teeth
Dysplastic, caries
Hematologic
Multifactorial anemia
RDEB–non-Hallopeau-Siemens—skin changes localized to acral bony prominences and fragility improves in adulthood; may be indistinguishable from DDEB; all other RDEB findings can occur but less severe

Dystrophic Epidermolysis Bullosa *(continued)*

Differential Diagnosis

Other forms of EB (pp. 204; 208)
Epidermolytic hyperkeratosis (p. 6)
Congenital erythropoietic porphyria (p. 226)
Staphylococcal scalded skin syndrome
Congenital syphilis
Neonatal HSV/bullous impetigo

Laboratory Data

Bacterial/viral cultures
Skin biopsy for light, electron microscopy; immunomapping; low threshold for skin biopsy to rule out squamous cell carcinoma
DNA analysis

Management

See EBS
Referral to symptom-specific subspecialist
Referral to nutritionist—vitamin, iron, protein supplementation, soft foods, mineral oil for chronic constipation
Referral to surgeons—repair mitten deformity, esophageal stenosis, excision of squamous cell carcinoma
Referral to dentist—soft toothbrush, pulsating water for hygiene
Systemic corticosteroids, phenytoin, retinoids, with only anecdotal success

Prognosis

DDEB
Blistering is debilitating, normal life span
RDEB
If mild, normal life span; if severe, marked morbidity and death within first three decades of life secondary to infection, anemia, malnutrition, squamous cell carcinoma; survivors markedly debilitated throughout life

Clinical Pearls (continued from Junctional EB)

As a general principle, patients with EB should be managed with a team of specialists that in addition to a dermatologist may include a gastroenterologist, nutritionist, ophthalmologist, orthopedic surgeon, hands surgeon, psychiatrist, and others, depending on the extent of the disease.

The general aims include avoidance of trauma, control of infections, and maintenance of appropriate nutritional status. If regular food intake is not able to sustain normal growth and development of the child with EB, direct gastric feeding through a button is most helpful. Infection prevention includes use of mild disinfectants in bath or whirlpool water and treatment of infections with topical Bactroban. Patients with severe recessive dystrophic EB with fusion of the digits are at special risks for development of aggressive squamous cell carcinomas which may start as early as late teens. Therefore, exercise vigilance in detecting and biopsying suspect lesions with signs of squamous metaplasia.

The website of the patient advocacy organizations DebRA of America and DEBRA International are most helpful: www.debra.org, www.debra-international. org *JU*

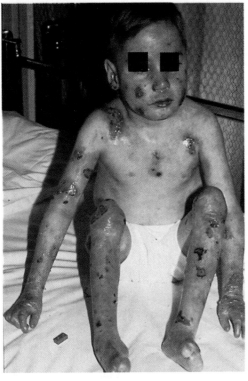

6.9. *Young boy with recessive dystrophic epidermolysis bullosa (RDEB) and generalized erosions, crusts, scarring, mitten deformity of the feet. (5)*

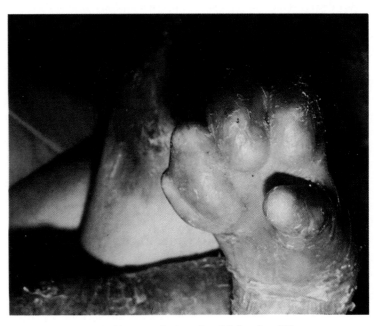

6.10. *Close-up of mitten-hand deformity. (20)*

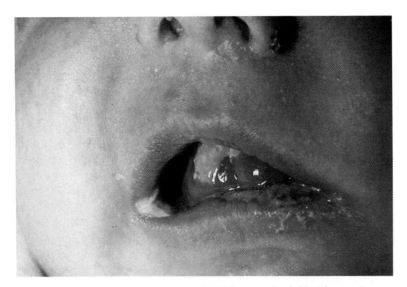

6.11. *Erosions and scarring on tongue and labial mucosa in child with recessive dystrophic epidermolysis bullosa (RDEB). (5)*

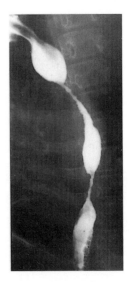

6.12. *Barium swallow demonstrating severe esophageal strictures at two sites in an 8-year-old girl with recessive dystrophic epidermolysis bullosa (RDEB). (85)*

RDEB

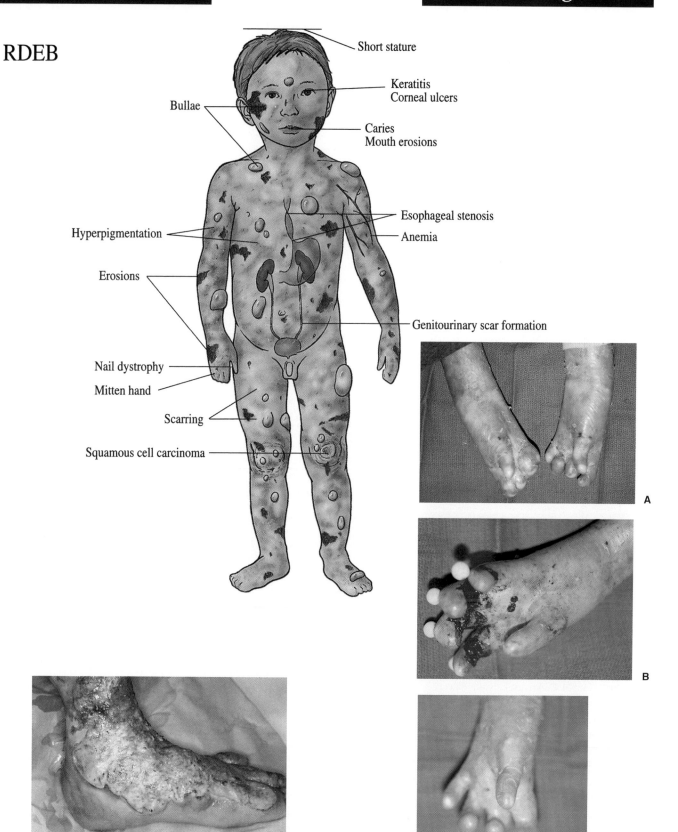

Short stature

Keratitis
Corneal ulcers

Bullae

Caries
Mouth erosions

Esophageal stenosis

Anemia

Hyperpigmentation

Erosions

Genitourinary scar formation

Nail dystrophy

Mitten hand

Scarring

Squamous cell carcinoma

A

B

C

6.13. *Squamous cell carcinoma developing in a patient with recessive dystrophic epidermolysis bullosa (RDEB). (86)*

6.14. *Surgical repair of mitten-hand deformity: preoperative, intraoperative, and postoperative views. (87)*

Suggested Reading

Epidermolysis Bullosa Simplex

Bonifas JM, Rothman AL, Epstein EH Jr. Epidermolysis bullosa simplex. Evidence in two families for keratin gene abnormalities. *Science* 1991;254:1202–1205.

Buchbinder LH, Lucky AW, Ballard E, et al. Severe infantile epidermolysis bullosa simplex. Dowling-Meara type. *Arch Dermatol* 1986;122:190–198.

Cao T, Longley MA, Wang XJ, Roop DR. An inducible mouse model for epidermolysis bullosa simplex. Implications for gene therapy. *J Cell Biol* 2001;152:651–656.

Chan Y, Anton-Lamprecht I, Yu QC, et al. A human keratin 14 "knockout": the absence of K14 leads to severe epidermolysis bullosa simplex and a function for an intermediate filament protein. *Genes Dev* 1994;8:2574–2587.

Chan YM, Yu QC, Fine JD, et al. The genetic basis of Weber-Cockayne epidermolysis bullosa simplex. *Proc Natl Acad Sci USA* 1993;90:7414–7418.

Coulombe PA, Fuchs E. Epidermolysis bullosa simplex. *Semin Dermatol* 1993;12:173–190.

Epstein EH Jr. Molecular genetics of epidermolysis bullosa. *Science* 1992;256:799–804.

Fine JD, Bauer EA, Briggaman RA, et al. Revised clinical and laboratory criteria for subtypes of inherited epidermolysis bullosa: a consensus report by the subcommittee on diagnosis and classification of the National Epidermolysis Bullosa Registry. *J Am Acad Dermatol* 1991;24:119–135.

Fontao L, Tasanen K, Huber M, et al. Molecular consequences of deletion of the cytoplasmic domain of bullous pemphigoid 180 in a patient with predominant features of epidermolysis bullosa simplex. *J Invest Dermatol* 2004;122:65–72.

Horn HM, Heiman MJ. The clinical spectrum of epidermolysis bullosa simplex. *Br J Dermatol* 2000;142:468.

Leigh IM, Lane EB. Mutations in the genes for epidermal keratins in epidermolysis bullosa and epidermolytic hyperkeratosis. *Arch Dermatol* 1993;129:1571–1577.

McLean WH, Pulkkinen L, Smith FJ, et al. Loss of plectin causes epidermolysis bullosa with muscular dystrophy: cDNA cloning and genomic organization. *Genes Dev* 1996;10:1724–1735.

McGrath JA, Ishida-Yamamoto A, Tidman MJ, et al. Epidermolysis bullosa simplex (Dowling-Meara). A clinicopathological review. *Br J Dermatol* 1992;126:421–430.

Paller AS. In this issue: the complexities of epidermolysis bullosa "simplex." *J Invest Dermatol* 2004;122:vi–vii.

Rugg EL, McLean WH, Lane EB, et al. A functional "knockout" of human keratin 14. *Genes Dev* 1994;8:2563–2573.

Schara U, Tucke J, Monier W, et al. Severe mucous membrane involvement in epidermolysis bullosa simplex with muscular dystrophy due to a novel plectin gene mutation. *Eur J Pediatr* 2004;163:218–222.

Schuilenga-Hut PH, Vlies P, Jonkman MF, et al. Mutation analysis of the entire keratin 5 and 14 genes in patients with epidermolysis bullosa simplex and identification of novel mutations. *Hum Mutat* 2003;21:447.

Shemanko CS, Horn HM, Keohane SG, et al. Laryngeal involvement in the Dowling-Meara variant of epidermolysis bullosa simplex with keratin mutations of severely disruptive potential. *Br J Dermatol* 2000;142:315–320.

Stephens K, Sybert VP, Wijsman EM, et al. A keratin 14 mutational hot spot for epidermolysis bullosa simplex, Dowling-Meara: implications for diagnosis. *J Invest Dermatol* 1993;101:240–243.

Stephens K, Zlotogorski A, Smith L, et al. An epidermolysis bullosa simplex patient with a keratin 5 homozygous defect. *J Invest Dermatol* 1994;102:609.

Weiner M, Stein A, Cash S, et al. Tetracycline and epidermolysis bullosa simplex: a double-blind, placebo-controlled, crossover randomized clinical trial. *Br J Dermatol* 2004;150:613–614.

Junctional Epidermolysis Bullosa

Aberdam D, Galliano M-F, Vailly J, et al. Herlitz's junctional epidermolysis bullosa is linked to mutations in the gene (LAMC2) for the T2 subunit of nicein/kalinin (LAMININ-5). *Nat Genet* 1994;6:299–304.

Allegra M, Gagnoux-Palacios L, Gache Y, et al. Rapid decay of alpha6 integrin caused by a mis-sense mutation in the propeller domain results in severe junctional epidermolysis bullosa with pyloric atresia. *J Invest Dermatol* 2003;121:1336–1343.

Anton-Lamprecht I. Prenatal diagnosis of genetic disorders of the skin by means of electron microscopy. *Hum Genet* 1981;59:392–405.

Bauer JW, Lanschuetzer C. Type XVII collagen gene mutations in junctional epidermolysis bullosa and prospects for gene therapy. *Clin Exp Dermatol* 2003;28:53–60.

Castiglia D, Posteraro P, Spirito F, et al. Novel mutations in the LAMC2 gene in non-Herlitz junctional epidermolysis bullosa: effects on Iaminin-5 assembly, secretion, and deposition. *J Invest Dermatol* 2001;117:731–739.

Cserhalmi-Friedman PB, Tang Y, Adler A, et al. Preimplantation genetic diagnosis in two families at risk for recurrence of Herlitz junctional epidermolysis bullosa. *Exp Dermatol* 2000;9:290–297.

Cserhalmi-Friedman PB, Baden H, Burgeson RE, et al. Molecular basis of non-lethal junctional epidermolysis bullosa: identification of a 38-base pair insertion and a splice site mutation in exon 14 of the LAMB3 gene. *Exp Dermatol* 1998;7:105.

Dessanti A, Di Benedetto V, Iannuccelli M, et al. Pyloric atresia: a new operation to reconstruct the pyloric sphincter. *J Pediatr Surg* 2004;39:297–301.

Falabella AF, Valencia IC, Eaglstein WH, et al. Tissue-engineered skin (Apligraf) in the healing of patients with epidermolysis bullosa wounds. *Arch Dermatol* 2000;136:1225–1230.

Fine JD. 19-DEJ-1, a monoclonal antibody to the hemidesmosome-anchoring filament complex, is the only reliable immunohistochemical probe for all major forms of junctional epidermolysis bullosa. *Arch Dermatol* 1990;126:1187–1190.

Hill JC, Grimwood RE, Parsons DS. Treatment of chronic erosions of junctional epidermolysis bullosa with human 184 epidermal allografts. *J Dematol Surg Oncol* 1992;18:396.

Holbrook KA, Christiano AM, Elias S, et al. Prenatal diagnosis of inherited epidermolysis bullosa: ultrastructural, antigenic and molecular approaches. In: Fine JD, Bauer EA, McGuire J Moshell A, eds. *Epidermolys¹s Bullosa: Clinical, Epidemiologic and Laboratory Advances and the Findings of the National Epidermolysis Bullosa Registry*. Baltimore: Johns Hopkins University Press, 1999:351–373.

Iacovacci S, Cicuzza S, Odorisio T, et al. Novel and recurrent mutations in the integrin beta 4 subunit gene causing lethal junctional epidermolysis bullosa with pyloric atresia. *Exp Dermatol* 2003;12:716–720.

Kivirikko S, McGrath JA, Pulkkinen L, et al. Mutational hotspots in the LAMBS gene in the lethal (Herlitz) type of junctional epidermolysis bullosa. *Hum Mol Genet* 1996;5:231–237.

Lestringant GG, Akel SR, Qayed KI. The pyloric atresia-junctional epidermolysis bullosa syndrome. Report of a case and review of the literature. *Arch Dermatol* 1992;128:1083–1086.

McGrath JA, Pulkkinen L, Christiano AM, et al. Altered laminin 5 expression due to mutations in the gene encoding the B3 chain (LAMB3) in generalized atrophic benign epidermolysis bullosa. *J Invest Dermatol* 1995;104:467–474.

Mellerio JE, Pulkkinen L, McMillan JR, et al. Pyloric atresia-junctional epidermolysis bullosa syndrome: mutations in the 134 gene (ITGB4) in two unrelated patients with mild disease. *Br J Dermatol* 1998;139:862–871.

Morrell DS, Fine JD. Junctional epidermolysis bullosa with pyloric stenosis. *Pediatr Dermatol* 2001;18:539–540.

Nakano A, Chao SC, Pulkkinen L, et al. Laminin 5 mutations in junctional epidermolysis bullosa: molecular basis of Herlitz vs non-Herlitz phenotypes. *Hum Genet* 2002;110:41–51.

Ortiz-Urda S, Lin Q, Yant SR, et al. Sustainable correction of junctional epidermolysis bullosa via transposon-mediated nonviral gene transfer. *Gene Ther* 2003;10:1099–1104.

Pulkkinen L, Christiano AM, Airenne T, et al. Mutations in the T2 chain gene

(LAMC2) of kalinin/laminin-5 in the junctional forms of epidermolysis bullosa. *Nat Genet* 1994;6:293–298.

Pulkkinen L, Uitto J. Hemidesmosomal variants of epidermolysis bullosa. Mutations in the alpha6beta4 integrin and the 180-kD bullous pemphigoid antigen/type XVII collagen genes. *Exp Dermatol* 1998;7:46–64.

Robbins PB, Lin Q, Goodnough JB, et al. In vivo restoration of laminin 5 β3 expression and function in junctional epidermolysis bullosa. *Proc Natl Acad Sci USA* 2001;98:5193–5198.

Robbins PB, Sheu SM, Goodnough JB, et al. Impact of laminin 5 beta3 gene versus protein replacement on gene expression patterns in junctional epidermolysis bullosa. *Hum Gene Ther* 2001;12:1443–1448.

Schofield OM, Fine JD, Verrando P, et al. GB3 monoclonal antibody for the diagnosis of junctional epidermolysis bullosa: results of a multicenter study. *J Am Acad Dermatol* 1990;23:1078–1083.

Seitz CS, Giudice GJ, Balding SD, et al. BP180 gene delivery in junctional epidermolysis bullosa. *Gene Ther* 1999;6:42–47.

Vailly J, Pulkkinen L, Miguel C, et al. Identification of a homozygous one-basepair deletion in exon 14 of the LAMB3 gene in a patient with Herlitz junctional epidermolysis bullosa and prenatal diagnosis in a family at risk for recurrence. *J Invest Dermatol* 1995;104:462–466.

Verrando P, Schofield D, Ishida-Yamamoto A, et al. Nicein (BM-600) in junctional epidermolysis bullosa: polyclonal antibodies provide new clues for pathogenic role. *J Invest Dermatol* 1993;101:738–743.

Vidal F, Aberdam D, Miquel C, et al. Integrin beta 4 mutations associated with junctional epidermolysis bullosa with pyloric atresia. *Nat Genet* 1995;10:229–234.

Wright JT, Johnson LB, Fine JD. Development defects of enamelin humans with hereditary epidermolysis bullosa. *Arch Oral Biol* 1993;38:945–955.

Dystrophic Epidermolysis Bullosa

Chen M, Costa FK, Lindvay CR, et al. The recombinant expression of full-length type VII collagen and characterization of molecular mechanisms underlying dystrophic epidermolysis bullosa. *J Biol Chem* 2002;277:2118–2124.

Christiano AM, Anhalt G, Gibbons S, et al. Premature termination codons in the type VII collagen gene (COL7A1) underlie severe, mutilating recessive dystrophic epidermolysis bullosa. *Genomics* 1994;21:160–168.

De Benedittis M, Petruzzi M, Favia G, et al. Oro-dental manifestations in Hallopeau-Siemens-type recessive dystrophic epidermolysis bullosa. *Clin Exp Dermatol* 2004;29:128–132.

Falabella AF, Valencia IC, Eaglstein WH, et al. Tissue-engineered skin (Apiigra) in the healing of patients with epidermolysis bullosa wounds. *Arch Dermatol* 2000;136:1225–1230.

Fine JD, Johnson LB, Suchindran C, et al. Cancer and inherited epidermolysis bullosa. Lifetable analyses of the national epidermolysis bullosa registry study population. In: Fine JD, Bauer EA, McGuire J, Moshell A, eds. *Epidermolysis Bullosa: Clinical, Epidemiologic and Laboratory Advances and the Findings of the National Epidermolysis Bullosa Registry*. Baltimore: Johns Hopkins University Press, 1999:175–192.

Fine JD, Fady RAJ, Bauer EA, et al. Revised classification system for inherited epidermolysis bullosa: report of the second international consensus meeting on diagnosis and classification of epidermolysis bullosa. *J Am Acad Dermatol* 2000;42:1051–1066.

Fine JD, Johnson LB, Weiner M, et al. Assessment of mobility, activities and pain in different subtypes of epidermolysis bullosa. *Clin Exp Dermatol* 2004;29:122–127.

Fine JD, Johnson LB, Weiner M, et al. Chemoprevention of squamous cell carcinoma in recessive dystrophic epidermolysis bullosa: results of a phase 1 trial of systemic isotretinoin. *J Am Acad Dermatol* 2004;50:563–571.

Fivenson DP, Scherschun L, Choucair M, et al. Graftskin therapy in epidermolysis bullosa. *J Am Acad Dermatol* 2003;48:886–892.

Fivenson DP, Scherschun L, Cohen LV. Apligraf in the treatment of severe mitten deformity associated with recessive dystrophic epidermolysis bullosa. *Plast Reconstr Surg* 2003;112:584–588.

Glicenstein J, Mariani D, Haddad R. The hand in recessive dystrophic epidermolysis bullosa. *Hand Clin* 2000;16:637–645.

Griffin RP, Mayou BJ. The anaesthetic management of patients with dystrophic epidermolysis bullosa. A review of 44 patients over a 10 year period. *Anaesthesia* 1993;48:810–815.

Hasegawa T, Suga Y, Mizoguchi M, et al. Clinical trial of allogeneic cultured dermal substitute for the treatment of intractable skin ulcers in 3 patients with recessive dystrophic epidermolysis bullosa. *J Am Acad Dermatol* 2004;50:803–804.

Hovnanian A, Christiana AM, Uitto J. The molecular genetics of dystrophic epidermolysis bullosa. *Arch Dermatol* 1993;129:1566–1570.

Hovnanian A, Hilal L, Blanchet-Bardon C, et al. DNA-based prenatal diagnosis of generalized recessive dystrophic epidermolysis bullosa in six pregnancies at risk for recurrence. *J Invest Dermatol* 1995;104:456–461.

Iohom G, Lyons B. Anaesthesia for children with epidermolysis bullosa: a review of 20 years' experience. *Eur J Anaesthesiol* 2001;18:745–754.

Ishiko A, Masunaga T, Ota T, et al. Does the position of the premature termination codon in COL7A1 correlate with the clinical severity in recessive dystrophic epidermolysis bullosa? *Exp Dermatol* 2004;13:229–233.

Kawasaki H, Sawarura D, Iwao F, et al. Squamous cell carcinoma developing in a 12-year-old boy with nonHallopeau-Siemens recessive dystrophic epidermolysis bullosa. *Br J Dermatol* 2003;148:1047–1050.

Lentz SR, Raish RJ, Orlowski EP, et al. Squamous cell carcinoma in epidermolysis bullosa. Treatment with systemic chemotherapy. *Cancer* 1990;66:1276–1278.

Masunaga T, Shimizu H, Takizawa Y, et al. Combination of novel premature termination codon and glycine substitution mutations in COL7A1 leads to moderately severe recessive dystrophic epidermolysis bullosa. *J Invest Dermatol* 2000;114:204–205.

Ortiz-Urda S, Lin Q, Green CL, et al. Injection of genetically engineered fibroblasts corrects regenerated human epidermolysis bullosa skin tissue. *J Clin Invest* 2003;111:251–255.

Pfendner EG, Nakano A, Pulkkinen L, et al. Prenatal diagnosis for epidermolysis bullosa: a study of 144 consecutive pregnancies at risk. *Prenat Diagn* 2003;23:447–456.

Pulkkinen L, Uitto J. Mutation analysis and molecular genetics of epidermolysis bullosa. *Matrix Biol* 1999;18:29–42.

Ryynanen M, Knowlton RG, Parente MG, et al. Human type VII collagen: genetic linkage of the gene (COL7A1) on chromosome 3 to dominant dystrophic epidermolysis bullosa. *Am J Hum Genet* 1991;49:797–803.

Serrano-Martinez MC, Bagan JV, Silvestre FJ, et al. Oral lesions in recessive dystrophic epidermolysis bullosa. *Oral Dis* 2003;9:264–268.

Terrill PJ, Mayou BJ, Pemberton J. Experience in the surgical management of the hand in dystrophic epidermolysis bullosa. *Br J Plast Surg* 1992;45:435–442.

Travis SP, McGrath JA, Turnbull AJ, et al. Oral and gastrointestinal manifestations of epidermolysis bullosa. *Lancet* 1992;340:1505–1506.

Weber F, Bauer JW, Sepp N, et al. Squamous cell carcinoma in junctional and dystrophic epidermolysis bullosa. *Acta Derm Venereol* 2001;81:189–192.

Wollina U, Konrad H, Fischer T. Recessive epidermolysis bullosa dystrophicans (Hallopeau–Siemens): improvement of wound healing by autologous epidermal grafts on an esterified hyaluronic acid membrane. *J Dermatol* 2001;28:217–220.

Wong WL, Entwisle K, Pemberton J. Gastrointestinal manifestations in the Hallopeau-Siemens variant of recessive dystrophic epidermolysis bullosa. *Br J Radiol* 1993;66:788–793.

Wong WL, Pemberton J. The musculoskeletal manifestations of epidermolysis bullosa: an analysis of 19 cases with a review of the literature. *Br J Radiol* 1992;65:480–484.

Chapter 7

Disorders of Porphyrin Metabolism

Clinical Pearls

Vincent DeLeo, M.D. (VD)

Porphyria Cutanea Tarda (PCT)

Inheritance
Autosomal dominant; Uroporphyrinogen (UROGEN) decarboxylase gene on 1p34—less common (20% of cases)
Sporadic/acquired—more common

Prenatal Diagnosis
DNA analysis in familial cases

Incidence
Most common porphyria; approximately 1:25,000 in North America; M=F

Age at Presentation
Usually third to fourth decade of life; some familial patients in first decade of life

Pathogenesis
UROGEN decarboxylase gene mutation leads to UROGEN decarboxylase deficiency in erythrocytes, hepatocytes, and 50% of all tissues in familial form; deficient enzyme in hepatocytes in sporadic form
Increased uroporphyrin (URO) in skin leads to photosensitization after absorbing light energy in soret band (400–410 nm)
Alcohol, estrogen, hepatic tumors precipitate all acquired forms and may unmask familial cases

Key Features
Skin
Delayed-type photosensitivity with bullae, erosions, skin fragility, facial hypertrichosis, hyperpigmentation; late changes include scarring, milia, sclerodermoid changes, subcutaneous calcification, alopecia
Gastrointestinal
Hepatocellular carcinoma (rare)
Liver hemosiderosis
Endocrine
Diabetes mellitus

Differential Diagnosis
Variegate porphyria (VP; p. 218)
Pseudoporphyria
Epidermolysis bullosa acquisita
Hereditary coproporphyria (p. 221)

Laboratory Data
Plasma porphyrin level and fluorescence spectrum—24-hour urine porphyrin level (≠URO) complete blood count (CBC), liver function tests, iron level, hepatitis panel, liver scan; in-office urine screen—coral pink fluorescence with Wood's light (high number of false-negatives)

Management
Phlebotomy—1 unit every 2 to 4 weeks until hemoglobin (Hb) 11 g/dL, hematocrit (Hct) 35
Antimalarials (low dose)
Eliminate alcohol, estrogen, iron exposure
Sun protection/physical-block sunscreens
Referral to dermatologist, internist, gastroenterologist

Prognosis
Normal life span with clinical and biochemical remission achievable with treatment; premature death with hepatocellular carcinoma

Clinical Pearls

I refer most of my patients to a hepatologist for work-up . . . Urine fluorescence in the office is a fun test, but certainly not an adequate screen given high number of false-negatives . . . Plasma porphyrin screens are useful in following patients therapeutically but I have had difficulty recently with plasma porphyrin analysis from the major labs around the country, so I am sticking to urine for follow-up . . . Some studies have shown extremely high levels of hepatitis C in patients with porphyria cutanea tarda (PCT) . . . I get a hepatitis panel . . . I recommend titanium dioxide or mexoryl containing sunscreens . . . Women usually have electrolysis or use depilatories for the hypertrichosis . . . First line therapy is phlebotomy as an outpatient if there are no contraindications . . . Clinical response lags behind biochemical response . . . I've taken care of at least 30 patients, and I've never seen a failure with phlebotomy . . . There is no evidence suggesting that by simply having PCT leads to liver damage . . . I would want my residents to know how to differentiate VP from PCT . . . They can have identical cutaneous findings . . . Once you have a positive porphyrin screen, you must rule out a seizure history, and check the ratio of URO to COPRO in the urine . . . In PCT, 8:1; in VP, 1:1 or COPRO > URO.   *VD*

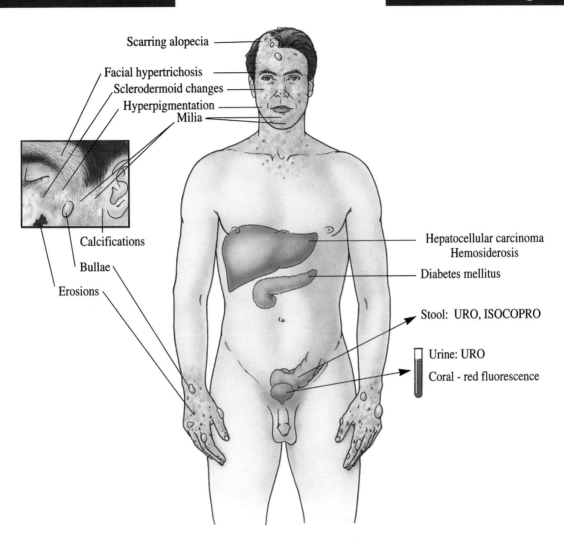

Scarring alopecia

Facial hypertrichosis

Sclerodermoid changes

Hyperpigmentation

Milia

Calcifications

Bullae

Erosions

Hepatocellular carcinoma
Hemosiderosis

Diabetes mellitus

Stool: URO, ISOCOPRO

Urine: URO

Coral - red fluorescence

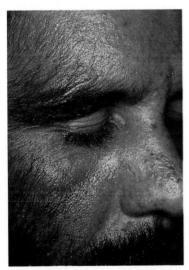

7.1. *Facial hypertrichosis with erosions and scarring on nose. (5)*

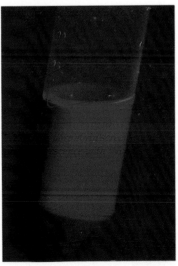

7.2. *Urine porphyrin screen-coral-pink fluorescence with Wood's light. (5)*

Variegate Porphyria (VP)

Inheritance
Autosomal dominant; protoporphyrinogen (*PROTOGEN*) oxidase gene on 1q22; severe forms associated with hemochromatosis gene on 6p21

Prenatal Diagnosis
DNA analysis

Incidence
Most common in South Africa—1:330 in white population
Elsewhere approximately 1:50,000 to 100,000; M=F

Age at Presentation
Usually begins after puberty in second to third decade of life

Pathogenesis
Mutation in *PROTOGEN* oxidase gene causes a 50% decrease in PROTOGEN oxidase activity
Acute attacks precipitated by drugs (barbiturates, estrogen, griseofulvin, sulfonamides), infection, fever, alcohol, pregnancy, decreased caloric intake
Increased Δ-aminolevulinic acid (ALA) synthetase with attacks

Key Features
Skin
Indentical to PCT with bullae, erosions, skin fragility, scarrring, millia, hypertrichosis, hyperpigmentation on photodistributed face, neck, and dorsum of hands
Acute Attacks (i.e., Acute Intermittent Porphyria and Hereditary Coproporphyra)
Gastrointestinal
Colicky abdominal pain, nausea, vomiting, constipation
Central Nervous System
Peripheral neuropathy with pain, weakness, paralysis; confusional state, anxiety, depression, delerium, seizures, coma
Cardiovascular
Tachycardia, hypertension

Differential Diagnosis
Porphyria cutanea tarda (p. 216)
Acute intermittent porphyria (AIP; p. 220)
Hereditary coproporphyria (HCP; p. 221)

Laboratory Data
Plasma porphyrin level
Plasma porphyrin fluorescence spectrum—626 nm is diagnostic
Twenty-four–hour urine porphyrin levels—coproporphyrin = or > uroporphyrin
Urinary ALA and porphobillinogen (PBG) levels increased during attacks
Fecal porphyrin levels—markedly elevated; protoporphyrin > coproporphyrin

Management
Glucose loading, hematin infusion during attacks
Avoid drug precipitators, severe dieting
Referral to dermatologist—opaque sunscreens, topical antibiotics, β-carotene
Referral to neurologist—antiseizure medication, pain control
Referral to nutritionist—small carbohydrate meals to maintain glucose levels

Prognosis
Acute attacks may be life threatening and may leave residual neurologic damage

Clinical Pearls

Still most common in the Dutch Afrikaners of South Africa . . . 50% with combination skin and neurologic, 15% just neurologic, 35% just skin . . . Don't bleed patients—you might rev up the cycle and lead to an attack . . . The trick is sun avoidance with titanium dioxide and mexoryl sunscreen . . . Need to work with neurologist who is aware of porphyria . . . Prior to surgery, the neurologist should talk with the anesthesiologist . . . Long periods of NPO (nothing by mouth) may be dangerous . . . Treat infection quickly . . . Hand patient "avoid these medications" list . . . Should they become pregnant?—tough question . . . Needs to be discussed with primary physician and obstetrician.   *VD*

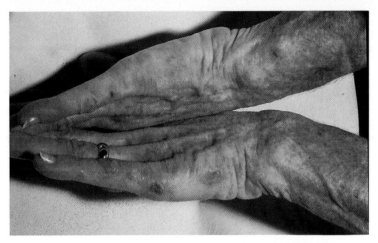

7.3. *Bullae, erosions scattered on dorsum of hands in patient with variegate porphyria (VP). (5)*

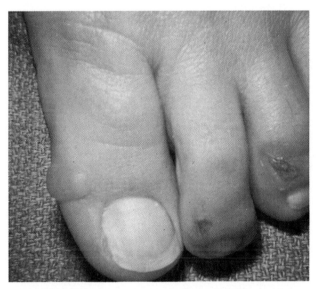

7.4. *Patient with variegate porphyria (VP) with bullae, erosions on toes. (5)*

Acute Intermittent Porphyria (AIP)

Inheritance	Autosomal dominant; Porphobilinogen deaminase (*PBGD*) gene on 11q23
Prenatal Diagnosis	Amniocentesis: porphobilinogen (PBG) deaminase deficiency in cultured amniotic fluid cells DNA analysis
Incidence	Approximately 1:66,000 worldwide; much higher in Scandinavia M:F=1:1.5
Age at Presentation	Third to fourth decade of life
Pathogenesis	*PBGD* gene mutation causes a deficiency in *PBGD* activity Acute attacks may be spontaneous or precipitated by drugs (see VP, p. 218), estrogen, infection, fever, decreased caloric intake, alcohol, pregnancy, menses Increased ALA synthetase with attacks Mechanism for attacks unknown
Key Features	**Acute Attacks** **Central Nervous System** Peripheral neuropathy with pain, weakness, paralysis; anxiety, depression, seizures, confusional state, delirium, coma; rarely, respiratory failure caused by paralysis **Gastrointestinal** Colicky abdominal pain, nausea, vomiting, constipation **Cardiovascular** Tachycardia, hypertension **Hematologic** Hyponatremia secondary to antidiuretic hormone (ADH) secretion
Differential Diagnosis	VP (p. 218) Hereditary coproporphyria (p. 221) Acute abdomen Organic neurologic/psychiatric disease
Laboratory Data	Enzyme assay—decreased *PBGD* in red blood cells Plasma porphyrin level and fluorescence spectrum Twenty-four–hour or spot urine—increased ALA and porphobilinogen during and between attacks; dark, port wine-colored urine CBC with differential (leukocytosis), chemical screen
Management	Glucose load, hematin infusion during acute attacks Referral to neurologist—antiseizure medication, pain control Avoid precipitators Referral to nutritionist—small carbohydrate meals to maintain glucose levels Fluid and electrolytes monitored Check family for carrier status with enzyme assay
Prognosis	Improved with avoidance of precipitators; acute attacks may be life threatening and leave residual neurologic deficits

Clinical Pearls

I can see these patients being labeled as having "chronic fatigue syndrome" . . . A lot of people end up having multiple exploratory laporatomies . . . They've seen multiple physicians including gastrointestinal, neurologic, and psychiatric . . . Many are thought to be crazy . . . Always give list of medicatoins to avoid . . . Pregnancy, surgical issues must be discussed with patients and their physicians . . . They can die from their attacks . . . But I don't think it's a high mortality rate at all . . . Like other seizure patients, they shouldn't swim alone.   *VD*

Hereditary Coproporphyria (HCP)

Inheritance	Autosomal dominant; coproporphyrinogen (*COPROGEN*) oxidase gene on 3q12
Prenatal Diagnosis	DNA analysis
Incidence	Rare—estimated 2 per million in Denmark; M=F; symptomatic M:F=1:2.5
Age at Presentation	Third to fourth decade of life
Pathogenesis	*COPROGEN* oxidase gene mutation causes the phenotype Acute attacks precipitated by same factors as AIP and VP Increased ALA synthetase with attacks

Key Features	**Skin (approximately 30% of symptomatic patients)**
	    Delayed photosensitivity changes similar to PCT and VP (see pp. 216, 218)
	Acute Attacks
	    Central Nervous System
	        Similar to AIP and VP (see p. 218, 220)
	    Gastrointestinal
	        Similar to AIP and VP (see p. 218, 220)

Differential Diagnosis	AIP (p. 220) VP (p. 218) PCT (p. 216)
Laboratory Data	Plasma porphyrin level and fluorescence spectrum Increased coproporphyrin levels in stool and urine Increased ALA and PBG in urine during attacks only
Management	See AIP (p. 220) and VP (p. 218)
Prognosis	Acute attacks may be life threatening; many gene carriers are asymptomatic throughout life

Clinical Pearls

Neurologic symptoms are more common than cutaneous . . . Clinical is the same for HCP and VP . . . Differentiation is based on porphyrin profiles . . . Again, hematin and glucose loading for attacks . . . β-carotene may help the skin problems . . . AIP can be differentiated with the PBGD enzyme assay.   *VD*

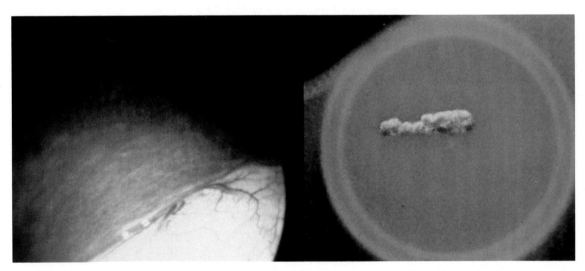

7.5. *Left. Laparoscopic exam reveals geographic pattern of gray-blue depressions on surface of liver in hereditary coproporphyria (HCP). (88) Right. Liver biopsy from depression fluoresces with ultraviolet light. (89)*

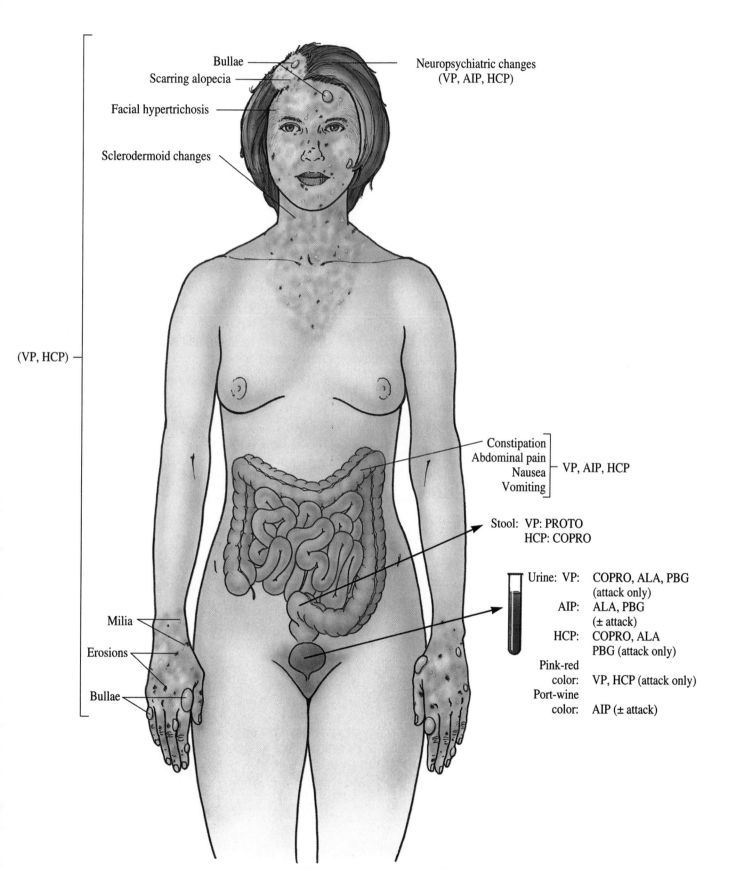

Bullae

Scarring alopecia

Facial hypertrichosis

Sclerodermoid changes

Neuropsychiatric changes
(VP, AIP, HCP)

(VP, HCP)

Constipation
Abdominal pain
Nausea
Vomiting
VP, AIP, HCP

Stool: VP: PROTO
HCP: COPRO

Urine: VP: COPRO, ALA, PBG
(attack only)
AIP: ALA, PBG
(± attack)
HCP: COPRO, ALA
PBG (attack only)

Pink-red
color: VP, HCP (attack only)
Port-wine
color: AIP (± attack)

Milia

Erosions

Bullae

Erythropoietic Protoporphyria (EPP)

Inheritance	Autosomal dominant; ferrochelatase (*FECH*) gene on 18q22
Prenatal Diagnosis	DNA analysis
Incidence	Most common erythropoietic porphyria—thousands of cases reported; M=F
Age at Presentation	Early childhood—average 4 years old
Pathogenesis	*FECH* gene mutation leads to ferrochelatase deficiency with excess protoporphyrin production and subsequent photosensitivity

Key Features	**Skin**
	  Early—Burning, stinging, erythematous plaques with edema in photodistribution on face, neck, back of hands during or shortly after exposure to UV light; rare vesicles/bullae
	  Late—waxy, thickened scarring over nose, face, back of hands; linear depressed scars periorally; shallow, elliptical scars on face
	Gastrointestinal
	  Cholelithiasis
	  Liver disease presenting as jaundice; may lead to cirrhosis, hepatic failure (rare)
	Hematologic
	  Mild anemia

Differential Diagnosis	Erythropoietic coproporphyria—clinically identical to EPP but increased coproporphyrin and protoporphyrin in red blood cells; enzyme defect unknown Polymorphic light eruption Hydroa vacciniforme Other porphyrias (pp. 216; 218; 220; 221) Solar urticaria
Laboratory Data	Plasma porphyrin level and fluorescence spectrum Increased free protoporphyrin in red blood cells, stool CBC, liver function tests Liver/gallbladder scans if symptomatic
Management	Referral to dermatologist—oral β-carotene, sunscreens Referral to gastroenterologist if symptomatic, elevated liver function tests Iron, red blood cell transfusion, hematin, cholestyramine, activated charcoal have all been tried with limited success; liver transplant if advanced disease Avoid alcohol, hepatotoxic drugs
Prognosis	If spared liver disease, normal life span

Clinical Pearls

Often kids can't verbalize that it's the sun that bothers them . . . They tell mom, "I don't want to go out" . . . The pain lasts for about 24 hours after outdoor exposure . . . They learn to put ice on skin to relieve burning and stinging . . . Their skin looks like the waxy lesions of lipoid proteinosis . . . They've cloned the gene for ferrochelatase . . . Like other porphyrias, there is a variable clinical presentation because a number of gene loci defects can cause the same enzyme deficiency . . . They can get gallstones at an early age . . . A very small percentage go on to fatal hepatic disease . . . Some patients have been transplanted . . . Get yearly plasma porphyrin screens and LFTs . . . Porphyrin levels will shoot up with liver failure . . . I don't know if there's anything to stop the liver disease once it starts . . . β-Carotene works for skin disease in 75% of cases . . . Orange palms don't bother patients . . . Critical to take synthetic and not natural carotene . . . Contaminants in the natural form may have caused hypervitaminosis A . . . Titanium dioxide and mexoryl sunscreens may help.   *VD*

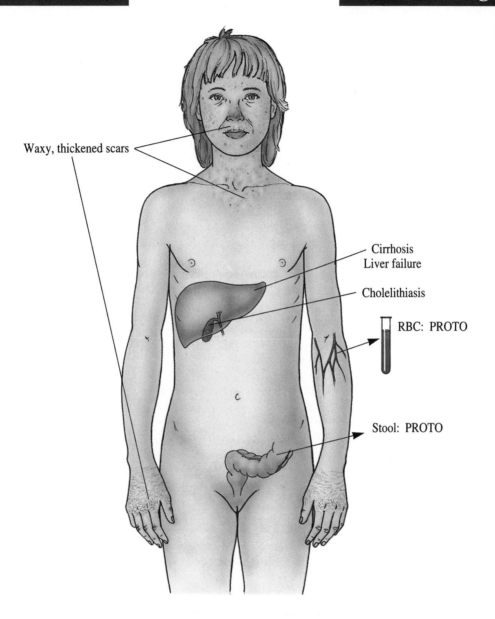

Waxy, thickened scars

Cirrhosis
Liver failure

Cholelithiasis

RBC: PROTO

Stool: PROTO

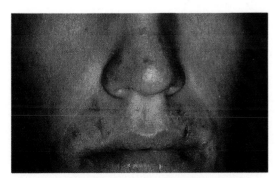

7.6. *Erosions, scars, and crusts on face. (90)*

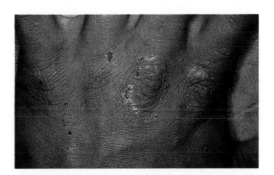

7.7. *Waxy, thickened scars, crusts on dorsum of hands. (90)*

Congenital Erythropoietic Porphyria (CEP)

Synonym	Günther's disease
Inheritance	Autosomal recessive; uroporphyrinogen III (*UROGEN III*) synthase gene on 10q25.2–q26
Prenatal Diagnosis	Amniocentesis: *UROGEN III* synthase activity decreased in cultured amniotic cells DNA analysis
Incidence	Very rare—less than 200 case reports; M=F
Age at Presentation	Infancy to early childhood
Pathogenesis	*UROGEN III* synthase gene mutations produce phenotype
Key Features	**Skin** **Early**—immediate photosensitivity with burning, edema, erythema, vesicles/bullae, erosions, infection **Late**—mutilating scar with deformation of nose, ears, fingers; scarring alopecia, hyper/hypopigmentation, sclerodermoid changes **Hair** Hypertrichosis with lanugo-like hair over face, neck, and extremities **Teeth** Red-brown staining of deciduous and permanent teeth; red-pink fluorescence with Wood's light **Eyes** Photophobia, ectropion, conjunctivitis **Hematology** Hemolyic anemia **Gastrointestinal** Splenomegaly
Differential Diagnosis	Hepatoerythropoietic porphyria (p. 228) Other porphyrias (pp. 216; 218; 220) Epidermolysis bullosa (p. 200) Xeroderma pigmentosum (p. 174) Bullous pemphigoid
Laboratory Data	Enzyme assay with red blood cells: uroporphyrinogen III synthetase level decreased; plasma porphyrin level and fluorescence spectrum; markedly increased uroporphyrin in red blood cells, plasma, and urine; increased coproporphyrin in stool; CBC
Management	Referral to dermatologist—avoidance of sun, physical-block sunscreens, wide-brimmed hats, photoprotective clothing, antibiotics for skin infections, β-carotene Referral to surgeon—splenectomy to improve hemolytic anemia Packed red blood cell transfusions, intravenous hematin, activated charcoal all have varying degrees of success and limited by side effects Referral to dentist—porcelain or acrylic crowns
Prognosis	If picked up early and closely followed with appropriate prophylactic measures, favorable life span; however, depending on severity, quality of life may be adversely affected

Clinical Pearls

Mom comes into the office with pink diapers . . . Babies cry and scream when outside . . . Can see red teeth in babies . . . Once again, variable severity depending on specific gene defect . . . It's a horrible disease . . . Treatment is avoidance, avoidance, avoidance of sun exposure . . . If they're well taken care of, normal life span . . . If severe, it may be a very difficult, mostly indoor life . . . Hats, titanium dioxide sunscreen, play tennis at night . . . May be set up for bone marrow transplant if severe enough . . . Nowadays, they are picked up early on . . . Those pictures of severe mutilation and scarring should be things of the past.   *VD*

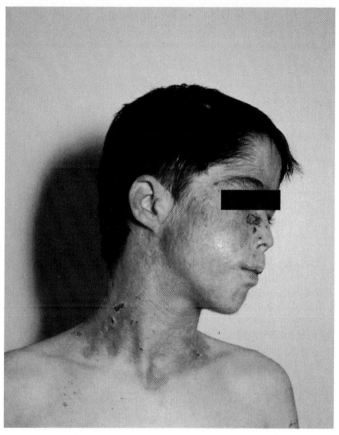

7.8. *Hypertrichosis, hyperpigmentation, mutilating scar with pinched nose, and erosions distributed on face, neck of patient with erythropoietic porphyria (CEP). Note sharp cut-off on neck demonstrating photodistribution. (48)*

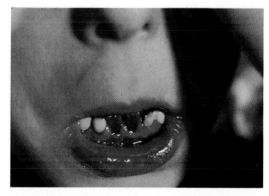

7.9. *Purple-brown stained teeth in child with erythropoietic porphyria (CEP). (5)*

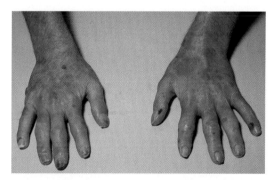

7.10. *Dorsum of hands with erosions, scarring in patient with CEP. (5)*

Hepatoerythropoietic Porphyria (HEP)

Inheritance	Autosomal dominant; uroporphyrinogen (*UROGEN*) decarboxylase gene on 1p34
Prenatal Diagnosis	DNA analysis
Incidence	Very rare; less than 20 case reports; M=F
Age at Presentation	Usually 1 year old
Pathogenesis	UROGEN decarboxylase markedly deficient due to a homozygous or compound heterozygote mutation in the *UROGEN* decarboxylase gene

Key Features	**Skin**
	  Similar to CEP with severe photosensitivity (see p. 226)
	  Photosensitivity diminishes with age
	Hematologic
	  Hemolytic anemia
	Gastrointestinal
	  Splenomegaly
	Genitourinary
	  Dark urine at birth

Differential Diagnosis	CEP (p. 226) Other porphyrias (pp. 216; 218; 220; 221)
Laboratory Data	Plasma porphyrin level and fluorescence spectrum Increased protoporphyrin in red blood cells (EP with increased uroporphyrin in red blood cells); increased urinary uroporphyrin, increased fecal coproporphyrin CBC
Management	Referral to dermatologist—avoidance of sun exposure, photoprotect with physical-block sunscreens, hats, clothing Referral to gastroenterologist, hematologist if symptomatic
Prognosis	Normal life span

Clinical Pearls

Patients resemble people with a mild Günther's . . . Differentiate from Günther's by looking at red cell porphyrins . . . For some ungodly reason, patients with HEP have proto in their red cells while patients with EP have uro . . . Less photosensitive than EP but more than EPP . . . The major treatment is avoidance, avoidance, avoidance of the sun . . . Titanium dioxide and mexoryl sunscreen.   *VD*

Skin

Associated Findings

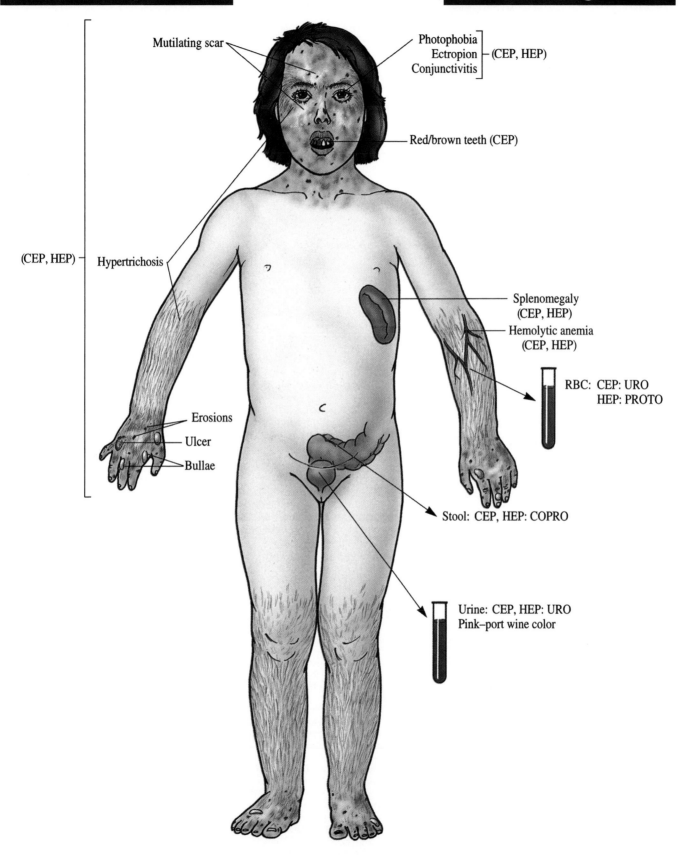

Mutilating scar

Photophobia
Ectropion — (CEP, HEP)
Conjunctivitis

Red/brown teeth (CEP)

(CEP, HEP) Hypertrichosis

Splenomegaly
(CEP, HEP)

Hemolytic anemia
(CEP, HEP)

RBC: CEP: URO
HEP: PROTO

Erosions
Ulcer
Bullae

Stool: CEP, HEP: COPRO

Urine: CEP, HEP: URO
Pink–port wine color

Suggested Reading

Porphyria Cutanea Tarda

Blauvelt A, Harris HR, Hogan DJ, et al. Porphyria cutanea tarda and human immunodeficiency virus infection. *Int J Dermatol* 1992;31:474–479.

Cappellini MD, Martinez di Montemuros F, et al. Seven novel point mutations in the uroporphyrinogen decarboxylase (UROD) gene in patients with familial porphyria cutanea tarda (f-PCT). *Hum Mutat* 2001;17:350.

Dubart A, Mattel MG, Raich N, et al. Assignment of human uroporphyrinogen decarboxylase (URO-D) to the p34 band of chromosome 1. *Hum Genet* 1986;73:277–279.

Enriquez de Salamanca R, Sepulveda P, Moran MJ, et al. Clinical utility of fluorometric scanning of plasma porphyrins for the diagnosis and typing of porphyrias. *Clin Exp Dermatol* 1993;18:128–130.

Fargion S, Fracanzani AL. Prevalence of hepatitis C virus infection in porphyria cutanea tarda. *J Hepatol* 2003;39:635–638.

Grossman ME, Bickers DR, Poh-Fitzpatrick, et al. Porphyria cutanea tarda: clinical features and laboratory findings in 40 patients. *Am J Med* 1979;67:277–286.

Grossman ME, Poh-Fitzpatrick MB. Porphyria cutanea tarda. Diagnosis, management and differentiation from other hepatic porphyrias. *Dermatol Clin* 1986;4:297–309.

Hitt RJ, Corrigall AV, Hancock V, et al. Porphyria cutanea tarda: the etiological importance of mutations in the HFE gene and viral infection is population-dependent. *Cell Mol Biol (Noisy-le-grand)* 2002;48:853–859.

Lacour JP, Bodokh I, Castanet J, et al. Porphyria cutanea tarda and antibodies to hepatitis C virus. *Br J Dermatol* 1993;128:121–123.

Lim HW, Mascaro JM. The porphyrias and hepatocellular carcinoma. *Dermatol Clin* 1995;13:135–142.

Martinez di Montemuros F, Tavazzi D, Patti E, et al. Human gene mutations. Gene symbol: UROD. Disease: porphyria, cutanea tardy. *Hum Genet* 2004;114:221.

Nagy Z, Koszo F, Par A, et al. Hemochromatosis (FIFE) gene mutations and hepatitis C virus infection as risk factors for porphyria cutanea tarda in Hungarian patients. *Liver Int* 2004;24:16–20.

Petersen CS, Thomsen K. High-dose hydroxychloroquine treatment of porphyria cutanea tarda. *J Am Acad Dermatol* 1992;26:614–619.

Phillips JD, et al. Functional consequences of naturally occurring mutations in human uroporphyrinogen decarboxylase. *Blood* 2001;98:3179.

Poh-Fitzpatrick MB. Is porphyria cutanea tarda a paraneoplastic disorder? *Clin Dermatol* 1993;11:119–124.

Sams H, Kiripolsk MG, Bhat L, et al. Porphyria cutanea tarda, hepatitis C, alcoholism, and hemochromatosis: a case report and review of the literature. *Cutis* 2004;73:188–190.

Siersema PD, ten Kate FJ, Mulder PG, et al. Hepatocellular carcinoma in porphyria cutanea tarda: frequency and factors related to its occurrence. *Liver* 1992;12:56–61.

Thunell S, Harper P. Porphyrins, porphyrin metabolism, porphyrias. III. Diagnosis, care and monitoring in porphyria cutanea tarda—suggestions for a handling programme. *Scand J Clin Lab Invest* 2000;60:561.

Variegate Porphyria

Corey TJ, DeLeo VA, Christianson H, et al. Variegate porphyria: clinical and laboratory features. *J Am Acad Dermatol* 1980;2:36–43.

D'Amato M, Bonuglia M, Barile S, et al. Genetic analysis of variegate porphyria (VP) in Italy: identification of six novel mutations in the protoporphyrinogen oxidase (PPOX) gene. *Hum Mutat* 2003;21:448.

Hift RJ, Davidson BP, Van Der Hooft C, et al. Plasma fluorescence scanning and fecal porphyrin analysis for the diagnosis of variegate porphyria: precise determination of sensitivity and specificity with detection of protoporphyrinogen oxidase mutations as a reference standard. *Clin Chem* 2004;50:915–923.

Lam H, Dragan L, Tsou HC, et al. Molecular basis of variegate porphyria: a de novo insertion mutation in the protoporphyrinogen oxidase gene. *Hum Genet* 1997;99:126.

Logan GM, Weimer MK, Ellefson M, et al. Bile porphyrin analysis in the evaluation of variegate porphyria. *N Engl J Med* 1991;324:1408–1411.

Muhlbauer JE, Pathak MA, Tishler PV, et al. Variegate porphyria in New England. *JAMA* 1982;247:3095–3102.

Palmer RA, Elder GH, Barrett DF, et al. Homozygous variegate porphyria: a compound heterozygote with novel mutations in the protoporphyrinogen oxidase gene. *Br J Dermatol* 2001;144:866–869.

Taketani S, Inazawa J, Abe T, et al. The human protoporphyrinogen oxidase gene (PPOX): organization and location to chromosome 1. *Genomics* 1995;29:698–703.

von und zu Fraunberg M, Tenhunen R, Kauppinen R. Expression and characterization of six mutations in the protoporphyrinogen oxidase gene among Finnish variegate porphyria patients. *Mol Med* 2001;7:320–328.

Whatley SD, Puy H, Morgan RR, et al. Variegate porphyria in Western Europe: identification of PPOX gene mutations in 104 families, extent of allelic heterogeneity, and absence of correlation between phenotype and type of mutation. *Am J Hum Genet* 1999;65:984–994.

Wiman A, Harper P, Floderus Y. Nine novel mutations in the protoporphyrinogen oxidase gene in Swedish families with variegate porphyria. *Clin Genet* 2003;64:122–130.

Acute Intermittent Porphyria

Gu XF, de Rooij F, Voortman G, et al. Detection of eleven mutations causing acute intermittent porphyria using denaturing gradient gel electrophoresis. *Hum Genet* 1994;93:47–52.

Kauppinen R. Molecular diagnostics of acute intermittent porphyria. *Expert Rev Mol Diagn* 2004;4:243–249.

Kauppinen R, Mustajoki P. Prognosis of acute porphyria: occurrence of acute attacks, precipitating factors, and associated diseases. *Medicine* 1992;71:1–13.

Lundin G, Wedell A, Thunell S, et al. Two new mutations in the porphobilinogen deaminase gene and a screening method using PCR amplification of specific alleles. *Hum Genet* 1994;93:59–62.

Mustajoki P, Nordmann Y. Early administration of heme arginate for acute porphyric attacks. *Arch Intern Med* 1993;153:2004–2008.

Namba H, Narahara K, Tsuji K, et al. Assignment of human porphobilinogen deaminase to 11q24. 1–g24.2 by in situ hybridization and gene dosage studies. *Cytogenet Cell Genet* 1991;57:105–108.

Sassa S, Kappas A. Molecular aspects of the inherited porphyrias. *J Intern Med* 2000;247:169.

Solis CS, Lopez-Echaniz I, Sefarty-Graneda D, et al. Gene symbol: H S. disease: acute intermittent porphyria. *Hum Genet* 2004;114:402.

Thunell S, Harper P, Brun A. Porphyrins, porphyrin metabolism and porphyrias. II. Diagnosis and monitoring in the acute porphyrias. *Scand J Clin Lab Invest* 2000;60:581–604.

von Brasch L, Zang C, Haverkamp T, et al. Molecular analysis of acute intermittent porphyria: mutation screening in 20 patients in Germany reveals 11 novel mutations. *Blood Cells Mol Dis* 2004;32:30–34.

Hereditary Coproporphyria

Andrews J, Erdjument H, Nicholson DC. Hereditary coproporphyria: incidence in a large English family. *J Med Genet* 1984;21:341–349.

Cacheux V, Martasek P, Fougerousse F, et al. Localization of the human coproporphyrinogen oxidase gene to chromosome band 3q12. *Hum Genet* 1994;94:557–559.

Fujita H, Kondo M, Taketani S, et al. Characterization and expression of cDNA encoding coproporphyrinogen oxidase from a patient with hereditary coproporphyria. *Hum Mol Genet* 1994;3:1807–1810.

Grandchamp B, Weil D, Nordmann Y, et al. Assignment of the human coproporphyrinogen oxidase to chromosome 9. *Hum Genet* 1983;64:180–183.

Lamoril J, Deybach JC, Puy H, et al. Three novel mutations in the coproporphyrinogen oxidase gene. *Hum Mutat* 1997;9:78–80.

Mandoki MW, Sumner GS. Psychiatric manifestations of hereditary coproporphyria in a child. *J Nerv Ment Dis* 1994;182:117–118.

Martasek P, Nordmann Y, Grandchamp B. Homozygous hereditary coproporphyria caused by a arginine to tryptophane substitution in coproporphyrinogen oxidase and common intragenic polymorphisms. *Hum Mol Genet* 1994;3:477–480.

Rosipal R, Lamoril J, Pu H, et al. Systematic analysis of coproporphyrinogen oxidase gene defects in hereditary coproporphyria and mutation update. *Hum Mutat* 1999;13:44–53.

Sassa S, Kondo M, Taketani S, et al. Molecular defects of the coproporphynnogen oxidase gene in hereditary coproporphyria. *Cell Mol Biol (Noisy-le-grand)* 1997;43:59–66.

Wiman A, Floderus Y, Harper P. Two novel mutations and coexistence of the 991C>T and the 1339C>T mutation on a single allele in the coproporphyrinogen oxidase gene in Swedish patients with hereditary coproporphyria. *J Hum Genet* 2002;47:407–412.

Erythropoietic Protoporphyria

DeLeo VA, Poh-Fitzpatrick M, Mathews-Roth MM, et al. Erythropoietic protoporphyria: 10 years experience. *Am J Med* 1976;60:8–22.

Di Pierre E, Moriondo V, Cappellini MD. Human gene mutations. Gene symbol: FECH. Disease: Porphyria, erythropoietic. *Hum Genet* 2004;114:221.

Fontanellas A, Mendez M, Mazurier F, et al. Successful therapeutic effect in a mouse model of erythropoietic protoporphyria by partial genetic correction and fluorescence-based selection of hematopoietic cells. *Gene Ther* 2001;8:618–626.

Goerz G, Bunselmeyer S, Bolsen K, et al. Ferrochelatase activities in patients with erythropoietic protoporphyria and their families. *Br J Dermatol* 1996;134:880–885.

Jacquemyn Y. Erythropoietic protoporphyria in pregnancy. *J Obstet Gynaeeol* 2003;23:196.

Johnson JA, Fusaro RM. Prognosis of liver transplantation in patients with erythropoietic protoporphyria. *Transplantation* 1989;48:175–176.

Krinksy NI. Antioxidant functions of carotenoids. *Free Radic Biol Med* 1989;7:617–635.

Lecha M. Erythropoietic protoporphyria. *Photodermatol Photoimmunol Photomed* 2003;19:142–146.

Lew W. A novel ferrochelatase gene mutation (IVS1-2 A—>C) in erythropoietic protoporphyria. *J Invest Dermatol* 2003;121:425–427.

Mathews-Roth MM, Michel JL, Wise RJ. Amelioration of the metabolic defect in erythropoietic protoporphyria by expression of human ferrochelatase in cultured cells. *J Invest Dermatol* 1995;104:497.

Mathews-Roth MM, Pathak MA, Fitzpatrick TB, et al. Beta-carotene as a photoprotective agent in erythropoietic protoporphyria. *N Engl J Med* 1970;282:1231–1234.

Meerman L, Veneer R, Slooff MJ, et al. Perioperative measures during liver transplantation for erythropoietic protoporphyria. *Transplantation* 1994;57:155–158.

Murphy GM. Diagnosis and management of the erythropoietic porphyrias. *Dermatol Ther* 2003;A6:57–64.

Nordmann Y. Erythropoietic protoporphyria and hepatic complications. *J Hepatol* 1992;16:4–6.

Pawliuk R, et al. Long-term cure of the photosensitivity of murine erythropoietic protoporphyria by preselective gene therapy. *Nat Med* 1999;5:768.

Risheg H, Chen FP, Bloomer JR. Genotypic determinants of phenotype in North American patients with erythropoietic protoporphyria. *Mol Genet Metab* 2003;80:196–206.

Rufener EA. Erythropoietic protoporphyria: a study of its psychosocial aspects. *Br J Dermatol* 1987;116:703–708.

Sarkany RP. Erythropoietic protoporphyria (EPP) at 40. Where are we now? *Photodermatol Photoimmunol Photomed* 2002;18:147–152.

Schneider-Yin X, Gouya L, Meier-Weinand A, et al. New insights into the pathogenesis of erythropoietic protoporphyria and their impact on patient care. *Eur J Pediatr* 2000;159:719–725

Thunell S, Harper P, Brun A. Porphyries, porphyrin metabolism and porphyries. IV. Pathophysiology of erythropoietic protoporphyria—diagnosis, care and monitoring of the patient. *Scand J Clin Lab Invest* 2000;60:581–604.

Wang X, Poh-Fitzpatrick M, Taketani S, et al. Screening for ferrochelatase mutations: molecular heterogeneity of erythropoietic protoporphyria. *Biochim Biophys Acta* 1994;1225:187–190.

Whitcombe DM, Carter NP, Albertson DG, et al. Assignment of the human ferrochelatase gene (EECH) and a locus for protoporphyria to chromosome 18g22. *Genomics* 1991;11:1152–1154.

Congenital Erythropoietic Porphyria

Aizencang G, Solis C, Bishop DF, et al. Human uroporphyrinogen-III synthase: genomic organization, alternative promoters, and erythroid-specific expression. *Genomics* 2000;70:223–231.

Astrin KH, Warner CA, Yoo HW, et al. Regional assignment of the human uroporphyrinogen III synthase (UROS) gene to chromosome 10q25. 2–q26. 3. *Hum Genet* 1991;87:18–22.

Dawe SA, Peters TJ, Du Vivier A, et al. Congenital erythropoietic porphyria: dilemmas in present day management. *Clin Exp Dermatol* 2002;27:680–683.

Fritsch C, Lang K, Bolsen K, et al. Congenital erythropoietic porphyria. *Skin Pharmacol Appl Skin Physiol* 1998;11:347–357.

Ged C, Moreau-Gaudry F, Taine L, et al. Prenatal diagnosis in congenital erythropoietic porphyria by metabolic measurement and DNA mutation analysis. *Prenat Diagn* 1996;16:83–86.

Ged C, Ozalla D, Herrero C, et al. Description of a new mutation in hepatoerythropoietic porphyria and prenatal exclusion of a homozygous fetus. *Arch Dermatol* 2002;138:957–960.

Harada FA, Shwayder TA, Desnick RJ, et al. Treatment of severe congenital erythropoietic porphyria by bone marrow transplantation. *J Am Acad Dermatol* 2001;45:279–282.

Kauffman L, Evans DI, Stevens RF, et al. Bone-marrow transplantation for congenital erythropoietic porphyria. *Lancet* 1991;337:1510–1511.

Kauppinen R, Glass IA, Aizencang G, et al. Congenital erythropoietic porphyria prolonged high-level expression and correction of the heme biosynthetic defect by retroviral-mediated gene transfer into porphyric and erythroid cells. *Mol Genet Metab* 1998;65:10–17.

Lazebnik N, Lazebnik RS. The prenatal presentation of congenital erythropoietic porphyria: report of two siblings with elevated maternal serum alpha-fetoprotein. *Prenat Diagn* 2004;24:282–286.

Pandhi D, Suman M, Khurana N, et al. Congenital erythropoietic porphyria complicated by squamous cell carcinoma. *Pediatr Dermatol* 2003;20:498–501.

Pimstone NR, Gandhi SN, Mukerji SK. Therapeutic efficacy of oral charcoal in congenital erythropoietic porphyria. *N Engl J Med* 1987;316:390–393.

Piomelli S, Poh-Fitzpatrick MB, Seaman C, et al. Complete suppression of the symptoms of congenital erythropoietic porphyria by long-term treatment with high-level transfusions. *N Engl J Med* 1986;314:1029–1031.

Poh-Fitzpatrick MB. The erythropoietic porphyrias. *Dermatol Clin* 1986;4:291–296.

Pollack SS, Rosenthal MS. Diaper diagnosis of porphyria. *N Engl J Med* 1994;330:114.

Shaw PH, Mancini AJ, McConnell JP, et al. Treatment of congenital erythropoietic porphyria in children by allogeneic stem cell transplantation: a case report and review of the literature. *Bone Marrow Transplant* 2001;227:101–105.

Ueda S, Rao GN, LoCascio JA, et al. Corneal and conjunctival changes in congenital erythropoietic porphyria. *Cornea* 1989;8:286–294.

Xu W, Warner CA, Desnick RJ. Congenital erythropoietic porphyria: identification and expression of 10 mutations in the uroporphyrinogen III synthase gene. *J Clin Invest* 1995;95:905–912.

Xu W, Astrin KH, Desnick RJ. Molecular basis of congenital erythropoietic porphyria: mutations in the human uroporphyrinogen III synthase gene. *Hum Mutat* 1996;7;187–192.

Hepatoerythropoietic Porphyria

Berenguer J, Blasco J, Cardenal C, et al. Hepatoerythropoietic porphyria: neuroimaging findings. *AJNR Am J Neuroradiol* 1997;18:1557–1560.

Bundino S, Topi GC, Zina AM, et al. Hepatoerythropoietic porphyria. *Pediatr Dermatol* 1987;4:229–233.

Czarnecki DB. Hepatoerythropoietic porphyria. *Arch Dermatol* 1980;116:307–311.

de Verneuil H, Bourgeois F, de Rooij F, et al. Characterization of a new mutation (R292G) and a deletion at the human uroporphyrinogen decarboxylase locus in two patients with hepatoerythropoietic porphyria. *Hum Genet* 1992;89:548–552.

de Verneuil H, Grandchamp B, Romeo PH, et al. Molecular analysis of uroporphyrinogen decarboxylase deficiency in a family with two cases of hepatoerythropoietic porphyria. *J Clin Invest* 1986;77:431–435.

de Verneuil H, Hansen J, Picat C, et al. Prevalence of the 281 (gly-to-glu) mutation in hepatoerythropoietic porphyria and porphyria cutanea tarda. *Hum Genet* 1988;78:101–102.

Ged C, Ozalla D, Herrero C, et al. Description of a new mutation in hepatoerythropoietic porphyria and prenatal exclusion of a homozygous fetus. *Arch Dermatol* 2002;138:957–960.

Horina JH, Wolf P. Epoetin for severe anemia in hepatoerythropoietic porphyria. *N Engl J Med* 2000;342:1294–1295.

Toback AC, Sassa S, Poh-Fitzpatrick MB, et al. Hepatoerythropoietic porphyria: clinical, biochemical, and enzymatic studies in a three-generation family lineage. *N Engl J Med* 1987;316:645–650.

Wang H, Long Q, Marty SD, et al. A zebrafish model for hepatoerythropoietic porphyria. *Nat Genet* 1998;20:239–243.

Chapter 8

Disorders With Photosensitivity

Clinical
Pearls

Moise Levy, M.D. (ML), Kurt Hirschhorn, M.D. (KH),
Judith Willner, M.D. (JW), and Leonard Milstone, M.D. (LM)

Bloom Syndrome

Inheritance	Autosomal recessive; *RecQL3* helicase gene on 15q26.1
Prenatal Diagnosis	Amniocentesis: amniotic fluid cell culture reveals high number of sister chromatid exchanges DNA analysis
Incidence	Over 100 case reports; increased frequency amongst Ashkenazi Jews from eastern Europe; M:F=1.3:1
Age at Presentation	First few months of life
Pathogenesis	A mutation in the *RecQL3* gene, encoding a DNA helicase responsible for unwinding DNA, interferes with DNA replication and repair leading to increased sister chromatid exchanges and chromosomal breaks, gaps, and rearrangement; shares helicase family mutation with Werner's syndrome, xeroderma pigmentosum (XP) B, XPD, and Rothmund-Thomson syndrome

Key Features

Skin
Photodistributed erythema with telangiectasias in butterfly distribution on nose and cheeks; eruption may involve the ears, forearms and dorsal hands; with/without bullae
Cheilitis
Café au lait macules

Craniofacial/Body Habitus
Long, narrow face with prominent nose, malar hypoplasia, small mandible; short stature

Ear-Nose-Throat
High-pitched voice

Immunology
Decreased immunoglobulin (Ig) A, IgM, with/without IgG with recurrent respiratory and gastrointestinal infections

Endocrine
Hypogonadism, infertility (males)

Neoplasia (20%)
Acute leukemia, lymphoma, and GI adenocarcinoma most common

Differential Diagnosis   Cockayne syndrome (p. 242)
Rothmund-Thomson syndrome (p. 238)
Lupus erythematosus
Erythropoietic protoporphyria (p. 224)

Laboratory Data   DNA analysis
Chromosome analysis
Immunoglobulin levels

Management   Referral to dermatologist—diagnosis, sun protection
Referral to pediatric infectious disease specialist, hematologist/oncologist, endocrinologist—antibiotics, carcinoma surveillance, short stature management respectively

Prognosis   Increased risk of premature death (second to third decade) due to malignancy; otherwise good general health with infections, skin changes decreasing with age

Clinical Pearls

In infancy, they have severe failure to thrive . . . In terms of nailing the diagnosis, the immunoglobulin abnormalities and a test for chromosome instability are most useful . . . There are labs set up to run the chromosome tests at the National Institutes of Health (NIH) and Armed Forces Institute of Pathology . . . They can be bothered by the facial erythema . . . I generally give families the names of cosmetic coverups and send them to our equivalent of Bloomingdale's . . . Photoprotect with sunscreens, hats, frogskin clothing.   *ML*

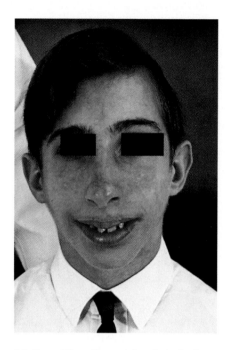

8.1. *Boy with erythema, telangiectasias in butterfly distribution on nose and cheeks with characteristic facies. (66)*

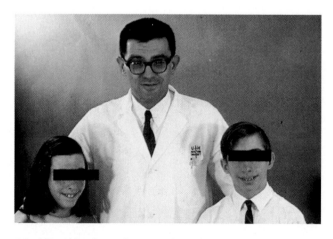

8.2. *Affected brother and sister with similar cutaneous changes and facies. (66)*

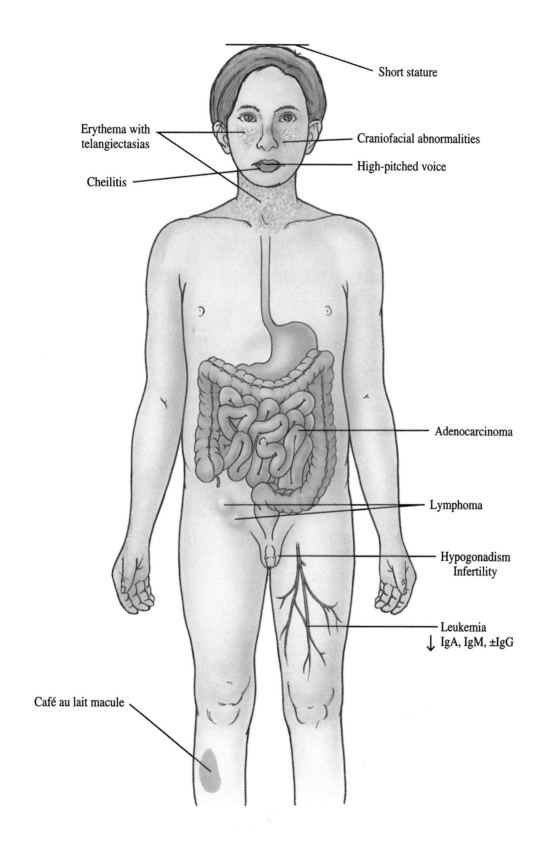

Short stature

Erythema with telangiectasias

Craniofacial abnormalities

Cheilitis

High-pitched voice

Adenocarcinoma

Lymphoma

Hypogonadism
Infertility

Leukemia
↓ IgA, IgM, ±IgG

Café au lait macule

Rothmund-Thomson Syndrome

Synonym	Poikiloderma congenitale
Inheritance	Autosomal recessive; *RecQL4* helicase gene on 8q24 in some cases
Prenatal Diagnosis	DNA analysis
Incidence	Over 130 cases reported; F>M; increased with consanguinity
Age at Presentation	Three to 6 months old (cutaneous changes)
Pathogenesis	A mutation in *RecQL4* helicase gene contributes to phenotype in some cases with predicted DNA repair problems and susceptibility to cancers as seen in Werner, Bloom and XPB, XPD (other helicase family gene mutation syndromes); otherwise unknown defect

Key Features

Skin
Initial erythema, edema on face rapidly replaced by red-brown reticulated patches associated with atrophy, hypopigmentation, telangiectasias on face, buttocks, extensor extremities
Photosensitivity with/without bullae
Acral verrucous keratoses after puberty—may precede squamous cell carcinoma

Hair
Alopecia of scalp, eyebrows, eyelashes

Nails
Dystrophic nails (25%)

Musculoskeletal
Short stature, small hands and feet, hypoplastic/absent thumbs, variety of skeletal abnormalities

Eyes
Juvenile cataracts (40% to 50%)—begins at 3 to 7 years old

Endocrine
Hypogonadism (25%)

Teeth
Dental dysplasia

Neoplasia (rare)
Reports of osteosarcoma, fibrosarcoma, and squamous cell carcinoma

Differential Diagnosis	Bloom syndrome (p. 234) Cockayne syndrome (p. 242) Werner syndrome (p. 158) Kindler syndrome
Laboratory Data	Long-bone x-rays
Management	Referral to dermatologist—diagnosis, photoprotection Referral to ophthalmologist—yearly screen and cataract management Referral to orthopedist, dentist, endocrinologist, hematologist/oncologist if symptomatic
Prognosis	If no malignancy then normal life span; usually normal intelligence

Clinical Pearls

Poikilodermatous changes are not necessarily confined to the sun-exposed areas . . . One patient I followed had striking involvement of the buttocks, another over the vulva . . . We had one child with such severe bowing of her distal tibias that the radiologist initially called and asked if the patient was wheelchair-bound . . . She had required multiple osteotomies to keep her mobile . . . Both of the patients referred to above have died from osteosarcoma. It is imperative to follow the bone changes for such degeneration. Malignant risks appear particularly marked in patients with documented *RECQL4* mutations . . . Have also seen many adults with hyperkeratosis involving palms/soles, which can be marked and clinically significant . . . Half the children have subtle learning disabilities . . . All the patients I follow have similar facies . . . Baseline ophthalmologist examination and then yearly . . . I counsel about photoprotection. *ML*

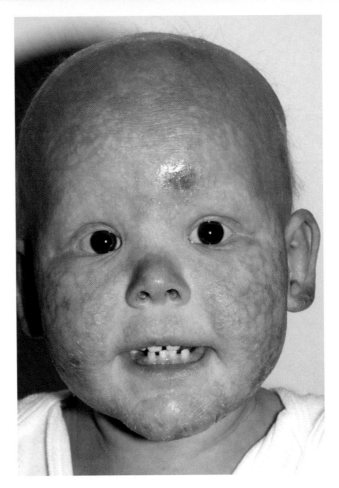

8.3. *Child with poikilodermatous changes of the face, forehead erosion, and dental dysplasia. (91)*

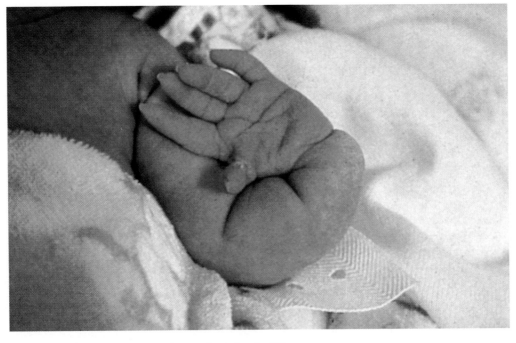

8.4. *Congenitally absent radius with hypoplastic thumb. (92)*

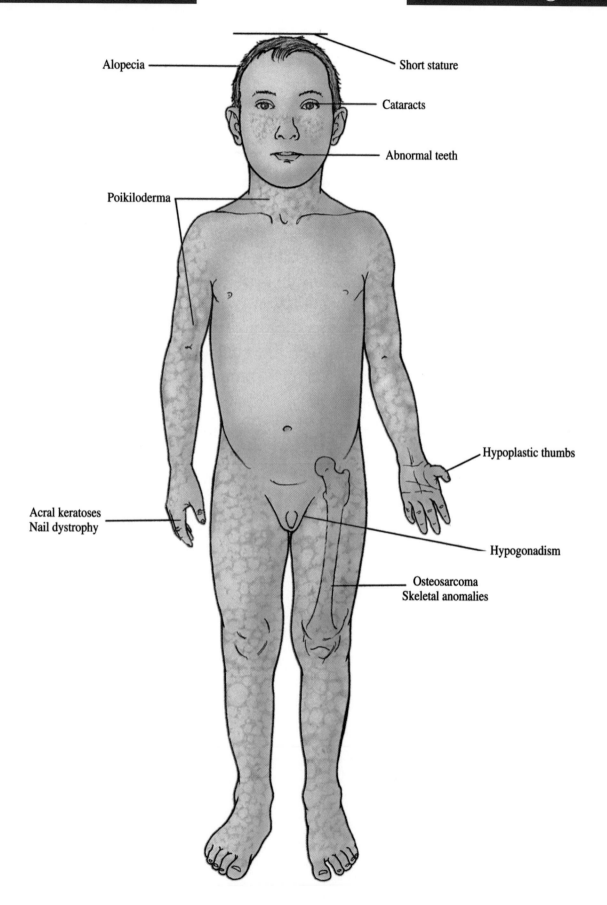

Alopecia

Short stature

Cataracts

Abnormal teeth

Poikiloderma

Hypoplastic thumbs

Acral keratoses
Nail dystrophy

Hypogonadism

Osteosarcoma
Skeletal anomalies

Cockayne Syndrome

Inheritance Autosomal recessive; Cockayne syndrome group A (CSA): *ERCC8* gene on chromosome 5
Cockayne syndrome group B (CSB): *ERCC6* gene on 10q11

Prenatal Diagnosis Amniocentesis/amniotic fluid cell culture—deficient RNA synthesis and increased cell death after UV irradiation
DNA analysis

Incidence Very rare; M=F; CSB most common (80% of cases)

Age at Presentation Birth to 2 years old; some later, into teens

Pathogenesis Mutations in *ERCC8* and *ERCC6* impairs DNA repair in active genes specifically, rendering the patient hypersensitive to UV and leads to progressive neurodegeneration; overlap of XPB, XPD, XPG with Cockayne exists in small number of patients

Key Features

Skin
Photosensitive eruption with erythema and scale in "butterfly" distribution on face—may resolve with hyperpigmentation and atrophy
Subcutaneous fat loss on face with resultant sunken eyes, aged appearance

Craniofacial/Body Habitus
Cachectic dwarf with microcephaly, thin nose, large ears ("Mickey Mouse" appearance); disproportionately long limbs with joint contractures; large, cold hands and feet

Nervous System
Diffuse demyelination of the central nervous sytem (CNS) and peripheral nerves with progressive neurologic deterioration; mental retardation; intracranial calcifications

Ear-Nose-Throat
Sensorineural deafness

Eyes
"Salt-and-pepper" retinal pigment, miotic pupils may be difficult to dilate, cataracts, optic atrophy

Teeth
Dental caries

Differential Diagnosis	Bloom syndrome (p. 234) Rothmund-Thomson syndrome (p. 238) Hartnup syndrome (p. 250) XP (p. 174) Progeria (p. 156)
Laboratory Data	DNA analysis Blood serum—UV irradiated cells with decreased DNA, RNA synthesis Brain computed tomography (CT)—calcifications; cortical atrophy
Management	Photoprotection with sunscreens, clothing, avoidance of sun Referral to neurologist, ophthalmologist, ear-nose-throat (ENT) specialist, dentist
Prognosis	Progressive, unremitting neurologic degeneration with death by second to third decade

Clinical Pearls

A child can have loss of milestones because the syndrome tends to be more of a neurodegenerative disease . . . Mental deficiency varies along a spectrum . . . I always have ophthalmology take a look as part of the workup . . . We currently follow a patient with strikingly deep-set eyes and periorbital pigmentation . . . Patients tend to be spindly. Very short stature; can be confused with the XP phenotype. *ML*

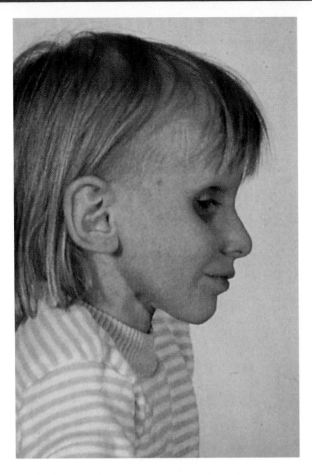

8.5. *Sunken eyes, large ears, and microcephaly. (5)*

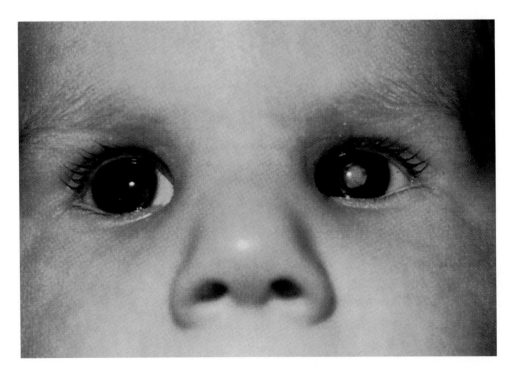

8.6. *Cataract in left eye of affected child. (93)*

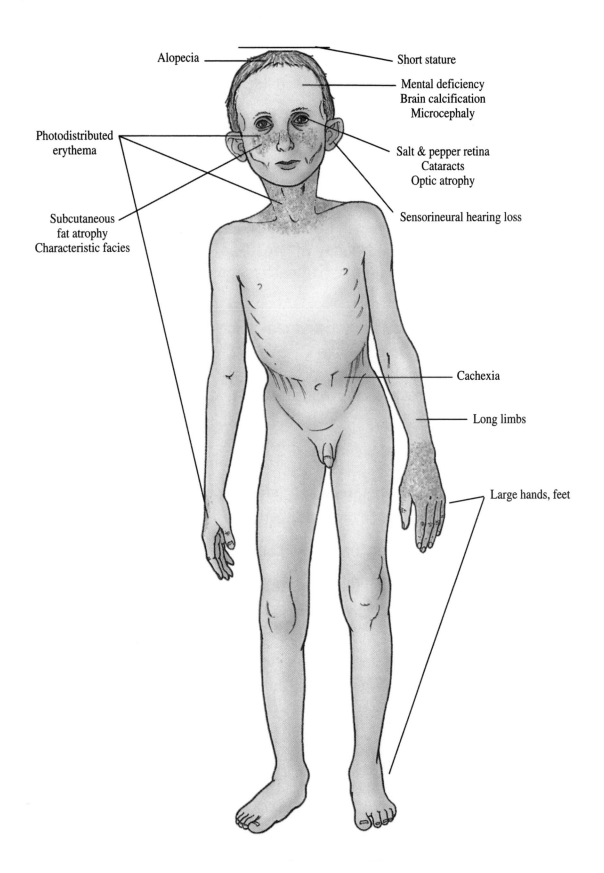

Alopecia

Short stature

Mental deficiency
Brain calcification
Microcephaly

Photodistributed
erythema

Salt & pepper retina
Cataracts
Optic atrophy

Subcutaneous
fat atrophy
Characteristic facies

Sensorineural hearing loss

Cachexia

Long limbs

Large hands, feet

Trichothiodystrophy

Synonym

(P)IBIDS—(**P**hotosensitivity), **i**chthyosis, **b**rittle Hair, **i**ntellectual impairment, **d**ecreased fertility, and **s**hort stature

Inheritance

Autosomal recessive; 50% with same complementation group as XPD with *ERCC2* gene defect on 19q13, all with photosensitivity
Less common XPB and TTD-A complementation groups

Prenatal Diagnosis

Amniocentesis/cultured amniotic fluid cells reveals reduction in unscheduled DNA synthesis in cases associated with XP-like DNA repair defect
DNA analysis

Incidence

Rare—less than 100 patients reported; M=F

Age at Presentation

Early infancy

Pathogenesis

Heterogeneous group of neuroectodermal disorders all sharing sulfur-deficient brittle hair; similar to XP and Cockayne syndrome, a mutation in DNA excision repair genes (*ERCC2*, *ERCC3*) leads to the photosensitive TTD phenotype—*ERCC2* defect (50% of cases) is same as in XP group D

Key Features

Skin
Photosensitivity (50% of cases) without signs of chronic actinic damage, no increase in skin cancer
Ichthyosis—variable severity; may resemble ichthyosis vulgaris, congenital ichthysiform erythroderma (CIE)
Hair
Short, sparse, brittle in scalp, eyebrows, eyelashes; alternating light and dark bands with polarizing microscope; trichoschisis; cyclical hair loss
Nails
Dystrophy
Central Nervous System
Intellectual impairment, ataxia
Eyes
Photosensitivity, cataracts
Genitourinary
Decreased fertility with hypogonadism
Musculoskeletal
Short stature, facial dysmorphism

Differential Diagnosis   Tay syndrome
XP (p. 174)
Cockayne syndrome (p. 242)
CIE (p. 12)
Netherton's syndrome (p. 24)

Laboratory Data   DNA analysis
Light and polarizing microscopy of hair shaft
Sulfur content of hairs

Management   Close follow-up with primary-care physician
Referral to dermatologist—emolliation, sun protection, diagnosis
Referral to symptom-specific specialist

Prognosis   Normal life span; quality of life dependent upon severity of symptoms

Clinical Pearls

Trichothiodystrophy (TTD) can be easy to diagnose but phenotypically quite variable and difficult to prognosticate. The ichthyosis, when present, often resembles mild CIE and requires minimal therapy. Polarizing microscopy on the hairs is easy to perform. Place one polarizing filter (or single lens from polarized sunglasses) over the microscope objective and the other over the light source. Rotate one lens 90 degrees and observe the bands. You will be immensely satisfied even if this office test succeeds only once in your career. Mutations in one gene, the XPD gene, cause TTD, xeroderma pigmentosum, and Cockayne syndromes. All patients with those diseases have DNA repair defects but, for unexplained reasons, TTD patients apparently do not have increased risk for skin cancers even if they are photosensitive. The XPD mutations in TTD also cause deficits in RNA transcription, resulting in various developmental deficits. To date, genotype/phenotype correlation only partially explains the phenotypic variability (e.g. IDS, IBIDS, PIBIDS).   *LM*

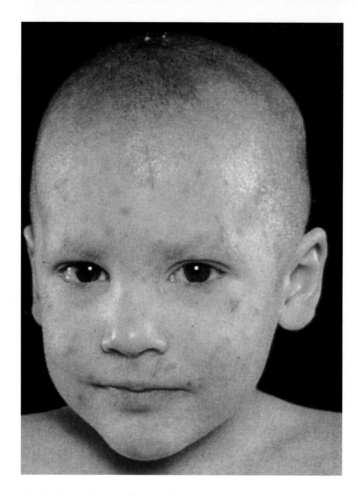

8.7. *Patient with sparse, brittle, short broken scalp, eyebrow, and eyelash hairs. (94)*

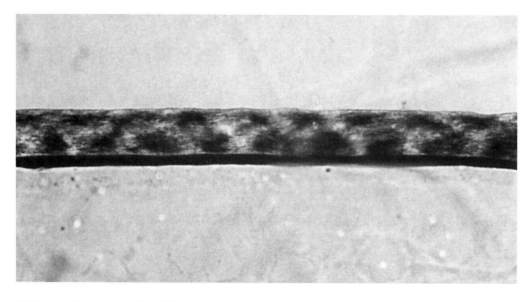

8.8. *Hair shaft under polarizing light microscopy demonstrating alternating light and dark bands.*

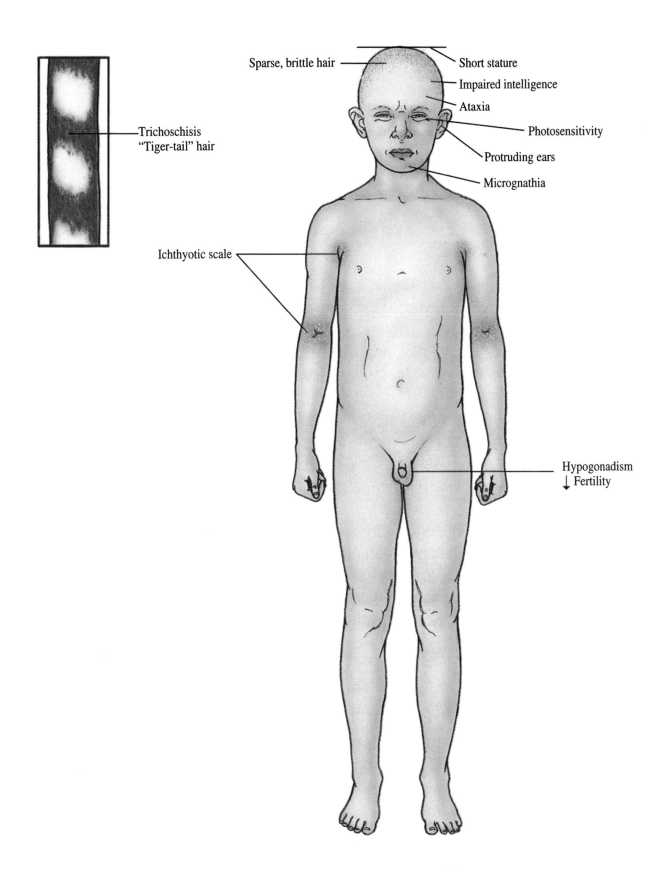

Trichoschisis "Tiger-tail" hair

Sparse, brittle hair

Short stature

Impaired intelligence

Ataxia

Photosensitivity

Protruding ears

Micrognathia

Ichthyotic scale

Hypogonadism
↓ Fertility

Hartnup Disease

Inheritance	Autosomal recessive; gene on 5p15
Prenatal Diagnosis	DNA analysis available in future
Incidence	Approximately 1:14,500 in Massachusetts survey; most cases asymptomatic in North America because of high nutritional standards offsetting lack of absorption (see Pathogenesis); M=F
Age at Presentation	First decade of life
Pathogenesis	Genetic defect in transport of neutral amino acids across brush border epithelium of intestine and kidney with resultant decreased absorption of tryptophan and pellagra-like syndrome (tryptophan necessary for nicotinic acid production)
Key Features	**Skin** Photodistributed erythema, scale, with/without bullae on forehead, cheeks, extensor arms, dorsum of hands **Central Nervous System** Cerebellar ataxia, mild mental retardation, psychiatric disturbances
Differential Diagnosis	Pellagra Cockayne syndrome (p. 242) Bloom syndrome (p. 234) Lupus erythematosus Erythropoietic protoporphyria (p. 224)
Laboratory Data	Urine screen for massive aminoaciduria and tryptophan derivatives
Management	Nicotinic acid (niacin) supplementation Good protein nutrition Referral to dermatologist, neurologist
Prognosis	Symptoms improve with supplementation and age; normal life span

Clinical Pearls

I've (KH) seen two in my whole life . . . Mainly because in the United States, the full-blown disorder is not seen . . . Kids get enough food . . . In third-world areas like Africa you'll see kids reeling around . . . Photosensitivity becomes a real problem there as well . . . When you get a kid with photosensitivity or cerebellar ataxia, take a look at the urine . . . In Massachusetts, because of Harvey Levy's interest, Hartnup is part of the neonatal screen.   *KH, JW*

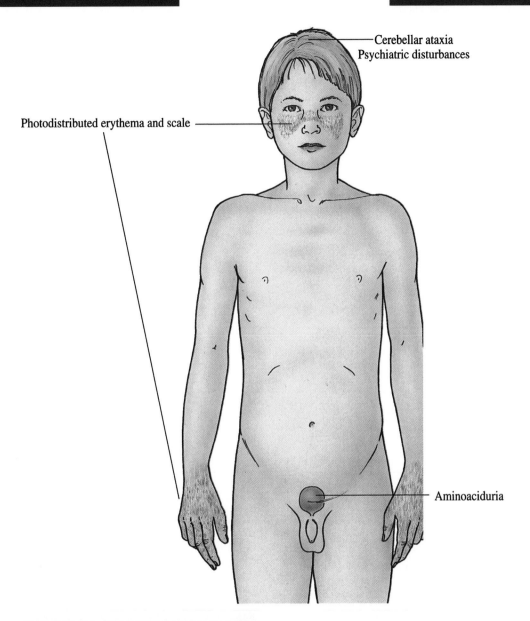

Cerebellar ataxia
Psychiatric disturbances

Photodistributed erythema and scale

Aminoaciduria

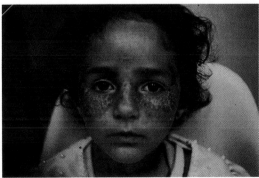

8.9. *Photodistributed butterfly erythema, hyperpigmentation and crust. (95)*

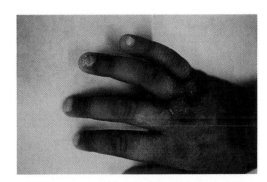

8.10. *Same patient with involvement of the dorsum of her hands. (95)*

Suggested Reading

Bloom Syndrome

Bhisitkul RB, Rizen M. Bloom syndrome: multiple retinopathies in a chromosome breakage disorder. *Br J Ophthalmol* 2004;88:354–357.

Hickson ID. RecQ helicases: caretakers of the genome. *Nat Rev Cancer* 2003;3:169–178.

Ellis NA, German J. Molecular genetics of Bloom's syndrome. *Hum Mol Genet* 1996;5(Spec No):1457–1463.

Ellis NA, Groden J, Ye TZ, et al. The Bloom's syndrome gene product is homologous to RecQ helicases. *Cell* 1995;83:655–666.

German J. Bloom syndrome: a mendelian prototype of somatic mutational disease. *Medicine* 1993;72:393–406.

German J, Passarge E. Bloom's syndrome. XII. Report from the Registry for 1987. *Clin Genet* 1989;35:57–69.

Gretzula JC, Hevia O, Weber PJ. Bloom's syndrome. *J Am Acad Dermatol* 1987;17:479–488.

Imamura O, Campbell JL. The human Bloom syndrome gene suppresses the DNA replication and repair defects of yeast dna2 mutants. *Proc Natl Acad Sci USA* 2003;100:8193–8198.

Janscak P, Garcia PL, Hamburger F, et al. Characterization and mutational analysis of the RecQ core of the Bloom syndrome protein. *J Mol Biol* 2003;330:29–42.

Karow JK, Chakraverty RK, Hickson ID. The Bloom's syndrome gene product is a 3'–5' DNA helicase. *J Biol Chem* 1997;272:30611–30614.

Langland G, Elliott J, Li Y, et al. The BLM helicase is necessary for normal DNA double-strand break repair. *Cancer Res* 2002;62:2766–2770.

Mohaghegh P, Hickson ID. DNA helicase deficiencies associated with cancer predisposition and premature aging disorders. *Hum Mol Genet* 2001;10:741–746.

Passarge E. Bloom's syndrome: the German experience. *Ann Genet* 1991;34:179–197.

Shahrabani-Gargir L, Shomrat R, Yaron Y, et al. High frequency of a common Bloom syndrome Ashkenazi mutation among Jews of Polish origin. *Genet Test* 1998;2:293.

Sirover MA, Vollberg TM, Seal G. DNA repair and the molecular mechanisms of Bloom's syndrome. *Crit Rev Oncol* 1990;2:19–33.

Wang W, Seki M, Narita Y, et al. Functional relation among RecQ family helicases RecQL1, RecQL5, and BLM in cell growth and sister chromatid exchange formation. *Mol Cell Biol* 2003;101:3527–3535.

Wu L, Hickson ID. The Bloom's syndrome helicase suppresses crossing over during homologous recombination. *Nature* 2003;426:870–874.

Rothmund-Thomson syndrome

Blaustein HS, Stevens AW, Stevens PD, et al. Rothmund-Thomson syndrome associated with annular pancreas and duodenal stenosis: a case report. *Pediatr Dermatol* 1993;10:59–163.

Drouin CA, Mongrain E, Sasseville D, et al. Rothmund-Thomson syndrome with osteosarcoma. *J Am Acad Dermatol* 1993;28:301–305.

Geronemus RG. Treatment of the cutaneous vascular component of the Rothmund-Thomson syndrome. *Pediatr Dermatol* 1996;13:175.

Kirkham TH, Werner EB. The ophthalmic manifestations of Rothmund's syndrome. *Can J Ophthalmol* 1975;10:1–14.

Kitao S, Shimamoto A, Goto M, et al. Mutations in RECQL4 cause a subset of cases of Rothmund-Thomson syndrome. *Nat Genet* 1999;22:82–84.

Lindor NM, Furuichi Y, Kitao S, et al. Rothmund-Thomson syndrome due to RECQ4 helicase mutations: report any clinical and molecular comparisons with Bloom syndrome and Werner syndrome. *Am J Med Genet* 2000;90:723-R.

Piquero-Casals J, Okubo AY, Nico MM. Rothmund-thomson syndrome in three siblings and development of cutaneous squamous cell carcinoma. *Pediatr Dermatol* 2002;19:312–316.

Potozkin JR, Geronemus RG. Treatment of the poikilodermatous component of the Rothmund-Thomson syndrome with the flashlamp-pumped pulsed dye laser: a case report. *Pediatr Dermatol* 1991;8:162–165.

Pujol LA, Erickson RP, Heidenreich RA, et al. Variable presentation of Rothmund-Thomson syndrome. *Am J Med Genet* 2000;95:204–207.

Wang LL, Gannavarapu A, Kozinetz CA, et al. Association between osteosarcoma and deleterious mutations in the RECQL gene in Rothmund-Thomson syndrome. *J Natl Cancer Inst* 2003;95:669–674.

Cockayne Syndrome

Cleaver JE, Thompson LH, Richardson AS, et al. A summary of mutations in the UV-sensitive disorders: xeroderma pigmentosum, Cockayne syndrome, and trichothiodystrophy. *Hum Mutat* 1999;14:9–22.

Greenhaw GA, Hebert A, Duke-Woodside ME, et al. Xeroderma pigmentosum and Cockayne syndrome: overlapping clinical and biochemical phenotypes. *Am J Hum Genet* 1992;50:677–689.

Lehmann AR, Francis AJ, Giannelli F. Prenatal diagnosis of Cockayne's syndrome. *Lancet* 1985;1:486–488.

Lehmann AR, Norris PG. DNA repair and cancer: speculations based on studies with xeroderma pigmentosum, Cockayne's syndrome and trichothiodystrophy. *Carcinogenesis* 1989;10:1353–1356.

Mallery DL, Tanganelli E, Colella S, et al. Molecular analysis of mutations in the CSB (ERCC6) gene in patients with Cockayne syndrome [published erratum appears in *Am J Hum Genet* 1999;64:1491]. *Am J Hum Genet* 1998;62:77–85.

Nance MA, Berry SA. Cockayne syndrome: review of 140 cases. *Am J Med Genet* 1992;42:68–84.

Ozdirim E, Topcu M, Ozon A, et al. Cockayne syndrome: review of 25 cases. *Pediatr Neurol* 1996;15:312–316.

Parris CN, Kraemer KH. Ultraviolet-induced mutations in Cockayne syndrome cells are primarily caused by cyclobutane dimer photoproducts while repair of other photoproducts is normal. *Proc Nail Acad Sci USA* 1993;90:7260–7264.

Traboulsi EL, De Becker I, Maumenee IH. Ocular findings in Cockayne syndrome. *Am J Ophthalmol* 1992;114:579–583.

Trichothiodystrophy

Broughton BC, Bernehurg M, Fawcett H, et al. Two individuals with features of both xeroderma pigmentosum and trichothiodystrophy highlight the complexity of the clinical outcomes of mutations in the XPD gene. *Hum Mol Genet* 2001;10:2539–2547.

Brusasco A, Restano L. The typical "tiger tail" pattern of the hair shaft in trichothiodystrophy may not be evident at birth. *Arch Dermatol* 1997;133:249.

Cleaver JE, Thompson LH, Richardson AS, et al. A summary of mutations in the UV-sensitive disorders: xeroderma pigmentosum, Cockayne syndrome, and trichothiodystrophy. *Hum Mutat* 1999;14:9–22.

de Boer J, Hoeijmakers JH. Nucleotide excision repair and human syndromes. *Carcinogenesis* 2000;21:453–460.

Itin PH, Pittelkow MR. Trichothiodystrophy: review of sulfur-deficient brittle hair syndromes and association with the ectodermal dysplasias. *J Am Acad Dermatol* 1990;22:705–717.

Itin PH, Sarasin A, Pittelkow MR. Trichothiodystrophy: update on the sulfur-deficient brittle hair syndromes. *J Am Acad Dermatol* 2001;44:891–920; quiz 921–924.

Johnson RT, Squires S. The XPD complementation group. Insights into xeroderma pigmentosum, Cockayne's syndrome and trichothiodystrophy. *Mutat Res* 1992;273:97–118.

Jorizzo JL, Atherton DJ, Crounse RG, et al. Ichthyosis; brittle hair, impaired intelligence, decreased fertility and short stature (IBIDS syndrome). *Br J Dermatol* 1982;106:705–710.

Lehmann AR. DNA repair-deficient diseases, xeroderma pigmentosum, Cockayne syndrome and trichothiodystrophy. *Biochimie* 2003;5:1101–1111.

Mondello C, Nardo T, Giliani S, et al. Molecular analysis of the XPD gene in Italian families with patients affected by trichothiodystrophy and xeroderma pigmentosum group D. *Mutat Res DNA Repair* 1994;314:159–165.

Price VH, Odom RB, Ward WH, et al. Trichothiodystrophy: sulfur-deficient brittle hair as a marker for a neuroectodermal symptom complex. *Arch Dermatol* 1980;116:1375–1384.

Rizzo R, Pavone L, Micali G, et al. Trichothiodystrophy: report of a new case with severe nervous system impairment. *J Child Neurol* 1992;7:300–303.

Sarasin A, Blanchet-Bardon C, Renault G, et al. Prenatal diagnosis in a subset of trichothiodystrophy patients defective in DNA repair. *Br J Dermatol* 1992;127:485–491.

Stefanini M, Vermeulen W, Weeda G, et al. A new nucleotide-excision-repair gene associated with the disorder trichothiodystrophy. *Am J Hum Genet* 1993;53:817–821.

Weeda G, Eveno E, Donker I, et al. A mutation in the XPB/ERCC3 DNA repair transcription gene, associated with trichothiodystrophy. *Am J Hum Genet* 1997;60:320–329.

Hartnup Disease

Broer A, Klingel K, Kowalezuk S, et al. Molecular cloning of mouse amino acid transport system BO, a neutral amine acid transporter related to hartnup disorder. *J Biol Chem* 2004; 279:24467–24476.

Erly W, Castillo M, Foosaner D, et al. Hartnup disease: MR findings. *Am J Neuroradiol* 1991;12:1026–1027.

Levy HL. Hartnup disorder. In: Scriver CR, Beaudet AL, Sly WS, Valle D, eds. *The Metabolic Basis of Inherited Disease.* 6th ed. New York: McGraw-Hill, 1989:2515–2527.

Levy HL, Madigan PM, Shih VE. Massachusetts metabolic screening program. I. Technique and results of urine screening. *Pediatrics* 1972;49:825–836.

Nozaki J, Dakeishi M, Ohura T, et al. Homozygosity mapping to chromosome 5p15 of a gene responsible for Hartnup disorder. *Biochem Biophys Res Commun* 2001;284:255–260.

Potter SJ, Lu A, Wileken B, et al. Hartnup disorder: polymorphisms identified in the neutral amino acid transporter SLC1A5. *J Inherit Metab Dis* 2002;25:437–448.

Schmidtke K, Endres W, Roscher A, et al. Hartnup syndrome, progressive encephalopathy and allo-albuminaemia. A clinico-pathological case study. *Eur J Pediatr* 1992;151:899–903.

Scriver CR, Mahon B, Levy HL, et al. The Hartnup phenotype: mendelian transport disorder, multifactorial disease. *Am J Hum Genet* 1987;40:401–412.

Symula DJ, Shedlovsky A, Guillery EN, et al. A candidate mouse model for Hartnup disorder deficient in neutral amino acid transport. *Mamm Genome* 1997;8:102–107.

Chapter 9

Disorders With Immunodeficiency

Clinical Pearls

Moise Levy, M.D. (ML)

Wiskott-Aldrich Syndrome

Inheritance	X-linked recessive; Wiskott-Aldrich Syndrome (WAS) gene on Xp11
Prenatal Diagnosis	DNA analysis Fetal blood sample in male fetus—abnormally small platelets
Incidence	1:250,000; males only
Age at Presentation	First few months of life with bleeding problems
Pathogenesis	Mutation in WAS gene that encodes WASp, a protein important in lymphocyte and megakaryocyte signal transduction and actin filament assembly, impairs T-cell activation and natural killer cell function

Key Features

Skin
Atopic dermatitis with increased involvement on scalp, face, flexures; secondary bacterial infection, eczema herpeticum, molluscum contagiosum, lichenification

Blood
Thrombocytopenia with petechiae, purpura, epistaxis, bloody diarrhea, hematemesis, intracranial hemorrhage

Infectious Disease
Recurrent bacterial infections (especially encapsulated organisms) with otitis media, pneumonia, meningitis, septicemia
Increased susceptibility to HSV (eczema herpeticum), *Pneumocystis carinii,* human papilloma virus

Immunology
Increased immunoglobulin (Ig) A, IgD, IgE, and decreased IgM
Impaired cell-mediated and humoral immune response
Increased IgE-mediated urticaria, food allergies, asthma

Neoplasm
Lymphoreticular malignancy (20%)—non-Hodgkin's lymphoma most common

Differential Diagnosis	Atopic dermatitis Severe combined immunodeficiciency (SCID) (p. 264) Hyper-IgE syndrome (p. 262) Chronic granulomatous disease (p. 258)
Laboratory Data	Complete blood count (CBC) with differential, platelets, mean platelet volume (MPV) Serum Ig levels Immunoblot/fluorescence-activated cell sorter analysis (FACS): WASp protein expression in mononuclear cells from peripheral blood DNA analysis
Management	Bone marrow transplant (BMT) Splenectomy with long-term antibiotic prophylaxis Appropriate antibiotics, intravenous immunoglobulin, plasma/platelet transfusions Topical corticosteroids, moisturizers, prophylactic oral acyclovir Referral to hematologist/oncologist, infectious disease specialist, and dermatologist
Prognosis	Frequently, premature death in first decade of life because of infection > hemorrhage > malignancy

Clinical Pearls

The bloody nature of the diarrhea may help distinguish from SCID. . . The big problem with platelet transfusions is that the patient may develop platelet antibodies, making subsequent transfusions less useful. . . Standard atopic care with vigorous use of moisturizers first and foremost. . . Defer topical steroids unless necessary. . . Crust with eczema can be hemorrhagic. . . Failure to thrive can be seen as with all primary immunodeficiencies in infancy. Often, early death without BMT although longer survival without BMT may occur. . . *ML*

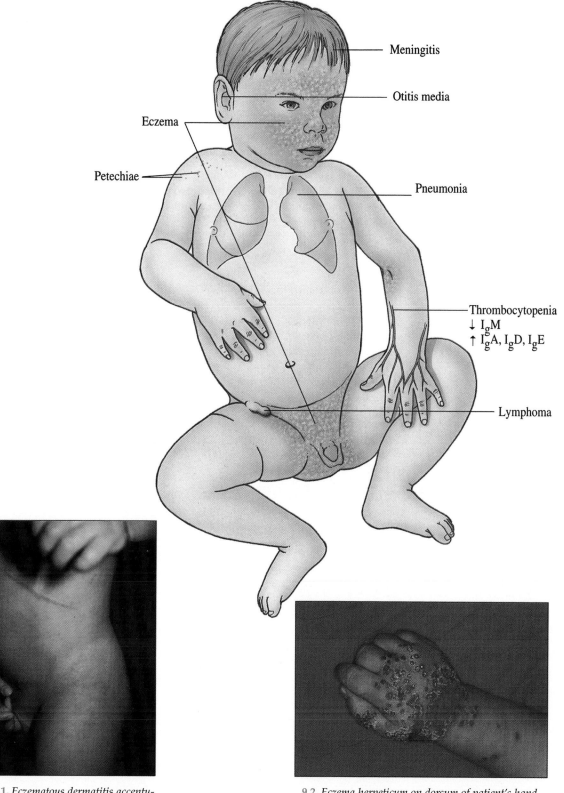

Meningitis

Otitis media

Eczema

Petechiae

Pneumonia

Thrombocytopenia
$\downarrow$ I$_g$M
$\uparrow$ I$_g$A, I$_g$D, I$_g$E

Lymphoma

9.1. *Eczematous dermatitis accentuated in flexures. Note splenectomy scar. (1)*

9.2. *Eczema herpeticum on dorsum of patient's hand.*

Chronic Granulomatous Disease

Inheritance

X-linked recessive (76%)—gp91-phox (phagocyte oxidase) gene on Xp21.1; autosomal recessive (24%)—p47 (more common), p67-phox genes on 7q11, 1q respectively

Prenatal Diagnosis

DNA analysis
Fetal blood sample—nitroblue tetrazolium (NBT) reduction assay of fetal leukocytes

Incidence

Approximately 1:250,000 to 500,000; M:F=9:1

Age at Presentation

Birth to 1 year old

Pathogenesis

Genetically heterogeneous group of immunodeficiency disorders caused by phox mutations in the nicotinamide dehydrogenase phosphate (NADPH) oxidase enzyme complex leading to an inability to produce a respiratory burst and defective killing of catalase positive organisms within phagocytic leukocytes; (respiratory burst occurs when NADPH oxidase acts as a catalyst for the production of superoxides and ultimately microbicidal oxidants)

Key Features

Skin
Recurrent pyoderma (*Staphyloccus aureus* most common), periorificial dermatitis with purulent drainage and regional lymphadenopathy, abcesses (perianal most common), granulomas
Mucous Membranes
Ulcerative stomatitis, chronic gingivitis
Lymph Nodes
Suppurative lymphadenitis with abscesses and fistulas (cervical nodes most common)
Lungs
Pneumonia with abscesses, cavitations, empyema (*Staphylococcus, Aspergillosis, Nocardia*)
Gastrointestinal Tract
Hepatosplenomegaly with granulomas, abscesses, chronic diarrhea, malabsorption
Musculoskeletal
Osteomyelitis (serratia marcescens most common), short stature

Chronic Granulomatous Disease *(continued)*

Differential Diagnosis   Hyper-IgE syndrome (p. 262)
SCID (p. 264)
Chédiak-Higashi syndrome (p. 62)
B-lymphocyte disorders

Laboratory Data   NBT reduction assay: leukocytes unable to reduce dye—no blue color change
CBC, erythrocyte sedimentation rate (ESR), immunoglobulin levels, chest x-ray, delayed hypersensitivity—skin test normal
Lungs, liver, bone imaging—locate occult inflammation; bacterial cultures
Immunoblot analysis of defective NADPH enzymes; DNA analysis

Management   Referral to infectious disease specialist—antibiotics
Referral to surgery—debridement, drainage, access to deeper infections; systemic steroids for obstructive visceral granulomas
Referral to dermatologist—topical and oral antibiotics, topical corticosteroids, antibacterial cleansers
Leukocyte transfusions, subcutaneous gamma interferon, BMT
Gene therapy for p47-phox form has been attempted with some persistence of corrected leukocytes at 6 months
Identify carriers and evaluate for lupus-like syndrome

Prognosis   Variable life span depending on control of infections; most with normal life span but poor quality of life

Clinical Pearls

A couple of kids have had resistant bacterial scalp infections. . . I have never seen the periorificial dermatitis. . . NBT is a simple test to do. . . Can be done right in the doctor's office. . . May pick up tender joints by observing the kid's positioning of the arms and legs. . . One-quarter of a cup of clorox to a full bath of water is a useful, cheap way to keep up with recurrent skin infections. . . I tend to not restrict patient's activity. . . Subcutaneous gamma interferon three times a week has provided clinical improvement. . . Patients with chronic granulomatous disease (CGD) tend to be better targets for prophylactic antibiotics. . .   *ML*

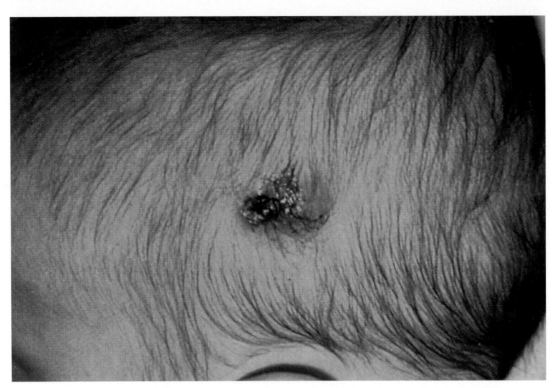

9.3. Three-month-old boy with granulomatous scalp nodule which grew serratia marcescens. (96)

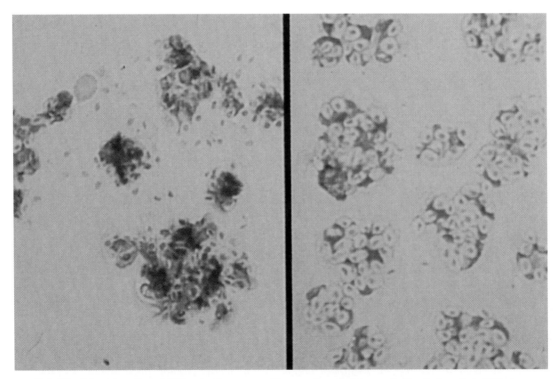

9.4. Left. Nitroblue tetrazolium (NBT) reduction assay with normal control demonstrating leukocytes' ability to reduce dye and produce blue color change. Right. Abnormal leukocytes in affected patient unable to reduce dye. (97)

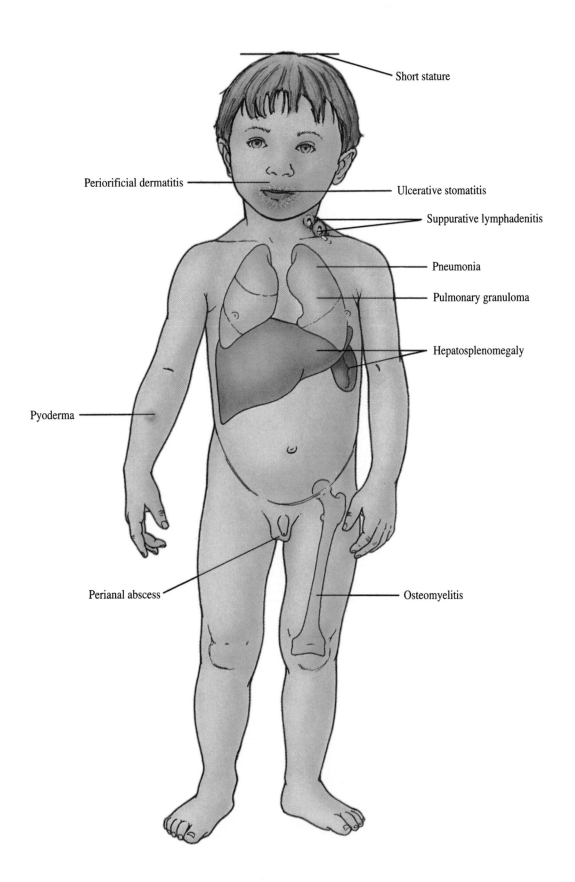

Short stature

Periorificial dermatitis

Ulcerative stomatitis

Suppurative lymphadenitis

Pneumonia

Pulmonary granuloma

Hepatosplenomegaly

Pyoderma

Perianal abscess

Osteomyelitis

Hyper-Immunoglobulin E Syndrome

Synonym Job syndrome thought to be a variant

Inheritance Autosomal dominant with variable expressivity; chromosome 4q21-gene unknown

Prenatal Diagnosis None

Incidence Rare—approximately 150 patients described; M=F

Age at Presentation First few months to first year of life

Pathogenesis Impaired regulation of IgE function and deficient neutrophil chemotaxis may play a role in susceptibility to infection

Key Features
Skin
　Excoriated papules, pustules, furuncles, cellulitis and abscesses (30% cold) on scalp, neck, axillae, groin, periorbital; paronychial infection; infected with *S. aureus* (most commonly); also *Candida, Streptococcus*
　Eczematous dermatitis increased in flexures, postauricular, hairline
Sinopulmonary
　Recurrent bronchitis, lung abscesses, pneumonia secondary to *S. aureus, Haemophilus influenzae;* pneumatoceles with bacterial/fungal superinfection, empyemas, recurrent otitis media, sinusitis
Craniofacial
　Coarse facies with broad nasal bridge, prominent nose
Musculoskeletal
　Osteopenia with secondary fractures (pelvis, long bones, ribs most common), scoliosis, hyperextensible joints
Dental
　Retained primary teeth, lack of development of secondary teeth

Differential Diagnosis Atopic dermatitis
Wiskott-Aldrich syndrome (p. 256)
DiGeorge syndrome

Laboratory Data IgE level markedly increased, IgD increased
Abnormal leukocyte/monocyte chemotaxis in some cases
Peripheral eosinophilia
Bacterial cultures

Management Long-term antistaphylococcal antibiotics for prophylaxis, therapy; incision/drainage of abscesses; antifungal therapy
Interferon-γ and γ-globulin—improve chemotaxis and decrease IgE levels, respectively
Cimetidine—immune modulation
Referral to thoracic surgeon—excision of persistent pneumatoceles

Prognosis Death may occur at early age if persistent bacterial or fungal infection of lungs exist; otherwise, with prophylaxis, prognosis is excellent

Clinical Pearls

I lump this syndrome with Job syndrome. . . You're talking about a child with diffuse dermatitis and deep-seated pyogenic infection. . . Not just your casual impetigo but deep-seated abscesses, chronic severe ear infections. . . Remember atopics can have IgE in the thousands as well. . . This is typically not a syndrome of infancy. . . Large pneumatoceles will be amenable to lobectomy. . .   *ML*

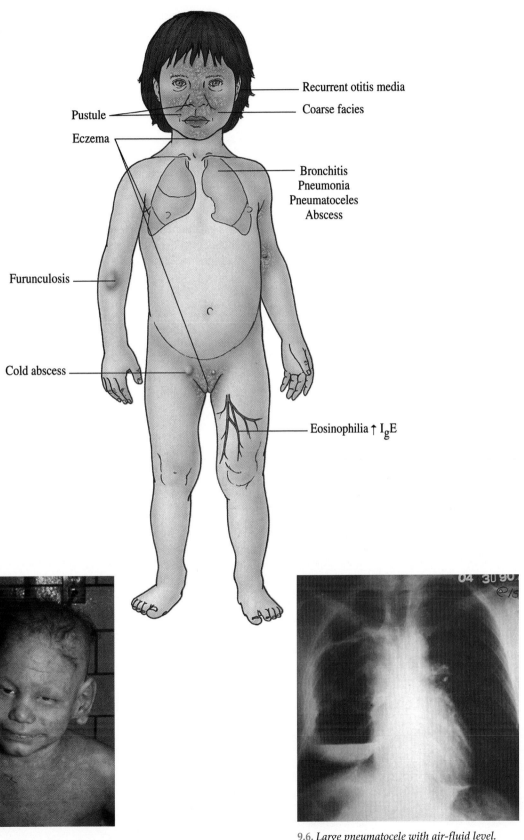

Recurrent otitis media

Coarse facies

Pustule

Eczema

Bronchitis
Pneumonia
Pneumatoceles
Abscess

Furunculosis

Cold abscess

Eosinophilia ↑ I$_g$E

9.5. *Coarse facies with broad nasal bridge, extensive dermatitis. (98)*

9.6. *Large pneumatocele with air-fluid level. Culture revealed Aspergillus fumigatus. (99)*

263

Severe Combined Immunodeficiency

Inheritance

X-linked recessive (most common)—γ chain (interleukin [IL]-2 receptor) gene on Xq13
Autosomal recessive—adenosine deaminase gene on 20q12–13 (approximately 20% of cases)
Autosomal recessive—JAK3 (Janus kinase3 in leukocytes) gene on 19p13

Prenatal Diagnosis

DNA analysis if gene defect known
Adenosine deaminase (ADA) assay in cultured amniocytes (in ADA deficiency only)

Incidence

1:100,000 to 1:500,000; approximately 80% males

Age at Presentation

First 6 months of life

Pathogenesis

Heterogeneous group of genetic disorders that share similar clinical and immunologic deficiencies; major defect in cell-mediated and humoral immunity; most lack antibody-dependent cellular cytotoxicity and natural killer (NK) cell function

Most common mutation is in the γ chain of the IL-2 receptor: important in signal transduction via JAK 3 (a tyrosine kinase) activation and is a receptor for other interleukins involved in T-cell activation; defective gamma chain leads to lack of T cells, NK cells, but normal B cells

A defect in the adenosine deaminase gene encoding an enzyme important in purine metabolism, leads to accumulation of adenosine which is toxic to immature lymphocytes; severe immunodeficiency with lack of T, B, NK cells ensues

Key Features

Skin
Candida albicans infection, S. aureus, Streptococcal pyogenes infection
May develop acute/chronic graft-versus host disease (GVHD) secondary to in utero maternal lymphocytes, nonirradiated transfused blood products, BMT—morbilliform to seborrheic-like dermatitis/lichen planus-like to sclerodermatous changes

Blood
Sepsis

Mouth
Oral candidiasis

Gastrointestinal
Chronic, viral-induced diarrhea, malabsorption with failure to thrive

Lungs
Pneumonia secondary to bacteria, Pneumocystis carinii, parainfluenza virus, cytomegalovirus (CMV)

Ear-Nose-Throat
Otitis media

Immunology
Lack tonsillar buds, lymphoid tissue despite infections

Differential Diagnosis	Acquired immune deficiency syndrome (AIDS) Hyper-IgE syndrome (p. 262) Histiocytosis Ommen's syndrome
Laboratory Data	DNA analysis FACS analysis of T, B, NK cells Immuno-cell–surface markers off peripheral blood smear ADA assay Human immunodeficiency virus (HIV) antibody titer Chest x-ray—absent thymic shadow, cupping and flaring of the costochondral junction in ADA deficiency; skin cultures, biopsy for GVHD
Management	BMT Protective isolation/vigorous antibiotic therapy Irradiate all blood products; avoid live vaccines Gene therapy: X-linked—retrovirus mediated gene transfer of gamma c gene has been successful with immunocompetency reestablished (serious drawback: two patients developed leukemia after retrovirus vector integrated with a protooncogene promoter in close proximity to gamma c) ADA deficiency—ADA replacement and gene therapy have been successful Recombinant IL-2 infusion
Prognosis	Death in 1 year without BMT

Clinical Pearls

Some cases may present with GVHD resulting from packed red blood cell transfusions or in neonates because of maternal-fetal transfusion. . . Most institutions are irradiating blood products. . . Ideally you'd see an absent thymic shadow on x-ray. . . Virtually every medical center in the United States will be able to do lymphocyte assays. . . A limited number will do ADA assays. . . ADA and gamma C have been targeted for gene therapy. . . BMT once diagnosis is made. . . Approximately 50% survival with transplant. . . Once the diagnosis is made, they are isolated with total reverse isolation. . . Like any chronic illness with kids, there are tremendous psychosocial issues. . . Multidisciplinary care centers with social workers and child-life workers are ideal. *ML*

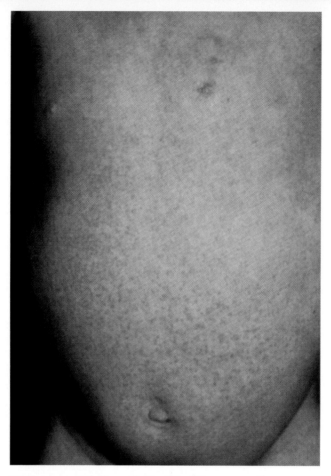

9.7. *Cutaneous infection with Candida albicans presenting as erythematous papules. (100)*

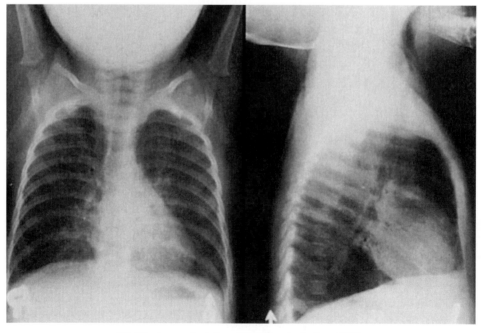

9.8. *Chest x-ray depicting absent thymic shadow. (101)*

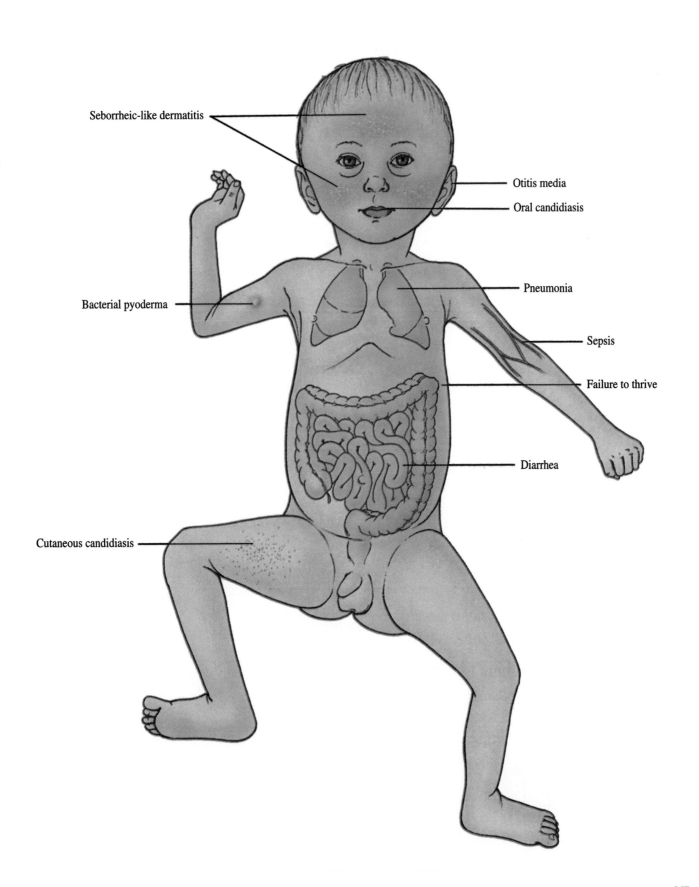

Seborrheic-like dermatitis

Otitis media

Oral candidiasis

Pneumonia

Bacterial pyoderma

Sepsis

Failure to thrive

Diarrhea

Cutaneous candidiasis

Hereditary Angioedema

Synonym	C1 esterase inhibitor deficiency Type I HAE, Type II HAE
Inheritance	Autosomal dominant with incomplete penetrance; both I and II involve C1INH gene on 11q13
Prenatal Diagnosis	DNA analysis
Incidence	1:150,000; 85% with type I HAE; 15% with type II HAE; M=F
Age at Presentation	Early childhood
Pathogenesis	Type I: C1 esterase inhibitor levels are less than 35% of normal secondary to heterogeneous mutations in the *C1INH* gene Type II: C1 esterase inhibitor levels are normal or elevated but dysfunctional secondary to a mutation at the active site of the *C1INH* gene Uncontrolled complement pathway activation, often induced by physical or emotional trauma Mechanism of edema formation is unknown
Key Features	**Skin** Angioedema without urticaria, pruritus, or pitting; with/without extension to mucous membranes Transient reticulated macular erythema Progressive presentation lasting from a few hours to 2 to 3 days **Ear-Nose-Throat** Laryngeal edema with airway obstruction **Gastrointestinal** Mucosal edema with secondary abdominal pain, vomiting, dysphagia
Differential Diagnosis	Acquired C1 esterase inhibitor deficiency secondary to monoclonal B-cell disease (i.e. lymphoma), cryoglobulinemia, other autoimmune disorders Urticaria Hypersensitivity reaction to medications, foods
Laboratory Data	C1 esterase inhibitor functional and quantitative serum assay C2, C4, levels decreased CH50, C3, and C1 normal
Management	Danazol/Stanazolol—stimulates production of functional C1 esterase inhibitor Fresh frozen plasma (FFP), antihistamines, epinephrine, corticosteroids—for severe, acute flares ε-Amino caproic acid (EACA)/tranexamic acid Medic alert bracelet—alert physicians and prevent unnecessary dental/ abdominal surgery Prophylactic use of FFP, EACA, or C1 INH concentrate if procedures necessary Evaluate family members
Prognosis	Ten percent to 30% die of airway compromise

Clinical Pearls

We have used Stanazolol to induce activity of the enzyme. . . It seems to have a shorter half-life and to be better tolerated by the patients than Danazol. . . Use with caution in growing children. . . Kids can start getting attacks at any time. . . To me, the classic occurrence is a fixed, indurated swelling of the lip without erythema. . . Angioedema is not responsive to histamines. . . These patients should be wearing medic alert bracelets. . . Death from laryngeal obstruction still occurs. *ML*

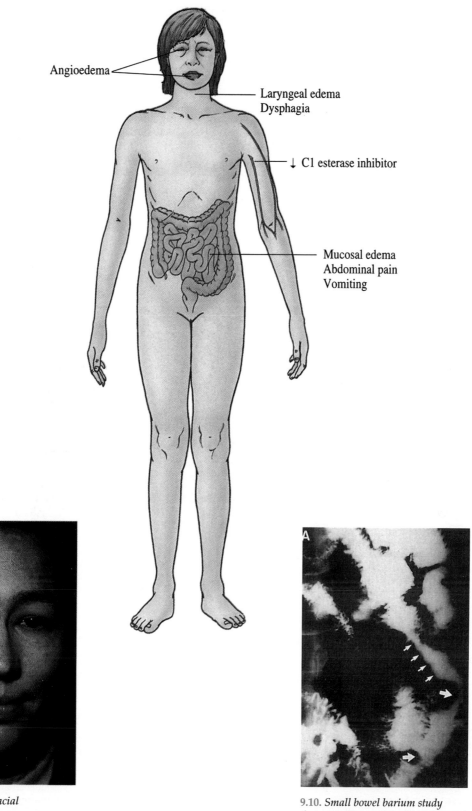

Angioedema

Laryngeal edema
Dysphagia

↓ C1 esterase inhibitor

Mucosal edema
Abdominal pain
Vomiting

9.9. Periorbital and facial angioedema. (102)

9.10. Small bowel barium study demonstrating mural edema (arrows) in the jejunum during acute episode of abdominal pain. (103)

Suggested Reading

Wiskott-Aldrich Syndrome

Brochstein JA, Gillio AP, Ruggiero M, et al. Marrow transplantation from human leukocyte antigen-identical or haploidentical donors for correction of Wiskott-Aldrich syndrome. *J Pediatr* 1991;119:907–912.

Derry JMJ, Ochs HD, Francke J. Isolation of a novel gene mutated in Wiskott-Aldrich syndrome. *Cell* 1994;78:635–644.

Giliani S, Fiorini M, Mella P, et al. Prenatal molecular diagnosis of Wiskott-Aldrich syndrome by direct mutation analysis. *Prenat Diagn* 1999;19:36–40.

Greer WL, Shehabeldin A, Schulman J, et al. Identification of WASP mutations, mutation hotspots and genotype-phenotype disparities in 24 patients with the Wiskott-Aldrich syndrome. *Hum Genet* 1996;198:685–690.

Imai K, Morio T, Zhu Y, et al. Clinical course of patients with WASP gene mutations. *Blood* 2004;103:456–464.

Lemahieu V, Gastier JM, Francke U. Novel mutations in the Wiskott-Aldrich syndrome gene and their effects on transcriptional, translational, and clinical phenotypes. *Hum Mutat* 1999;14:54–66.

Kwan S-P, Lehner T, Hagemann T, et al. Localization of the gene for the Wiskott-Aldrich syndrome between two flanking markers, TIMP and DXS255, on Xp11. 22–Xp11.3. *Genomics* 1991;10:29–33.

Lenarsky C, Parkman R. Bone marrow transplantation for the treatment of immune deficiency states. *Bone Marrow Transplant* 1990;6:361–369.

Litzman J, Jones A, Hann I, et al. Intravenous immunoglobulin, splenectomy, and antibiotic prophylaxis in Wiskot-Aldrich syndrome. *Arch Dis Child* 1996;75:436–439.

Ochs HD. The Wiskott-Aldrich syndrome. *Isr Med Assoc J* 2002;4:379–384.

Peacocke M, Siminovitch KA. The Wiskott-Aldrich syndrome. *Semin Dermatol* 1993;12:247–254.

Peacocke M, Siminovitch KA. Wiskott-Aldrich syndrome: new molecular and biochemical insights. *J Am Acad Dermatol* 1992;27:507–519.

Remold-O'Donnell E, Rosen FS. Sialophorin (CD43) and the Wiskott-Aldrich syndrome. *Immunodefic Rev* 1990;2:151–174.

Snapper SB, Rosen FS. The Wiskott-Aldrich syndrome protein (WASP): roles in signaling and cytoskeletal organization. *Annu Rev Immunol* 1999;17:905–929.

Sullivan KE, Mullen CA, Blaese RM, et al. A multiinstitutional survey of the Wiskott-Aldrich syndrome. *J Pediatr* 1994;125:876–885.

Thrasher AJ, Kinnon C. The Wiskott-Aldrich syndrome. *Clin Exp Immunol* 2000;120:2.

Chronic Granulomatous Disease

Babior BM. The respiratory burst oxidase and the molecular basis of chronic granulomatous disease. *Am J Hematol* 1991;37:263–266.

Chinen J, Puck JM. Successes and risks of gene therapy in primary immunodeficiencies. *J Allergy Clin Immunol* 2004;113:595–603.

Curnutte JT. Conventional versus interferon-gamma therapy in chronic granulomatous disease. *J Infect Dis* 1993;167:S8–S12.

Dinauer MC, Orkin SH. Chronic granulomatous disease. *Annu Rev Med* 1992;43:117–124.

Ding C, Kume A, Bjorgvinsdottir H, et al. High-level reconstitution of respiratory burst activity in a human X-linked chronic granulomatous disease (X-CGD). Cell line and correction of murine X-CGD bone marrow cells by retroviral-mediated gene transfer of human gp91 phox. *Blood* 1996;88:1834–1840.

Ezekowitz RAB, Dinauer MC, Jaffe HS, et al. Partial correction of the phagocyte defect in patients with X-linked chronic granulomatous disease by subcutaneous interferon gamma. *N Engl J Med* 1988;319:146–151.

Fischer A, Segal AW, Seger R, et al. The management of chronic granulomatous disease. *Eur J Pediatr* 1993;152:896–899.

Goebel WS, Dinauer MC. Gene therapy for chronic granulomatous disease. *Acta Haematol* 2003;110:86–92.

Gorlin JB. Identification of (CA/GT)n polymorphisms within the X-linked chronic granulomatous disease (X-CGD) gene: utility for prenatal diagnosis. *J Pediatr Hematol Oncol* 1998;20:112–119.

Ho CM, Vowels Mr, Lockwood L, et al. Successful bone marrow transplantation in a child with X-linked chronic granulomatous disease. *Bone Marrow Transplant* 1996;18:213–215.

Malech HL, Mapels PB, Whiting-Theoblad N, et al. Prolonged production of NADPH oxidase-corrected granulocytes after gene therapy of chronic granulomatous disease. *Proc Nat Acad Sci USA* 1997;94:12133–12138.

Mouy R, Veber R, Blanche S, et al. Long-term itroconazole prophylaxis against Aspergillus infections in thirty-two patients with chronic granulomatous disease. *J Pediatr* 1994;125:998–1003.

Nathan DG, Baehner RL, Weaver DK. Failure of nitro blue tetrazolium reduction in the phagocytic vacuoles of leukocytes in chronic granulomatous disease. *J Clin Invest* 1969;48:1895–1904.

Pogrebniak HW, Gallin JI, Malech HL, et al. Surgical management of pulmonary infections in chronic granulomatous disease of childhood. *Ann Thorac Surg* 1993;55:844–849.

Rosenzweig SD, Holland SM. Phagocyte immunodeficiencies and their infections. *J Allergy Clin Immunol* 2004;113:620–626.

Sahn EE, Migliardi RT. Crusted scalp nodule in an infant. Chronic granulomatous disease of childhood (CGD). *Arch Dermatol* 1994;130:105–108.

Segal BH, Leto TL, Gaiiin JI, et al. Genetic, biochemical, and clinical features of the chronic granulomatous disease. *Medicine* 2000;79:170.

Tauber AL, Borregaard N, Simons E, et al. Chronic granulomatous disease: a syndrome of phagocyte oxidase deficiencies. *Medicine* 1983;62:286–309.

Winkelstein JA, Marino MC, Johnston RB Jr, et al. Chronic granulomatous disease. Report on a national registry of 368 patients. *Medicine (Baltimore)* 2000;79:155–169.

Zambrano E, Esper F, Rosenberg R, et al. Chronic granulomatous disease. *Pediatr Dev Pathol* 2003;6:577–581.

Hyper-Immunoglobulin E Syndrome

Borges WG, Augustine NH, Hill HR. Defective interleukin-12/interferon-g pathway in patients with hyperimmunoglobulinemia E syndrome. *J Pediatr* 2000;136:176–180.

Donabedian H, Gallin JI. Mononuclear cells from patients with the hyperimmunoglobulin E-recurrent-infection syndrome produce an inhibitor of leukocyte chemotaxis. *J Clin Invest* 1982;69:1155–1163.

Donabedian H, Gallin JI. The hyperimmunoglobulin E recurrent-infection (Job's) syndrome: a review of the NIH experience and the literature. *Medicine* 1983;62:195–208.

Erlewyn-Lajeunesse MD. Hyperimmunoglobulin-E syndrome with recurrent infection: a review of current opinion and treatment. *Pediatr Allergy Immunol* 2000;11:133–141.

Garraud O, Mollis SN, Holland SM, et al. Regulation of immunoglobulin production in hyper-IgE (Job's) syndrome. *J Allergy Clin Immunol* 1999;103:333.

Grimbacher B, Schaffer AA, Holland SM, et al. Genetic linkage of hyper-IgE syndrome to chromosome 4. *Am J Hum Genet* 1999;65:735–744.

Grimbacher B, Holland SM, Gallin JI, et al. Hyper-IgE syndrome with recurrent infections—an autosomal dominant multisystem disorder. *N Engl J Med* 1999;340:692–702.

Ito R, Mori M, Katakura S, et al. Selective insufficiency of IFN-gamma secretion in patients with hyper-IgE syndrome. *Allergy* 2003;58:329–336.

Jeppson JD, Jaffe HS, Hill HR. Use of recombinant human interferon gamma to enhance neutrophil chemotactic responses in Job syndrome of hyperimmunoglobulinemia E and recurrent infections. *J Pediatr* 1991;118:383–387.

Kamei R, Honig PJ. Neonatal Job's syndrome featuring a vesicular eruption. *Pediatr Dermatol* 1988;5:75–82.

Lavoie A, Rottem M, Grodofsky MP, et al. Anti-Staphylococcus aureus IgE antibodies for diagnosis of hyperimmunoglobulinemia-E recurrent infection syndrome in infancy. *Am J Dis Child* 1989;143:1038–1041.

Shamberger RC, Wohl ME, Perez-Atayde A, et al. Pneumatocele complicating hyperimmunoglobulin E syndrome (Job's syndrome). *Ann Thorac Surg* 1992;54:1206–1208.

Shemer A, Weiss G, Confino Y, et al. The hyper-IgE syndrome. Two cases and review of the literature. *Int J Dermatol* 2001;40:622–628.

Van Eendenburg JP, Smitt JH, Weening RS. Hyperimmunoglobulin E recurrent infection (Job's) syndrome. *Br J Dermatol* 1991;125:397.

Severe Combined Immunodeficiency

Aiuti A. Advances in gene therapy for ADA-deficient SCID. *Curr Opin Mol Ther* 2002;4:515–522.

Buckley RH, Schiff SE, Schiff RI, et al. Haploidentical bone marrow stem cell transplantation in human severe combined immunodeficiency. *Semin Hematol* 1993;30:92–101.

Cournoyer D, Caskey CT. Gene therapy of the immune system. *Annu Rev Immunol* 1993;11:297–329.

De Raeve L, Song M, Levy J, et al. Cutaneous lesions as a clue to severe combined immunodeficiency. *Pediatr Dermatol* 1992;9:49–51

Fischer A, Hacein-Bey S, Le Deist F, et al. Gene therapy of severe combined immunodeficiencies. *Immunol Rev* 2000;178:13–20.

Fischer A. Severe combined immunodeficiencies (SCID). *Clin Exp Immunol* 2000;122:143.

Frucht DM, Gadina M, Jagadeesh GJ, et al. Unexpected and variable phenotypes in a family with JAK3 deficiency. *Genes Immunol* 2001;2:422–432.

Gaspar HB, et al. Severe combined immunodeficiency: molecular pathogenesis and diagnosis. *Arch Dis Child* 2001;84:169.

Gennery AR, Cant AJ. Diagnosis of severe combined immunodeficiency. *J Clin Pathol* 2001;54:191–195.

Hacein-Bey-Abina S, Fischer A, Cavazzana-Calvo M. Gene therapy of X-linked severe combined immunodeficiency. *Int J Hematol* 2002;76:295–298.

Hacein-Bey-Abina S, Le Deist F, Carlier F, et al. Sustained correction of X-linked severe combined immunodeficiency by ex vivo gene therapy. *N Engl J Med* 2002;346:1185–1193.

Hacein-Bey-Abina S, Von Kalle C, Schmidt M, et al. LMO2-associated clonal T cell proliferation in two patients after gene therapy for SCID-Xl [published erratum appears in *Science* 200324;302:568]. *Science* 2003;302:415–419.

Hirschhorn R. In vivo reversion to normal of inherited mutations in humans. *J Med Genet* 2003;40:721–728.

Hirschhorn R. Overview of biochemical abnormalities and molecular genetics of adenosine deaminase deficiency. *Pediatr Res* 1993;33:S35–S41.

Hirschhorn R. Severe combined immunodeficiency and adenosine deaminase deficiency. *N Eng J Med* 1975;292:714–719.

Leonard WJ, Noguchi M, Russell SM, et al. The molecular basis of X-linked severe combined immunodeficiency: the role of the interleukin-2 receptor gamma chain as a common gamma chain, gamma c. *Immunol Rev* 1994;138:61–86.

McCormack MP, Forster A, Drynan L, et al. The LMO2 T-cell oncogene is activated via chromosomal translocations or retroviral insertion during gene therapy but has no mandatory role in normal T-cell development. *Mol Cell Biol* 2003;23:9003–9013.

Ortiz-Urda S, Thyagarajan B, Keene DR, et al. Stable nonviral genetic correction of inherited human skin disease [published erratum appears in *Nat Med* 2003;9:237]. *Nat Med* 2002;8:1166–1170.

Postigo Llorente C, Ivars Amoros J, Ortiz de Frutos FJ, et al. Cutaneous lesions in severe combined immunodeficiency: two case reports and a review of the literature. *Pediatr Dermatol* 1991;8:314–321.

Roberts JL, Lengi A, Brown SM, et al. Janus kinase 3 (JAK3) deficiency: clinical, immunologic, and molecular analyses of 10 patients and outcomes of stem cell transplantation. *Blood* 2004;103:2009–2018.

Hereditary Angioedema

Cicardi M, Bergamaschini L, Cugno M, et al. Pathogenetic and clinical aspects of C1 inhibitor deficiency. *Immunobiology* 1998;199:366–376.

Cicardi M, Bergamaschini L, Marasini B, et al. Hereditary angioedema: an appraisal of 104 cases. *Am J Med Sci* 1982;284:2–9.

Cooper KD. Urticaria and angioedema: diagnosis and evaluation. *J Am Acad Dermatol* 1991;25:166–174

Cumming SA, Halsall DJ, Ewan PW, et al. The effect of sequence variations within the coding region of the C1 inhibitc gene on disease expression and protein function in families with hereditary angio-oedema. *J Med Genet* 2003;40:e114.

Freiberger T, Kolarova L, Mejstrik P, et al. Five novel mutations in the C1 inhibitor gene (C1NH) leading to a premature stop codon in patients with type I hereditary angioedema. *Hum Mutat* 2002;19:461.

Gelfand JA, Boss GR, Conley CL, et al. Acquired C1 esterase inhibitor deficiency and angioedema: a review. *Medicine* 1979;58:321–328.

Gelfand JA, Sherins RJ, Ailing DW, et al. Treatment of hereditary angioedema with danazol: reversal of clinical and biochemical abnormalities. *N Engl J Med* 1976;295:1444–1448.

Grace RJ, Jacob A, Mainwaring CJ, et al. Acquired C1 esterase inhibitor deficiency as manifestation of T-cell lymphoproliferative disorder. *Lancet* 1990;336:118.

Greaves M, Lawlor F. Angioedema: manifestations and management. *J Am Acad Dermatol* 1991;25:155–161.

Hellmann G, Schneider L, Krieg T, et al. Efficacy of danazol treatment in a patient with the new variant of hereditary angio-oedema (HAE III). *Br J Dermatol* 2004;150:157–158.

Nzeako UC, Frigas E, Tremaine WJ. Hereditary angioedema: a broad review for clinicians. *Arch Intern Med* 2001;161:2417–2429.

Sekijima Y, Hashimoto T, Kawachi Y, et al. A novel RNA splice site mutation in the C1 inhibitor gene of a patient with type I hereditary angioedema. *Intern Med* 2004;43:253–255.

Stoppa-Lyonnet D, Tosi M, Laurent J, et al. Altered C1 inhibitor genes in type I hereditary angioedema [published erratum appears in *N Engl J Med* 1987;317:641]. *N Engl J Med* 1987;317:1–6.

Theriault A, Whaley K, McPhaden AR, et al. Regional assignment of the human C1-inhibitor gene to 11q11–q13. 1. *Hum Genet* 1990;84:477–479.

Waytes AT, Rosen FS, Frank MM. Treatment of hereditary angioedema with a vapor-heated C1 inhibitor concentrate. *N Engl J Med* 1996;334:1666–1667.

Weinstock LB, Kothari T, Sharma RN, et al. Recurrent abdominal pain as the sole manifestation of hereditary angioedema in multiple family members. *Gastroenterology* 1987;93:1116–1118.

Winnewisser J, Rossi M, Spath P, et al. Type I hereditary angio-oedema: variability of clinical presentation and course within two large kindreds. *J Int Med* 1007;241:39–46.

Chapter 10

Disorders of Hair and Nails

Clinical Pearls

David Whiting, M.D. (DW), Bernice Krafchik, M.D. (BK),
Richard Scher, M.D. (RS), Kurt Hirschhorn, M.D. (KH), and
Judith Willner, M.D. (JW)

Menkes' Syndrome

Synonym	Menkes kinky hair syndrome Occipital horn syndrome (OHS)
Inheritance	X-linked recessive; *MKN* or *ATP7A* gene on Xq13
Prenatal Diagnosis	DNA analysis Amniocentesis/chorionic villus sampling (CVS)—increased incorporation of copper by cultured amniotic fluid cells
Incidence	1:35,000 in Australia, 1:300,000 in Europe; males only; approximately 90% with classic, severe form, 10% with milder OHS
Age at Presentation	First few months of life
Pathogenesis	Mutations in *MKN* or *ATP7A*, a gene encoding the copper-binding enzyme adenosine triphosphatase (ATPase), leads to defective copper transport and metabolism with subsequent low levels of serum copper; phenotype reflects deficiency of copper-dependent enzyme activity in various systems

Key Features

Hair
Pili torti most common; trichorrhexis nodosa, monilethrix described; hypopigmented, sparse, short, brittle, "steel-wool" quality; sparse, broken horizontal eyebrows; sparse eyelashes

Skin
Hypopigmented, "doughy" consistency with laxity, pudgy cheeks, Cupid's bow upper lip

Central Nervous System
Progressive deterioration with lethargy, seizures, mental and motor retardation, hypertonia, hypothermia

Musculoskeletal
Failure to thrive, frontal bossing, wormian bones in sagittal and lambdoid sutures, metaphyseal widening with spurs in long bones, fractures

OHS: occipital horns (exostosis at insertion of trapezius and sternocleidomastoid muscles), abnormal facies, short flat clavicles, elbow deformities secondary to radial subluxation

Cardiovascular
Tortuous arteries (especially brain)

Genitourinary
Variety of anomalies

Differential Diagnosis	Battered child syndrome Argininosuccinic aciduria (p. 278) Björnstad syndrome (p. 276)
Laboratory Data	Serum copper, ceruloplasmin levels DNA analysis
Management	Parenteral copper histidine if initiated first 8 weeks of life may be of benefit Antiseizure medications, pamidronate has been helpful in preventing fractures in one study
Prognosis	Progressive deterioration with death by 2–3 years of age associated with pneumonia

Clinical Pearls

Can have an awful lot of trichorrhexis nodosa as well. . . They live only about a year or two. . . Female carriers can have pili torti. . . Genetic counseling should be stressed. *DW*

Skin

Associated Findings

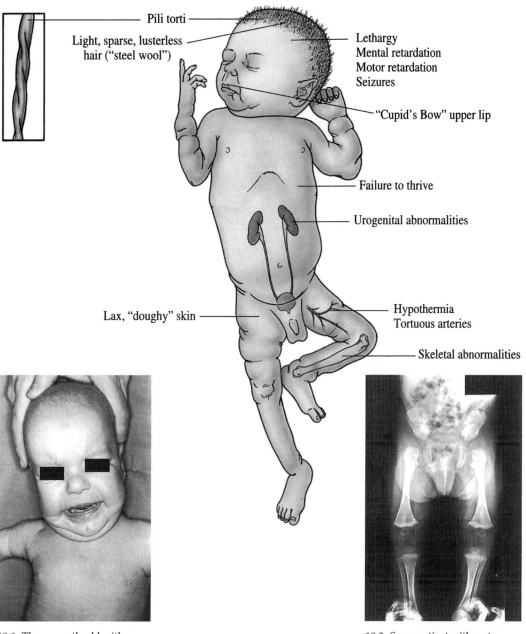

Pili torti
Light, sparse, lusterless hair ("steel wool")
Lethargy
Mental retardation
Motor retardation
Seizures
"Cupid's Bow" upper lip
Failure to thrive
Urogenital abnormalities
Lax, "doughy" skin
Hypothermia
Tortuous arteries
Skeletal abnormalities

10.1. *Three-month-old with doughy, lax skin and "pudgy" face, sparse hair. (104)*

10.2. *Same patient with metaphysical widening of femur and tibia and femoral spurs. Note osteoporosis. (104)*

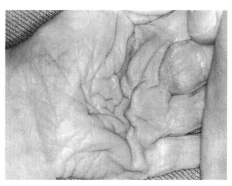

10.3. *Doughy redundant skin on palm. (104)*

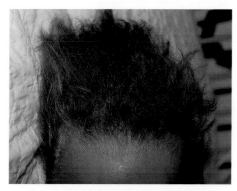

10.4. *"Steel-wool" hair (105)*

Björnstad Syndrome

Inheritance	Autosomal recessive; 2q34–q36 gene locus
Prenatal Diagnosis	None
Incidence	Very rare—approximately 25 cases reported; M=F
Age at Presentation	By 2 years old
Pathogenesis	Unknown

Key Features	**Hair**
	  Pili torti with/without alopecia of scalp; eyebrows, eyelashes unaffected
	Ear-Nose-Throat
	  Bilateral sensorineural deafness

Differential Diagnosis	Crandall syndrome (pili torti, deafness, hypogonadism) Menkes' syndrome (p. 274)
Laboratory Data	Auditory testing
Management	Referral to audiologist
Prognosis	Normal intelligence, life span; hearing loss mild to severe with increased severity associated with more severe hair defects

Clinical Pearls

If you diagnose pili torti in a child, send them all to an audiologist early on to prevent potential speech deficits. . . They get "classic" pili torti as a rule.   *DW*

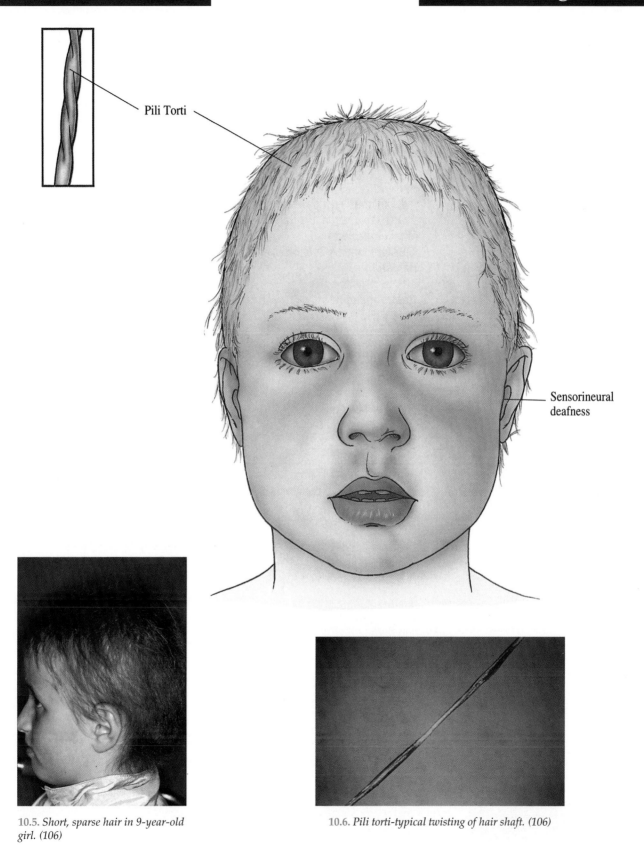

Pili Torti

Sensorineural
deafness

10.5. *Short, sparse hair in 9-year-old girl. (106)*

10.6. *Pili torti-typical twisting of hair shaft. (106)*

Argininosuccinic Aciduria

Inheritance	Autosomal recessive; argininosuccinate lyase (ASL) gene on 7cen-q11.2
Prenatal Diagnosis	Amniocentesis—argininosuccinase assay in cultured amniotic fluid cells DNA analysis
Incidence	1:70,000 U.S. births; M=F
Age at Presentation	Neonate (neonatal form) or second year of life (late-onset form)
Pathogenesis	Mutation in *ASL* leads to a deficiency in argininosuccinate lyase—second most common urea cycle defect Mechanism of hair defect unknown
Key Features	**Hair** Trichorrhexis nodosa (approximately 50% affected)—increased with late-onset disease; dull, dry, matted and fragile; increased in occipital region **Musculoskeletal** Failure to thrive (neonatal) **Hematologic** Hyperammonemia **Gastrointestinal** Vomiting Hepatomegaly (neonatal) **Central Nervous System** Seizures Lethargy, coma (neonatal) Ataxia, severe mental retardation (late-onset)
Differential Diagnosis	Citrullinemia Familial trichorrhexis nodosa Acquired trichorrhexis nodosa
Laboratory Data	Enzyme assay—argininosuccinase deficiency in red blood cells and cultured fibroblasts High-voltage electrophoresis or ion-exchange chromatography—increased blood, urine, or cerebrospinal fluid (CSF) argininosuccinic acid levels Increased ammonia levels in blood
Management	Restricted protein diet (1.0 to 1.5 g/kg per day) with arginine supplementation (3 to 5 mmol/kg per day) Referral to dermatologist, neurologist Liver transplant
Prognosis	If survival beyond the neonatal period, most will be mentally retarded; late-onset cases are severely mentally retarded

Clinical Pearls

One child we took care of actually received a liver transplant in Pittsburgh, which is the only available therapy. . . Unfortunately, she died of fungal sepsis 1 year later. . . Prenatal linkage studies could not be done on the family. . . An enormous rarity.
KH, JW

Trichorrhexis nodosa is caused by trauma and is often seen in metabolic disorders with brittle hair. *DW*

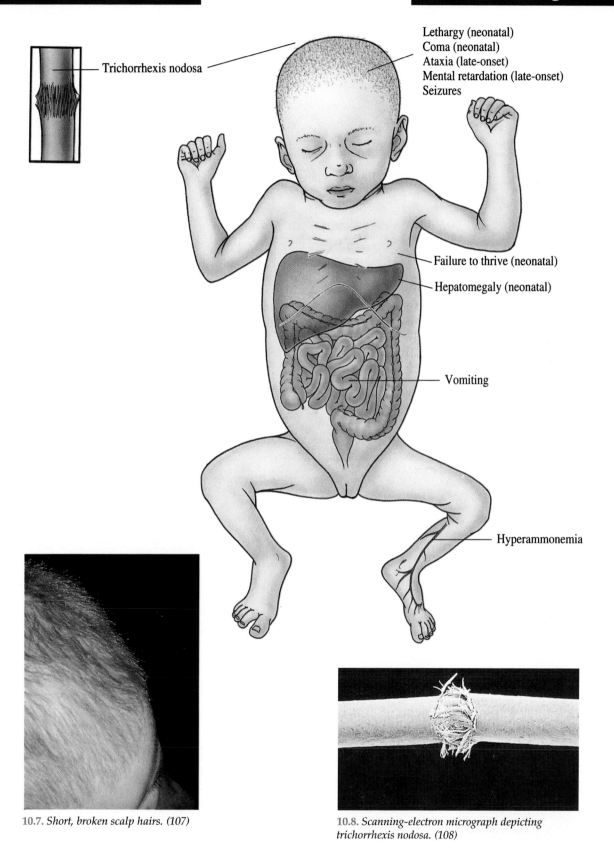

Trichorrhexis nodosa

Lethargy (neonatal)
Coma (neonatal)
Ataxia (late-onset)
Mental retardation (late-onset)
Seizures

Failure to thrive (neonatal)
Hepatomegaly (neonatal)

Vomiting

Hyperammonemia

10.7. *Short, broken scalp hairs.* (107)

10.8. *Scanning-electron micrograph depicting trichorrhexis nodosa.* (108)

Monilethrix

Inheritance	Autosomal dominant; human basic type II hair keratin genes, hHb1 and hHb6 on 12q13
Prenatal Diagnosis	None
Incidence	Rare; M=F
Age of Presentation	First few months of life
Pathogenesis	Mutations in human hair keratin genes expressed in cortical trichocytes of the hair shaft, leads to defect in many cases
Key Features	**Hair**
	Structural defect: elliptical nodes along shaft (0.7 to 1.0 mm apart) with undulating variation in diameter; "beaded" appearance under the light microscope; breaks at internodes
	Dry, brittle, lusterless, sparse, short
	Scalp most common, but may occur on eyelashes, eyebrows, and body
	Skin (most common association)
	Keratosis pilaris on upper back, nape of neck, arms
	Nails
	Brittle
	Eyes
	Cataracts (rare)
	Mouth
	Teeth abnormalities
	Central Nervous System
	Mental retardation (rare)
Differential Diagnosis	None
Laboratory Data	Light microscopy of hair shaft
Management	Referral to dermatologist—avoid hair trauma, retinoids, topical minoxidil
	Referral to symptom-specific specialist
Prognosis	May improve with pregnancy and at puberty

Clinical Pearls

You can try isotretinoin or acitretin. . . I saw a family at a meeting in San Antonio a few years ago where the sons had severe alopecia, while the father had mild alopecia. . . His had been severe as a boy. . . Associations not that common. . . Occasional case reports.   *DW*

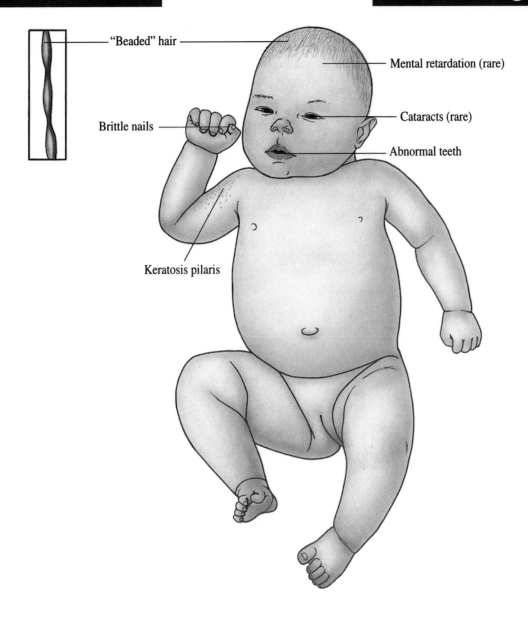

"Beaded" hair

Mental retardation (rare)

Brittle nails

Cataracts (rare)

Abnormal teeth

Keratosis pilaris

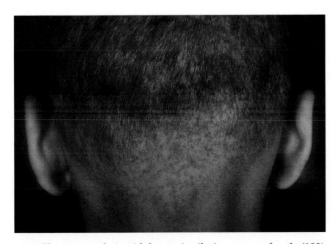

10.9. Short, sparse hair with keratosis pilaris on nape of neck. (109)

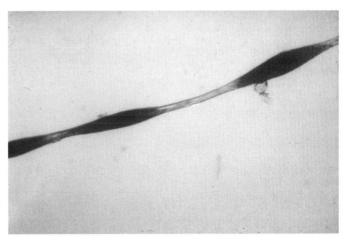

10.10. Monilethrix- "beaded" appearance under light microscopy (110)

Uncombable Hair Syndrome

Synonym	Pili trianguli et canaliculi Spun-glass hair
Inheritance	Autosomal dominant in some cases; gene locus unknown
Prenatal Diagnosis	None
Incidence	Approximately 50 cases reported; M=F
Age at Presentation	Usually in infancy
Pathogenesis	Unknown

Key Features	**Hair**
	   Blonde, dry, shiny hair—unable to comb into place, not fragile
	   Eyelashes, eyebrows unaffected

Differential Diagnosis	None
Laboratory Data	Electron microscopy—canal-like groove along shaft of a triangular-shaped hair
Management	Biotin 0.3 mg three times per day may help
Prognosis	May improve with age

Clinical Pearls

Doesn't always improve with age, but it may. . . Not fragile hair. . . Just difficult to comb. . . Walter Shelley has found that biotin helped to manage the hair in one case. . . He sent me hair from the case, and I found the structural defect unchanged. . . Looking under the light microscope, I had no problem finding longitudinal grooves. . . No common associations.   *DW*

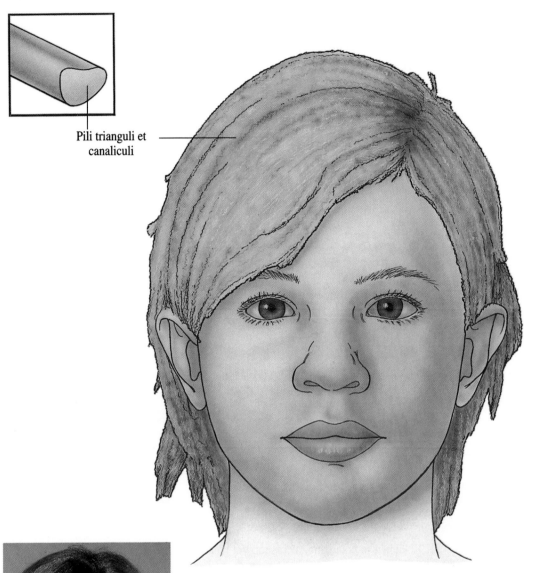

Pili trianguli et
canaliculi

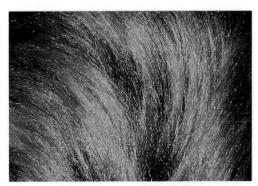

10.11. Shiny, "spun glass" hair. Note
normal eyebrows, eyelashes. (111)

10.12. Close-up of scalp hair. (111)

Hypohidrotic Ectodermal Dysplasia

Synonym	Anhidrotic ectodermal dysplasia Christ-Siemens-Touraine syndrome
Inheritance	X-linked recessive—ectodysplasin (*EDA*) gene on Xq12–q13 Autosomal dominant, recessive and other x-linked (NEMO mutations) cases described but rare
Prenatal Diagnosis	DNA analysis Fetoscopy (20 weeks)—skin biopsy with absent pilosebaceous units
Incidence	Approximately 1:100,000; >90% males; female carriers partially affected
Age at Presentation	Infancy to early childhood
Pathogenesis	Mutation in ectodysplasin, a member of the tumor necrosis family, leads to defective regulation of ectodermal structures

Key Features

Skin
Smooth, soft, dry, fine wrinkles with pigmentation periorbitally; hypoanhidrosis with hyperpyrexia; increased frequency of atopic dermatitis
Newborn: may have collodion membrane, marked scaling

Hair
Hypopigmented, fine, short, sparse scalp and body hair; longitudinal groove on electron microscopy; eyebrows, eyelashes fine to absent

Nails
Slight dystrophy (much less common and insignificant compared to hidrotic ectodermal dysplasia)

Craniofacial
Frontal bossing, saddle nose, prominent supraorbital ridges, everted thick lips, hypoplastic midface, abnormal ears

Teeth
Hypo-anodontia, peg-shaped/conical incisors and canines; molars with hooked cusps; deciduous and permanent affected; hypoplastic gum ridges noted early on

Sinopulmonary (less common)
Atrophic rhinitis with thick, foul-smelling discharge; increased bronchopulmonary infection, asthma

Differential Diagnosis	Other ectodermal dysplasias
Laboratory Data	Skin biopsy of palmar skin—lack of eccrine units Jaw film DNA analysis
Management	Avoid overheating with limits on physical activity, exercise, "cool suit," appropriate occupation, air conditioning, cool baths, avoid warm climates; close monitoring for infection with early antibiotic intervention, antipyretics Methyl cellulose 1% drops for dry mucosa of eyes, nose—avoid antihistamines; skin emolliation Referral to pediatric dentist—dentures, implants Referral to plastic surgery—facial cosmesis, wig Referrral to ear-nose-throat (ENT) specialist—manage recurrent infection, asthma Examine first-degree relatives
Prognosis	May have stunted development, febrile convulsions; rarely fatal early on with improvement in late childhood; otherwise normal life span

Clinical Pearls

Most importantly, avoid overheating. . . Air conditioning, cool temperatures, light clothing. . . I have to write to schools and tell them the kids should be in an air-conditioned environment. . . One infant used to drag himself across the marble floor to keep cool. . . Kids find out for themselves what their exercise limitations are. . . Our dentist does beautiful work using plates early on and implants as they get older. . . Avoid extracting teeth so that the alveolar ridge can be maintained. . . Early acquaintance with the dentist. . . Difficult diagnosis in nursery but may be recognized by the typical wrinkles around the eye. . . Look at mother carefully. . . Carriers often have dry hair, skin, and missing teeth. . . Nail changes do not occur. . . They all start to resemble one another. . . *BK*

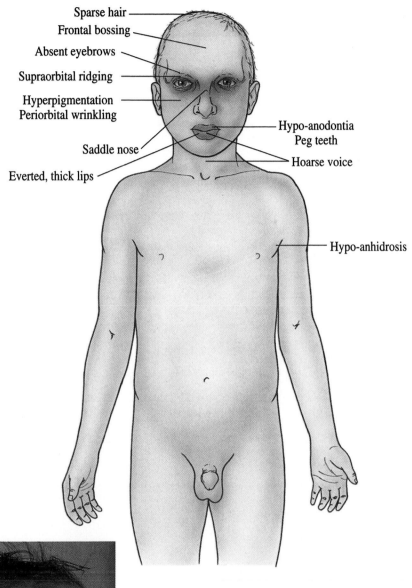

Sparse hair
Frontal bossing
Absent eyebrows
Supraorbital ridging
Hyperpigmentation
Periorbital wrinkling
Saddle nose
Everted, thick lips

Hypo-anodontia
Peg teeth
Hoarse voice

Hypo-anhidrosis

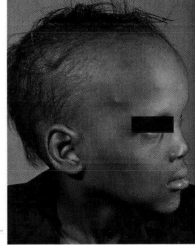

10.13. Indian male with fine, short,
sparse hair, frontal bossing, saddle nose,
prominent supraorbital ridge, periorbital
pigmentation, and thick everted lips. (5)

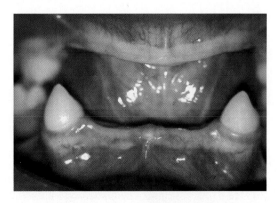

10.14. Anodontia and conical canines. (112)

Hidrotic Ectodermal Dysplasia

Synonym	Clouston syndrome
Inheritance	Autosomal dominant; connexin 30 (*GJB6*) gene on 13q11–12
Prenatal Diagnosis	None
Incidence	Rare; most common in French-Canadian and French population; M=F
Age at Presentation	Birth to neonatal period
Pathogenesis	Mutation in connexin 30 leads to defective ectodermal development and maintenance

Key Features

Skin
Palmoplantar keratoderma with transgradiens

Nails
Dystrophy—thickened, milky white early on, micronychia, hyperconvex, longitudinal striations, discolored, brittle, absent
Paronychial infections with/without nail matrix destruction

Hair
Scalp—normal early on but often becomes thin, wiry, brittle, pale, sparse, or absent after puberty
Body, eyelashes, eyebrows—sparse to absent; secondary conjunctivitis, blepharitis

Musculoskeletal
Tufting of terminal phalanges and thickened skull bones may occur

Differential Diagnosis	Other palmoplantar keratodermas Pachyonychia congenita
Laboratory Data	None
Management	Referral to dermatologist—diagnosis, keratolytics, surgical debridement, antibiotics (paronychia), wigs and nail sculpturing/bonding for cosmesis; nail matrix ablation to relieve pain
Prognosis	Normal life span

Clinical Pearls

Not exclusively French-Canadians. . . Blacks, Chinese, and most other groups have been described. . . A little girl I saw had complete alopecia. . . Interestingly, her family members grew hair when they became older. . . A wig is about the only thing to help the hair loss. . . The swollen, tufted terminal phalanges can be far more helpful than the nondiagnostic nail findings in establishing the syndrome. . . The skin on the palms and soles can get very calloused and thickened presenting as a keratoderma. . . I send them to a podiatrist for paring. . . Nail changes are common. . .   *BK*

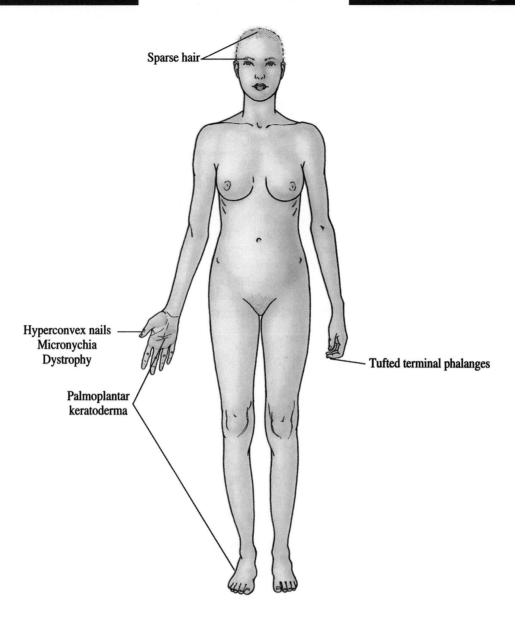

Sparse hair

Hyperconvex nails
Micronychia
Dystrophy

Tufted terminal phalanges

Palmoplantar
keratoderma

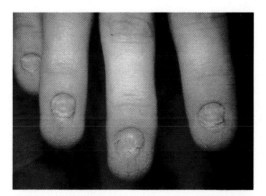

10.15. *Nail dystrophy with micronychia, partial
anonychia, and hyperconvexity of nail plate. (113)*

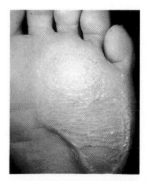

10.16. *Focal plantar keratoderma. (113)*

287

EEC Syndrome

Synonym	**E**ctrodactyly-**E**ctodermal Dysplasia-**C**left lip/palate syndrome
Inheritance	Autosomal dominant; three gene loci identified: EEC 1 on 7q11–21; EEC2 on chromosome 19, and EEC3, the p63 gene on 3q27 (majority of cases)
Prenatal Diagnosis	DNA analysis
Incidence	Rare; approximately 150 cases reported; M=F
Age at Presentation	Birth
Pathogenesis	Mutations in the p63 gene, a tumor suppressor gene required for normal limb, craniofacial, and epidermal morphogenesis, are responsible for the majority of cases; gene on chromosome 19 may be a modifying gene that modulates the phenotypic expression of p63 mutations

Key Features

Skin
Dry, scaling; thickening of palms, soles; normal sweat
Hair
Coarse, blonde, dry, can be sparse; axillary, pubic hair sparse
Nails
Dystrophic (even on unaffected fingers)
Teeth
Hypodontia, premature loss of permanent teeth, problems related to cleft
Musculoskeletal
Ectrodactyly (80% to 100%)—abnormal development of the median rays of feet > hands—"lobster-claw deformity"; cleft palate with/or without lip (70% to 100%)
Ear-Nose-Throat
Chronic otitis media, secondary conductive hearing loss (50%)
Genitourinary
Hydronephrosis, structural malformations (approximately 30%)
Ophthalmologic
Lacrimal gland/duct abnormalities

Differential Diagnosis	AEC syndrome (p. 290) Aplasia cutis congenita with limb defects (p. 160) Limb-mammary syndrome
Laboratory Data	Films to evaluate cleft, limbs Renal ultrasound
Management	Referral to plastic surgeon—cleft repair team Referral to orthopedist—limb repair Referral to ENT—antibiotics, follow for hearing loss Referral to dentist after cleft repair Referral to ophthalmologist, urologist based on signs, symptoms
Prognosis	Early intervention will improve overall outcome

Clinical Pearls

The ectodermal dysplasia is usually mild, some only showing sparsity and discoloration of the hair. May have problems with lacrimal ducts. I have seen genitourinary problems but this is rare. Syndrome varies from mild to severe. *BK*

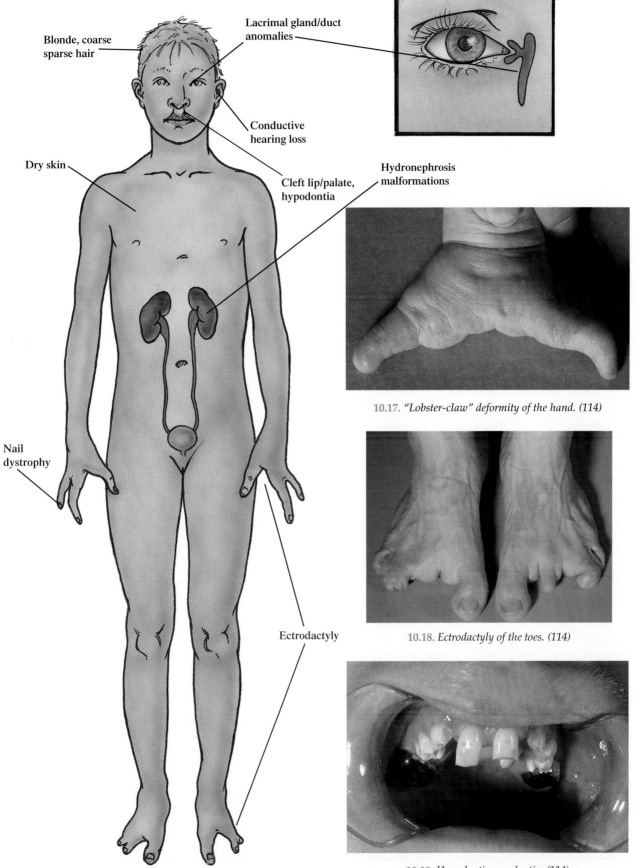

Skin

Blonde, coarse sparse hair

Dry skin

Nail dystrophy

Lacrimal gland/duct anomalies

Conductive hearing loss

Cleft lip/palate, hypodontia

Hydronephrosis malformations

Ectrodactyly

Associated Findings

10.17. *"Lobster-claw" deformity of the hand. (114)*

10.18. *Ectrodactyly of the toes. (114)*

10.19. *Hypodontia, anodontia. (114)*

AEC Syndrome

Synonym

Ankyloblepharon filiforme adenatum-**E**ctodermal dysplasia-**C**left palate-Hay-Wells syndrome

Inheritance

Autosomal dominant; p63 gene on 3q27

Prenatal Diagnosis

DNA analysis
Ultrasound

Incidence

Rare; M=F

Age at Presentation

Birth

Pathogenesis

Heterozygous missense mutations in the sterile alpha motif (SAM) domain of the p63 tumor suppressor gene contribute to phenotype in many cases

Key Features

Skin
  Birth
    Collodion membrane-like with erythroderma, scale, erosions; sheds to reveal dry, thin skin
  Scalp
    Chronic erosive dermatitis with granulation tissue, crusting, bacterial superinfection
Hair
  Scalp hair is sparse, wiry, light color, scarring alopecia
  Sparse body hair, eyelashes, eyebrows
Nails
  Dystrophic, absent
Eyes
  Ankyloblepharon (fusion of eyelids with strands of skin) (70%); lacrimal duct atresia/obstruction with secondary conjunctivitis, blepharitis
Head/Neck
  Cleft palate with/or without lip (80%), anodontia/hypodontia, malformed ears, chronic otitis with secondary hearing loss

Differential Diagnosis

EEC syndrome (p. 288)
Rapp-Hodgkin syndrome
CIE (p. 12)
Epidermolysis bullosa (p. 200)

Laboratory Data
Bacterial cultures of skin
Head films
DNA analysis

Management
Referral to plastic surgeon—cleft repair team
Referral to ophthalmology—surgical lysis of ankyloblepharon, general ophthalmologic care
Referral to dermatologist—emolliation, infection surveillance, gentle scalp care

Prognosis
Early intervention will lead to improved outcome

Clinical Pearls

The major problem with these infants relates to the scalp dermatitis, which may be extremely severe and requires constant care; secondary bacterial infection of the scalp is common. The scalp skin is thin and red with the veins evident through the skin. Despite dressing changes management is difficult. Cooperation between the plastic surgeons and dermatologists is helpful to parents who need a great deal of emotional support. The skin on the body is thin and often quite eroded. A typical facies can be recognized. *BK*

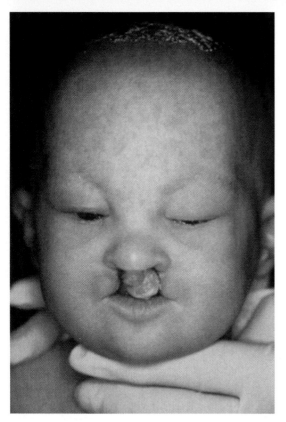

10.20. *Complete bilateral cleft lip/palate with sparse hair growth. (115)*

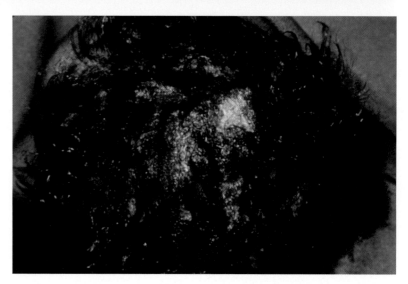

10.21. *Alopecia of scalp with erythema, pustules, crusting. (116)*

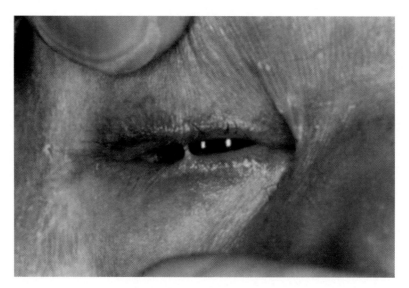

10.22. *Ankyloblepharon filiforme adenatum with single band of tissue connecting upper and lower eyelids. (117)*

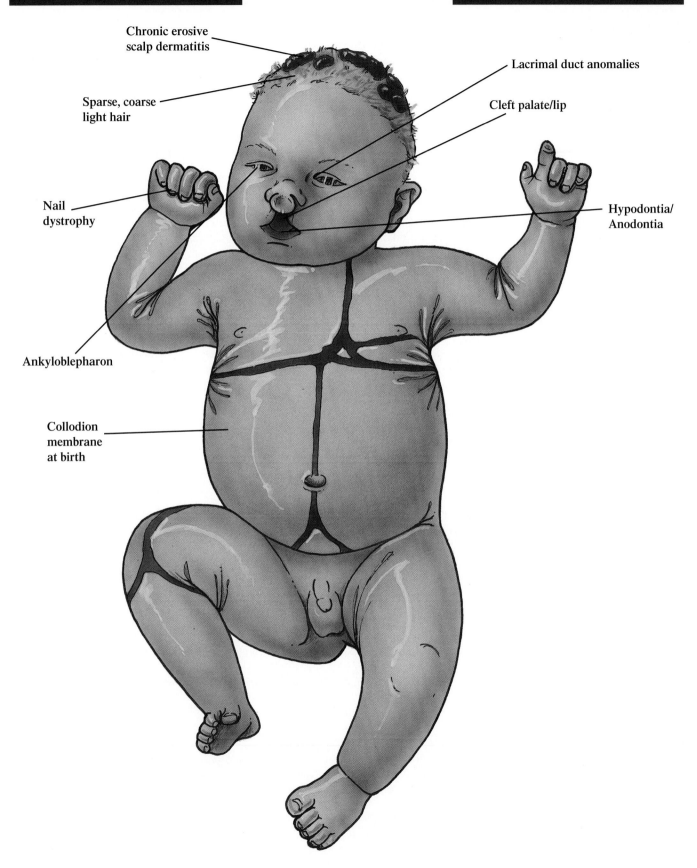

Chronic erosive scalp dermatitis

Sparse, coarse light hair

Nail dystrophy

Ankyloblepharon

Collodion membrane at birth

Lacrimal duct anomalies

Cleft palate/lip

Hypodontia/ Anodontia

Pachyonychia Congenita

Synonym	Jadassohn-Lewandowsky syndrome, PC-1 Jackson-Lawler, PC-2
Inheritance	PC-1: autosomal dominant; K16 and K6a gene on 17q12–21 and 12q13, respectively PC-2: autosomal dominant; K17 and K6b gene on 17q12–21 and 12q13, respectively
Prenatal Diagnosis	DNA analysis
Incidence	Over 100 case reports; increased in Slavic and Jewish population; M>F
Age at Presentation	Birth (if natal teeth); otherwise first few months of life
Pathogenesis	Keratin gene defects disrupt normal intermediate filament assembly and may play a role when frictional stressors are applied to epithelial cells
Key Features	**Nails** All 20 nails affected—fingers > toes; subungual hyperkeratosis with increased transverse curvature ("pincer nail effect") and distal elevation of nail plate; brownish-yellow discoloration; painful paronychial infection with *Candida, Staphylococcus;* may shed nail plate **Skin** Focal symmetric palmoplantar keratoderma with/without hyperhidrosis, pain, bullae Follicular hyperkeratosis of elbows, knees, extensor extremities Steatocystoma multiplex (PC-2), epidermoid cysts (PC-2) **Mouth** Natal teeth (PC-2) Oral leukokeratosis (PC-1, not premalignant)—tongue, buccal mucosa **Eyes (less common)** Corneal dystrophy, cataracts
Differential Diagnosis	Dyskeratosis congenita (p. 180) Other palmoplantar keratodermas Weber-Cockayne syndrome (p. 242) Psoriasis Onychomycosis
Laboratory Data	Oral biopsy (if diagnosis equivocal) Nail biopsy
Management	Referral to dermatologist/podiatrist—nail paring with electric file, urea or salicylic acid in petrolatum under occlusion to nail plate, avulsion with matrix destruction, antibiotics, orthotics; keratolytics, emolliation to hyperkeratotic lesions
Prognosis	Lesions persist throughout life; rarely blindness secondary to corneal dystrophy

Clinical Pearls

Babies can suffer from recurrent painful staphylococcal paronychia. . . Treat infection promptly. . . Dental filers work well in paring the nail. . . Podiatrist can be tremendous help. . . I've seen a few adults attending the EB clinic who were misdiagnosed. . . The presence of natal teeth and nail changes is very suggestive of pachyonchia congenita. . . It is important to remember the type that begins after birth called the tardive variety. . . *BK*

The nail defect markedly affects function making it difficult to pick up small objects and impairs fine touch. . . Most patients have been male. . . Although there's not a lot to offer them, you may try 40% urea in petrolatum applied to nail plate for 7 to 10 days under occlusion with subsequent physical debridement. . . Total nail avulsion surgically may be necessary. . . *RS*

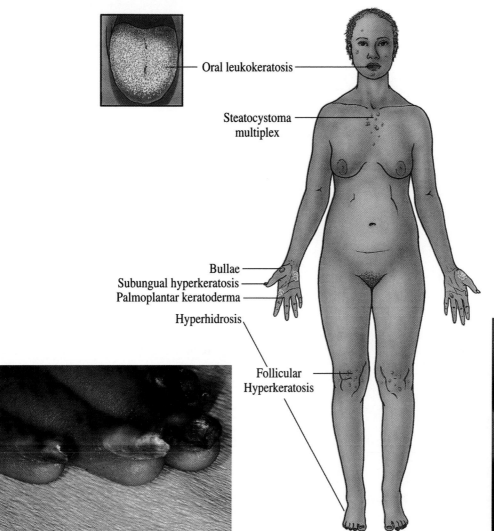

Oral leukokeratosis

Steatocystoma multiplex

Bullae

Subungual hyperkeratosis

Palmoplantar keratoderma

Hyperhidrosis

Follicular Hyperkeratosis

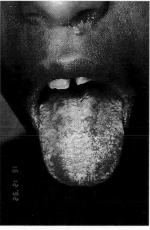

10.23. *Fingernails with yellow-brown discoloration, marked subungual hyperkeratosis, increased transverse curvature, and distal elevation of nail plate. (20)*

10.24. *Benign oral leukokeratosis on tongue. (20)*

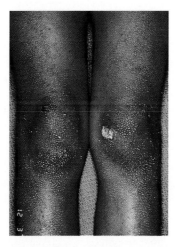

10.25. *Follicular hyperkeratosis on knees. (20)*

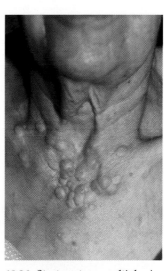

10.26. *Steatocystoma multiplex in patient with PC-2. (1)*

Nail-Patella Syndrome

Synonym	Hereditary osteo-onychodysplasia
Inheritance	Autosomal dominant; *LMX1B* gene on 9q34
Prenatal Diagnosis	DNA analysis Ultrasound
Incidence	1:50,000; M=F
Age at Presentation	Birth (nail defects); often in childhood
Pathogenesis	Mutation in *LMX1B* gene, encoding for a LIM homeodomain protein involved in dorsal/ventral limb patterning, contributes to phenotype; *LMX1B*'s proximity to COL5A1(type V collagen is a major component of glomerular basement membrane zones) on 9q34 may help describe how renal and musculoskeletal defects converge in this syndrome

Key Features

Nails
Triangular lunulae, micronychia with hemionychia, anonychia, longitudinal fissures (thumb > index finger > other fingers; rare on toes)
Skin
Palmoplantar hyperhidrosis
Musculoskeletal
Absent or hypoplastic patella with secondary pain, gait bnormalities, osteoarthritis, posterior iliac horns, radial head subluxation, thickened scapulae, scoliosis
Kidney
Glomerulonephritis, renal dysplasia, renal failure
Eye
Lester iris-hyperpigmentation of pupillary margin of iris, cataracts, heterochromia irides, glaucoma

Differential Diagnosis

Nails
Anonychia
Lichen planus
Idiopathic atrophy

Laboratory Data

Bone films (knee, elbow, pelvis)
Urinalysis

Management

Referral to orthopedist—management of knee, elbows; adjust physical activity
Referral to nephrologist—manage kidney failure, renal transplant
Referral to dermatologist—nail evaluation
Referral to ophthalmologist—regular eye examinations

Prognosis

Renal disease rarely fatal; osteoarthritis, joint limitation without intervention

Clinical Pearls

The triangular lunula is pathognomonic. . . Apex of triangle points distally. . . Great opportunity for the dermatologist to make the diagnosis. . . No great nail treatment. . . My first patient with nail-patella (NP) syndrome sort of waddled into the office with the presumptive diagnosis of fungal infection of the nail. . . Observe their gait closely. . . Their arms are often deviated laterally with difficulty in pronation and supination. . . I refer to orthopedics to do the films and manage the bony problems. . . Screen with a urinalysis. . . I have seen a number of patients, and none has had renal disease. *RS*

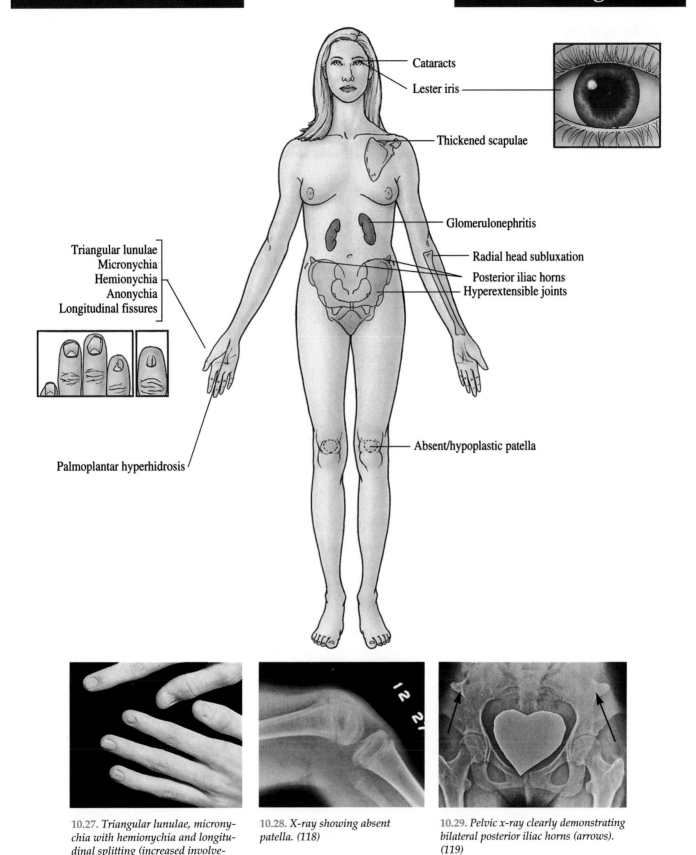

Cataracts

Lester iris

Thickened scapulae

Glomerulonephritis

Radial head subluxation

Posterior iliac horns

Hyperextensible joints

Triangular lunulae
Micronychia
Hemionychia
Anonychia
Longitudinal fissures

Absent/hypoplastic patella

Palmoplantar hyperhidrosis

10.27. Triangular lunulae, micronychia with hemionychia and longitudinal splitting (increased involvement of thumbs and index fingers).
(118)

10.28. X-ray showing absent
patella. (118)

10.29. Pelvic x-ray clearly demonstrating
bilateral posterior iliac horns (arrows).
(119)

297

Suggested Reading

Menkes' Syndrome

Ambrosini L, Mercer JF. Defective copper-induced trafficking and localization of the Menkes protein in patients with mild and copper-treated classical Menkes disease. *Hum Mol Genet* 1999;8:1547–1555.

Brownstein JN, Primosch RE.Oral manifestations of Menkes' kinky hair syndrome. *J Clin Pediatr Dent* 2001;25:317–321.

Christodoulou J, Danks DM, Sarkar B, et al. Early treatment of Menkes disease with parenteral copper-histidine: long-term follow-up of four treated patients. *Am J Med Genet* 1998;76:154–164.

Cobbold C, Coventry J, Ponnambalam S, et al. Actin and microtubule regulation of trans-Golgi network architecture, and copper-dependent protein transport to the cell surface. *Mol Membr Biol* 2004;21:59–66.

Gu YH, Kodama H, Murata Y, et al. ATP7A gene mutations in 16 patients with Menkes disease and a patient with occipital horn syndrome. *Am J Med Genet* 2001;99:217–222.

Horn M, Tonnesen T, Turner Z. Menkes disease: an x-linked neurological disorder of the copper metabolism. *Brain Pathol* 1992;2:351–362.

Kaler SG. Menkes disease. *Adv Pediatr* 1994;41:263.

Menkes JH. Kinky hair disease: twenty-five years later. *Brain Dev* 1988;10:77–79.

Menkes JH, Alter M, Steigleder GK, et al. A sex-linked recessive disorder with retardation of growth, peculiar hair and focal cerebral and cerebellar degeneration. *Pediatrics* 1962;29:764–779.

Møller LB, Tümer Z, Lund C, et al. Similar splice-site mutations of the ATP7A gene lead to different phenotypes: classical Menkes disease or occipital horn syndrome. *Am J Hum Genet* 2000;66:1211–1220.

Pascale MC, Franceschelli S, Moltedo O, et al. Endosomal trafficking of the Menkes copper ATPase ATP7A is mediated by vesicles containing the Rab7 and Rab5 GTPase proteins. *Exp Cell Res* 2003;291:377–385.

Pase L, Voskoboinik I, Greenough M, et al. Copper stimulates trafficking of a distinct pool of the Menkes copper ATPas (ATP7A) to the plasma membrane and diverts it into a rapid recycling pool. *Biochem J* 2004;378:1031–1037.

Peterson J, Drolet BA, Esterly NB. What syndrome is this? Menkes' kinky-hair syndrome. *Pediatr Dermatol* 1998;15.137–139.

Tümer Z, Horn N, Tonnesen T, et al. Early copper-histidine treatment for Menkes disease. *Nat Genet* 1996;12:11–13.

Vulpe C, Levinson B, Whitney S, et al. Isolation of a candidate gene for Menkes disease and evidence that it encodes a copper-transporting ATPase. *Nat Genet* 1993;3:7–13.

Wesenberg RL, Gwinn JL, Barnes GR Jr. Radiological findings in the kinky-hair syndrome. *Radiology* 196;92:500–506.

Whiting DA. Hair shaft defects. In: Olsen EA, ed. *Disorders of Hair Growth: Diagnosis and Treatment*. New York: McGraw-Hill, 2003.

Björnstad Syndrome

Björnstad R. Pili torti and sensory-neural loss of hearing. Proceedings of the 7th Meeting of the Northern Dermotologic Society, Copenhagen. May 17–29, 1965.

Loche F, Bayle-Lebey P, Carriere JP, et al. Pili torti with congenital deafness (Björnstad syndrome): a case report . *Pediatr Dermatol* 1999;16:220–221.

Lubianca Netoa JF, Lu L, Eavey RD, et al. The Björnstad syndrome (sensorineural hearing loss and pili torti) disease gene maps to chromosome 2q34–36. *Am J Hum Genet* 1998;62:1107–1112.

Petit A, Dontenwille MM, Bardon CB, et al. Pili torti with congenital deafness (Björnstad's syndrome)—report of three cases in one family, suggesting autosomal dominant transmission. *Clin Exp Dermatol* 1993;18:94–95.

Richards KA, Mancini AJ. Three members of a family with pili torti and sensorineural hearing loss: the Björnstad syndrome. *J Am Acad Dermatol* 2002;46:301–303.

Scott MJ Jr, Bronson DM, Esterly NB. Björnstad syndrome and torti. *Pediatr Dermatol* 1983;1:45–50.

Selvaag E. Pili torti and sensorineural hearing loss: a follow-up of Børnstad's original patients and a review of the literature. *Eur J Dermatol* 2000;10:91–97.

Van Buggenhout G, Trommelen J, Hamel B, et al. Björnstad syndrome in a patient with mental retardation. *Genet Couns* 1998;9:201–204.

Voigtlander V. Pili torti with deafness (Björnstad syndrome). Report of a family. *Dermatologica* 1979;159:50–54.

Whiting DA. Structural abnormalities of the hair shaft. *J Am Acad Dermatol* 1987;16:1–25.

Argininosuccinic Aciduria

Gerrits GP, Gabreels FJ, Monnens LA, et al. Argininosuccinic aciduria: clinical and biochemical findings in three children with the late onset form, with special emphasis on cerebrospinal fluid findings of amino acids and pyrimidines. *Neuropediatrics* 1993;24:15–18.

Kleijer WJ, Garritsen VH, Linnebank M, et al. Clinical, enzymatic, and molecular genetic characterization of a biochemical variant type of argininosuccinic aciduria: prenatal and postnatal diagnosis in five unrelated families. *J Inherit Metab Dis* 2002;25:399–410.

Kvedar JC, Baden HP, Baden LA, et al Dietary management reverses grooving and abnormal polarization of hair shafts in argininosuccinase deficiency. *Am J Med Genet* 1991;40:211–213.

Linnebank M, Tschiedel E, Haberle J, et al. Argininosuccinate lyase (ASL) deficiency: mutation analysis in 27 patients and a completed structure of the human ASL gene. *Hum Genet* 2002;111:350–359.

Parsons HG, Scott RB, Pinto A, et al. Argininosuccinic acidurias: long-term treatment with arginine. *J Inherit Metab Dis* 1987;10:152–161.

Pijpers L, Kleijer WJ, Reuss A, et al. Transabdominal chorionic villus sampling in a multiple pregnancy at risk of argininosuccinic aciduria: a case report. *Am J Med Genet* 1990;36:449–450.

Potter JL, Timmons GD, et al. Arginosuccinicaciduria: the hair shaft abnormality revisited. *Am J Dis Child* 1980;134:1095–1096.

Reid Sutton V, Pan Y, Davis EC, et al. A mouse model of argininosuccinic aciduria: biochemical characterization. *Mol Genet Metab* 2003;78:11–16.

Widhalm K, Koch S, Scheibenreiter S, et al. Long-term follow-up of 12 patients with the late-onset variant of argininosuccinic acid lyase deficiency: no impairment of intellectual and psychomotor development during therapy. *Pediatrics* 1992;89:1182–1184.

Monilethrix

Birch-Machin MA, Healy E, Turner R, et al. Mapping of monilethrix to the type II keratin gene cluster at chromosome 12q13 in three new families, including one with variable expressivity. *Br J Dermatol* 1997;137:339–343.

Bray DW, Smith SB, Elston DM. What is your diagnosis? Monilethrix. *Cutis* 2003;72:431, 453–454.

de Berker D, Dawber RP. Monilethrix treated with oral retinoids. *Clin Exp Dermatol* 1991;16:226–228.

de Berker DA, Ferguson DJ, Dawber RP. Monilethrix: a clinicopathological illustration of a cortical defect. *Br J Dermatol* 1993;128:327–331.

Despontin K, Krafchik B. What syndrome is this? Monilethrix syndrome. *Pediatr Dermatol* 1993;10:192–194.

Djabali K, Panteleyev AA, Lalin T, et al. Recurrent missense mutations in the hair keratin gene hHb6 in monilethrix. *Clin Exp Dermatol* 2003;28:206–210.

Gebhart M, Fischee T, Claussen U, et al. Monilethrix—improvement by hormonal influences? *Pediatr Dermatol* 1999;16:297–300.

Horev L, Djabali K, Green J, et al. De novo mutations in monilethrix. *Exp Dermatol* 2003;12:882–885.

Horev L, Glaser B, Metzker A, et al. Monilethrix: mutational hotspot in the helix termination motif of the human hair basic keratin 6. *Hum Hered* 2000;50:325–330.

Khandpur S, Bairwa NK, Reddy BS, et al. A study of phenotypic correlation with the genotypic status of HTM regions of

KRTHB6 and KRTHB1 genes in monilethrix families of Indian origin. *Ann Genet* 2004;47:77–84.

Korge BP, Hamm H, Jury CS, et al. Identification of novel mutations in basic hair keratins hHb1 and hHb6 in monilethrix: implications for protein structure and clinical phenotype. *J Invest Dermatol* 1999;113:607–612.

Landau M, Brenner S, Metzker A. Medical Pearl: an easy way to diagnose severe neonatal monilethrix. *J Am Acad Dermatol* 2002;46:111–112.

Richard G, Itin P, Lin JP, et al. Evidence for genetic heterogeneity in monilethrix. *J Invest Dermatol* 1996;107:812–814.

Rogers M. Hair shaft abnormalities Part I. *Australas J Dermatol* 1995;36:179–186.

Winter H, Clark RD, Tarras-Wahlberg C, et al. Monilethrix: a novel mutation (Glu402Lys) in the helix termination motif of the type II hair keratin hHb6. *J Invest Dermatol* 1999;113:263–266.

Whiting DA. Hair shaft defects. In: Olsen EA, ed. *Disorders of Hair Growth: Diagnosis and Treatment.* New York: McGraw-Hill, 2003.

Uncombable Hair Syndrome

Ang P, Tay YK. What syndrome is this? Uncombable hair (pili trianguli et canaliculi). *Pediatr Dermatol* 1998;15:475–476.

Fritz TM, Trueb RM. Uncombable hair with angel shaped phalango-epiphyseal dysplasia. *Pediatr Dermatol* 2000;17:21–24.

Hebert AA, Charrow J, Esterly NB, et al. Uncombable hair (pili trianguli et canaliculi): evidence for dominant inheritance with complete penetrance based on scanning electron microscopy. *Am J Med Genet* 1987;28:185–193.

Hicks J, Mary DW, Barrish J, et al. Uncombable hair (cheveux incoiffables, pili trianguli et canaliculi) syndrome: brief review and role of scanning electron, microscopy in diagnosis. *Ultrastruct Pathol* 2001;25:99–103.

Itin PH, Buhler U, Buchner SA, et al. Pili trianguli et canaliculi: a distinctive hair shaft defect leading to uncombable hair. *Dermatology* 1993;187:296–298.

Mallon ME, Dawber RP, De Berker D, et al. Cheveux incoiffables—diagnostic, clinical and hair microscopic findings, and pathogenic studies. *Br J Dermatol* 1994;131:608–614.

Matis WL, Baden H, Green R, et al. Uncombable hair syndrome. *Pediatr Dermatol* 1987;4:215–219.

McCullum N, Sperling LC, Vidmar D. The uncombable hair syndrome. *Cutis* 1990;46:479–481.

Mortimer PS. Unruly hair. *Br J Dermatol* 1985;113:467–473.

Rest EB, Fretzin DF. Quantitative assessment of scanning electron microscope defects in uncombable-hair syndrome. *Pediatr Dermatol* 1990;7:93–96.

Shelley WB, Shelley ED. Uncombable hair syndrome: observations on response to biotin and occurrence in siblings with ectodermal dysplasia. *J Am Acad Dermatol* 1985;13:97–102.

Whiting DA. Hair shaft defects. In: Olsen EA, ed. *Disorders of Hair Growth: Diagnosis and Treatment.* New York: McGraw-Hill, 2003.

Zanca A, Zanca A. Ancient observations of "uncombable hair syndrome." *Int J Dermatol* 1993;32:707.

Hypohidrotic Ectodermal Dysplasia

Berg D, Weingold DH, Abson KG, et al. Sweating in ectodermal dysplasia syndromes. A review. *Arch Dermatol* 1990;126:1075–1079.

Cunniff C. Hypohidrotic ectodermal dysplasia. *Pediatr Dermatol* 1990;7:235–236.

Doffinger R, Smahin A, Bessia C, et al. X-linked anhidrotic ectodermal dysplasia with immunodeficiency is caused by impaired NF-kB signaling. *Nat Genet* 2001;27:277–285.

Dunn WJ. Hypohidrotic ectodermal dysplasia: a review and case report. *Gen Dent* 2003;51:346–348.

Gilgenkrantz S, Blanchet-Bardon C, Nazzaro V, et al. Hypohidrotic ectodermal dysplasia: clinical study of a family of 30 over three generations. *Hum Genet* 1989;81:120–122.

Guckes LAD, Brahim JS, McCarthy GR, et al. Using endosseousdentai implants for patients with ectodermal dysplasia. *J Am Dent Assoc* 1991;122:59–62.

Headon DJ, Emmal SA, Ferguson BM, et al. Gene detect to ectodermal dysplasia implicates a death domain adaptor in development. *Nature* 2001;414:913–916.

Ho L, Williams MS, Spritz RA. A gene for autosomal dominant hypohidrotic ectodermal dysplasia (EDA3) maps to chromosome 2q11–q13. *Am J Hum Genet* 1999;62:1102–1106.

Kere J, Srivastava AK, Montonen O, et al. X-linked anhidrotic (hypohidrotic) ectodermal dysplasia is caused by a mutation in a novel transmembrane protein. *Nat Genet* 1996;13:409–416.

Monreal AW, Ferguson BM, Headon DJ, et al. Mutations in the human homologue of mouse dl cause autosomal recessive and dominant hypohidrotic ectodermal dysplasia. *Nat Genet* 1999;22:366–369.

Munoz F, Lestringant G, Sybert V, et al. Definitive evidence for an autosomal recessive form of hypohidrotic ectodermal dysplasia clinically indistinguishable from more common X-linked disorder. *Am J Hum Genet* 1997;61:94–100.

Puel A, Picard C, Ku CL, et al. Inherited disorders of NF-kappaB-mediated immunity in man. *Curr Opin Immunol* 2004;16:34–41.

Rogers M. The "bar code phenomenon": a microscopic artifact seen in patients with hypohidrotic ectodermal dysplasia. *Pediatr Dermatol* 2000;17:329–330.

Siegel MB, Potsic WP. Ectodermal 'dysplasia: the otolaryngologic manifestations and management. *Int J Pediatr Otorhinolaryngol* 1990;19:265–271.

Skrinjaric I, Skrinjaric K, Vranic DN, et al. Craniofacial anthropometric pattern profile in hypohidrotic ectodermal dysplasia—application in detection of gene carriers. *Coll Antropol* 2003;27:753–759.

Tanner BA. Psychological aspects of hypohidrotic ectodermal dysplasia. *Birth Defects* 1988;24:263–275.

Vincent MC, Biancalana V, Ginisty D, et al. Mutational spectrum of the EDI gene in X-linked hypohidrotic ectodermal dysplasia. *Eur J Hum Genet* 2001;9:355–363.

Hidrotic Ectodermal Dysplasia

Ando Y, Tanaka T, Horiguchi Y, et al. Hidrotic ectodermal dysplasia: a clinical and ultrastructural observation. *Dermatologica* 1988;176:205–211.

Common JE, Becker D, Di WL, et al. Functional studies of human skin disease- and deafness-associated connexin 30 mutations. *Biochem Biophys Res Commun* 2002;298:651–656.

Fraser FC, Der Kaloustian VM. A man, a syndrome, a gene: Clouston's hidrotic ectodermal dysplasia (HED) [published erratum appears in *Am J Med Genet* 2001;102:394]. *Am J Med Genet* 2001;100:164–168.

Lamartine J, Munhoz Essenfelder G, Kibar Z, et al. Mutations in GJB6 cause hidrotic ectodermal dysplasia. *Nature Genet* 2000;26:142–144.

Smith FJ, Morley SM, McLean WH. A novel connexin 30 mutation in Clouston syndrome. *J Invest Dermatol* 2002;118:530–532.

van Steensel MA, Jonkman ME, van Geel M, et al. Clouston syndrome can mimic pachyonychia congenita. *J Invest Dermatol* 2003;121:1035–1038.

Zhang XJ, Chen JJ, Yang S, et al. A mutation in the connexin 30 gene in Chinese Han patients with hidrotic ectodermal dysplasia. *J Dermatol Sci* 2003;32:11–17.

EEC Syndrome

Barrow LL, van Bokhoven H, Daack-Hirsch S, et al. Analysis of the p63 gene in classical EEC syndrome, related syndromes, and non-syndromic orofacial clefts. *J Med Genet* 2002;39:559–566.

Bigata X, Bielsa I, Artigas M, et al. The ectrodactyly-ectodermal dysplasia-clefting syndrome (EEC): report of five cases. *Pediatr Dermatol* 2003;20:113–118.

Buss PW, Hughes HE, Clarke A. Twenty-four cases of the EEC syndrome: clinical presentation and management. *J Med Genet* 1995;32:716–723.

Celli J, Duijf P, Hamel BC, et al. Heterzozygous germline mutations in the p53 homolog p63 are the cause of EEC syndrome. *Cell* 1999;99:143–153.

Fernandez B, Ruas E, Machado A, et al. Ectrodactyly-ectodermal dysplasia-clefting syndrome (EEC): report of a case: with perioral papiliomatosis. *Pediatr Dermatol* 2002;19:330–332.

Fosko SW, Stenn KS, Bolognia JL. Ectodermal dysplasias associated with clefting: significance of scalp dermatitis. *J Am Acad Dermatol* 1992;27:249–256.

Glorio R, Haas R, Jaimovich L. Ectrodactyly, ectodermal dysplasia and clefting (EEC) syndrome. *J Eur Acad Dermatol Venereol* 2003;17:356–358.

Mills AA, Zheng B, Wang XJ, et al. p63 is a p53 homologue required for limb and epidermal morphogenesis. *Nature* 1999;398:708–713.

Roelfsema NM, Cobben JM. The EEC syndrome: a literature study. *Clin Dysmorphol* 1996;5:115–127.

Trueb RM, Bruckner-Tudoman L, Wyss M, et al. Scalp dermatitis, distinctive hair abnormalities and atopic disease in the ectrodactyly-ectodermal dysplasia-clefting syndrome. *Br J Dermatol* 1995;132:621–625.

Trueb RM, Tsambaos D, Spycher MA, et al. Scarring folliculitis in the ectrodactyly-ectodermal dysplasia-clefting syndrome. *Dermatology* 1997;194:191–194.

Van Bolchaven H, Hamel BC, Bamshad M, et al. p63 gene mutations in EEC syndrome, limb-mammary syndrome and isolated split hand—split foot malformation suggest a genotype-phenotype correlation. *Am J Hum Genet* 2001;69:481–492.

Wessagowit V, Mellerio JE, Pernbroke AC, et al. Heterozygous germline missense mutation in the p63 gene underlying EEC syndrome. *Clin Exp Dermatol* 2000;25:441–443.

AEC Syndrome

Fosko SW, Stenn KS, Bolognia JL. Ectodermal dysplasias associated with clefting: significance of scalp dermatitis. *J Am Acad Dermatol* 1992;27(2 Pt 1):249–256.

Hay RJ, Wells RS. The syndrome of ankyloblepharon, ectodermal defects and cleft lip and palate: an autosomal dominant condition. *Br J Dermatol* 1976;94:277–289.

Mancini AJ, Faller AS. What syndrome is this? Ankyloblepharon-ectroderal defects-cleft lip and palate (Hay–Wells) syndrome. *Pediatr Dermatol* 1997;14:403–405.

McGrath JA, Duijf PH, Doetsch V, et al. Hay-Wells syndrome is caused by heterozygous missense mutations in the SAM domain of p63. *Hum Mol Gene* 2001;10:221–229.

Rule DC, Shaw MJ. The dental management of patients with ankyloblepharon (AEC) syndrome. *Br Dent J* 1988;164:215–218.

Satoh K, Tosa Y, Ohtsuka S, et al. Anky-loblepharon, ectodermal dysplasia, cleft lip and palate (AEC) syndrome: surgical corrections with an 18-year follow-up including maxillary osteotomy. *Plast Reconstr Surg* 1994;93:590–594.

Tsutsui K, Asai Y, Fujimoto A, et al. A novel p63 sterile alpha motif (SAM) do-main mutation in a Japanese patient with ankyloblepharon, ectodermal defects and cleft lip and palate (AEC) syn-drome without ankyloblepharon. *Br J Dermatol* 2003;149:395–399.

Vanderhooft SL, Stephan MJ, Sybert VP. Severe skin erosions and scalp infec-tions in AEC syndrome. *Pediatr Derma-tol* 1993;10:334–340.

Pachyonychia Congenita

Bowden PE, Haley J, Kansky A, et al. Mutation of a type II keratin gene (K6a) in pachyonychia congenita. *Nat Genet* 1995;10:363–365.

Elston DM. What is your diagnosis? Pachyonychia congenita. *Cutis* 2003;72:104, 143–144.

Feinstein A, Friedman J, Schewach-Millet M. Pachyonychia congenita. *J Am Acad Dermatol* 1988;19:705–711.

Feng YG, Xiao SX, Ren XR, et al. Keratin 17 mutation in pachyonychia congenita type 2 with early onset sebaceous cysts. *Br J Dermatol* 2003;148:452–455.

Fitzgerald BJ, Sanders LJ. Pachyonychia congenita: a four generation pedigree. *Cutis* 1990;46:435–439.

Hersh SP. Pachyonychia congenita. Manifestations for the otolaryngologist. *Arch Otolaryngol Head Neck Surg* 1990;116:732–734.

Oriba HA, Lo JS, Bergfeld WF. Callused feet, thick nails, and white tongue. Pachyonychia congenita. *Arch Dermatol* 1991;127:113–114,116–117.

Rohold AE, Brandup F. Pachyonychia congenita: therapeutic and immunologic aspects. *Pediatr Dermatol* 1990;7:307–309.

Smith FJ, Fisher MP, Healy E, et al. Novel keratin 16 mutations and protein expression studies in pachyonychia congenita type 1 and focal palmoplantar keratoderma. *Exp Dermatol* 2000;9:170–177.

Smith FJ, Jonkman MF, van Goor H, et al. A mutation in human keratin K6b produces a phenocopy of the K17 disorder pachyonychia congenita type 2. *Hum Mel Genet* 1998;7:1143–1148.

Su WE, Chun SI, Hammond DE, et al. Pachyonychia congenita: a clinical study of 12 cases and review of the literature. *Pediatr Dermatol* 1990;7:33–38.

Terrinoni A, Smith FJ, Didona B, et al. Novel and recurrent mutations in the genes encoding keratins K6a, K16 and K17 in 13 cases of pachyonychia congenita. *J Invest Dermatol* 2001;117:1391–1396.

Thomsen RJ, Zuehlke RL, Beckman BI. Pachyonychia congenita: surgical management of the nail changes. *J Dermatol Surg Oncol* 1982;8:24–28.

Ward KM, Cook-Bolden FE, Christiano AM, et al. Identification of a recurrent mutation in keratin 6a in a patient with overlapping clinical features of pachyonychia congenita types 1 and 2. *Clin Exp Dermatol* 2003;28:434–436.

Nail-Patella Syndrome

Beguiristain JL, de Rada PD, Barriga A. Nail-patella syndrome: long term evolution. *J Pediatr Orthop B* 2003;12:13–16.

Bongers EM, Gubler MC, Knoers NV. Nail-patella syndrome. Overview on clinical and molecular findings. *Pediatr Nephrol* 2002;17:703–712.

Browning MC, Weidner N, Lorentz WB Jr. Renal histopathology of the nail-patella syndrome in a 2 year old boy. *Clin Nephrol* 1988;29:210–213.

Buddin D, Loomis C, Shwayder T, et al. What syndrome is this? Nail-patella syndrome. *Pediatr Dermatol* 2002;19:454–456.

Chan PC, Chan KW, Cheng IK, et al. Living related renal transplantation in a patient with nail-patella syndrome. *Nephron* 1988;50:164–166.

Daniel CR III, Osment LS, Noojin RO. Triangular lunulae. A clueto nail-patella syndrome. *Arch Dermatol* 1980;116:448–449.

Dryer SD, Zhou G, Baldini A, et al. Mutations in LMX1B cause abnormal skeletal patterning and renal dysplasia in nail-patella syndrome. *Nat Genet* 1988;19:47–50.

Gubler MC, Levy M. Prenatal diagnosis of nail-patella syndrome by intrauterine kidney biopsy [letter; comment]. *Am J Med Genet* 1993;47:122–124.

Guidera KJ, Satterwhite Y, Ogden JA, et al. Nail patella syndrome: a review of 44 orthopaedic patients. *J Pediatr Orthop* 1991;11:737–742.

Hamlington JD, Jones C, McIntosh I. Twenty-two novel LMX1B mutations identified in nail patella syndrome (NPS) patients. *Hum Mutat* 2001;18:458.

Heidet L, Bongers EM, Sich M, et al. In vivo expression of putative LMX1B targets in nail-patella syndrome kidneys. *Am J Pathol* 2003;163:145–155.

Knoers NV, Bongers EM, van Beersum SE, et al. Nail-patella syndrome: identification of mutations in the LMX1B gene in Dutch families. *J Am Soc Nephrol* 2000;11:1762–1766.

Looij BJ Jr, Slaa RL, Hogewind BL, et al. Genetic counselling in hereditary osteo-onychodysplasia (HOOD, nail-patella syndrome) with nephropathy. *J Med Genet* 1988;25:682–686.

Morello R, Zhou G, Dreyer SD, et al. Regulation of glomerular basement membrane collagen expression by LMX1B contributes to renal disease in nail patella syndrome. *Nat Genet* 2001;27:205–208.

Ogden JA, Cross GL, Guidera KJ, et al. Nail patella syndrome. A 55-year follow-up of the original description. *J Pediatr Orthop* 2002;11:333–338.

Rohr C, Protel J, Heidet L, et al. The LIM-homeodomain transcription factor Lmx1b plays a crucial role in podocytes. *J Clin Invest* 2002;109:1073–1082.

Schulz-Butulis BA, Welch MD, Norton SA. Nail-patella syndrome. *J Am Acad Dermatol* 2003;49:1086–1087.

Sty JR, Wells RG, Gregg DC. Nail-patella syndrome. Image correlation. *Clin Nucl Med* 1992;17:977–978.

Chapter 11

Disorders of Metabolism

Clinical Pearls

Kurt Hirschhorn, M.D. (KH) and Judith Willner, M.D. (JW)

Alkaptonuria

Synonym	Ochronosis
Inheritance	Autosomal recessive; homogentisate 1,2-dioxygenase (*HGO*) gene on 3q21–q23
Prenatal Diagnosis	DNA analysis
Incidence	1:250,000; increased in Dominican Republic, Slovakia; M=F
Age at Presentation	Childhood (dark cerumen, black-stained underwear) to adulthood (skin pigment, arthropathy)
Pathogenesis	Mutations in the HGO gene leads to deficiency of homogentisic acid oxidase with secondary accumulation of homogentisic acid in connective tissue

Key Features

Skin
Blue-gray pigmentation increased on nose, cheeks, forehead, axillae; blue-gray pigmented cartilage and tendons visualized through skin on ears, nose tip, extensor hands, costochondral junctions; brown/black cerumen, sweat

Eyes
Blue-gray scleral pigment

Musculoskeletal
Severe arthropathy involving larger joints including hip, knee, shoulder, spine; intervertebral disc calcification

Genitourinary
Dark urine with pH above 7.0 (diapers, clothing discolored after cleansing with alkaline soaps)

Cardiovascular
Mitral and aortic valvulitis; increased incidence of myocardial infarction later in life

Differential Diagnosis	Exogenous ochronosis (antimalarials, hydroquinone) Argyria Chrysoderma Amiodarone administration
Laboratory Data	Enzyme assay: measurement of urinary homogentisic acid Darkening of urine with addition of NaOH Spine films Electrocardiogram (ECG) in older patients
Management	Analgesics, physical therapy, joint replacement for arthropathy Supplemental vitamin C up to 1 g per day for older children and adults Reduction of phenylalanine and tyrosine may help reduce homogentisate excretion
Prognosis	Normal life span with persistent pigmentation changes and unremitting arthropathy; older patients with increased incidence of myocardial infarction

Clinical Pearls

With advent of disposable diapers, noticing dark-stained cloth diapers after washing no longer helps make the diagnosis. . . Most of the time, parents/patients never notice black urine. . . Degenerative surfaces and narrowing of joint space on x-ray. . . Historically, this syndrome is very important because it is the first biochemical disease described by Garrod. . . He is the man who invented biochemical genetics, termed the words "inborn errors of metabolism," and came up with the idea that we're all biochemically different. . . Interestingly, the diagnosis has been made in Egyptian mummies with black cartilage. *KH, JW*

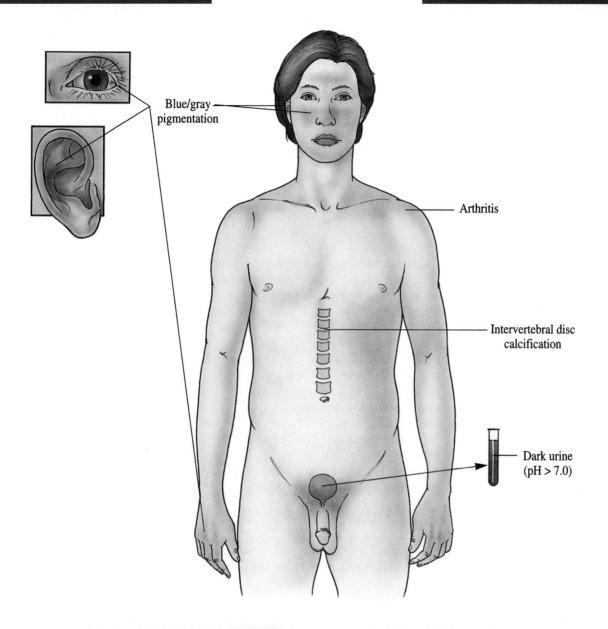

Blue/gray pigmentation

Arthritis

Intervertebral disc calcification

Dark urine (pH > 7.0)

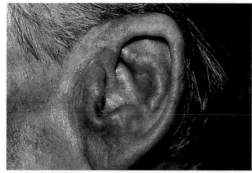

11.1. *Blue-gray pigmentation involving ear cartilage. (120)*

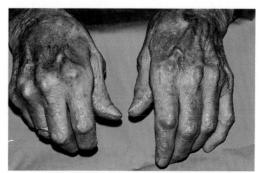

11.2. *Similar pigmentation on patient's hands. (120)*

Fabry Disease

Synonym	Angiokeratoma corporis diffusum
Inheritance	X-linked recessive; α-galactosidase A (*GLA*) gene on Xq21.33–q22
Prenatal Diagnosis	Chorionic villus sampling (CVS)/amniocentesis—α-galactosidase A enzyme assay DNA analysis
Incidence	Approximately 1:40,000 males; female heterozygotes reported with marked variability in expression
Age at Presentation	Childhood to adolescence
Pathogenesis	Mutation in *GLA* leads to defective activity of α-galactosidase A and accumulation of neutral glycosphingolipids with preferential deposition in vascular endothelium resulting in ischemia and infarction; also deposits within most tissues of the body, including heart and kidney

Key Features

Skin
Angiokeratomas—dark red to blue-black papules with/without overlying hyperkeratosis concentrated symmetrically between the umbilicus and knees, increase in number and size with age; hypoanhidrosis

Mucous Membranes
Angiokeratomas—oral mucosa, conjunctiva

Peripheral Nervous System
Painful crises—most severe on hands and feet but can spread proximally; exercise, fever, climate/temperature changes, emotional stress may trigger episode
Acroparesthesias—constant discomfort of hands and feet with burning, tingling paresthesias

Cardiovascular
Angina, myocardial infarction, conduction defects, mitral insufficiency

Kidney
Progressive renal deterioration with proteinuria, birefringent lipid globules ("maltese crosses") seen with polarizing microscopy, renal failure

Central Nervous System
Peripheral neuropathy, cerebrovascular accidents

Eyes
Characteristic corneal opacities with whorl-like configuration, lenticular opacities, dilated and tortuous conjunctival and retinal vessels

Differential Diagnosis

Rheumatic fever
Mercury/heavy metal poisoning
Erythromelalgia
Other angiokeratomas: angiokeratoma of Fordyce, fucosidosis, sialidosis, β-galactosidase deficiency, aspartylglucosaminuria

Laboratory Data

DNA analysis
Enzyme assay—deficient α-galactosidase A activity
Skin, bone marrow biopsy
Urinary sediment examination with polarizing microscopy
Slit-lamp ophthalmologic examination
ECG

Management

α-Galactosidase A intravenous replacement therapy
Diphenylhydantoin, carbamazepine—pain crises
Symptomatic care of cardiac, central nervous system (CNS), and ocular manifestations
Long-term hemodialysis, renal transplantation
Advise physical education teachers/occupational advice—minimize physical/emotional stresses

Prognosis

Premature death during fifth decade secondary to myocardial infarction, cerebrovascular accidents, and renal failure; enzyme replacement therapy, hemodialysis, renal transplantation may extend life span

Clinical Pearls

Acral pain and paresthesias are very specific findings. . . You virtually never see them except in mercury/heavy metal poisoning. . . Pain is so severe that patients develop very peculiar behavior to help deal with it. . . Such as dunking their hands and feet in cold toilet water. . . The kid is often labeled "nuts" by parents and medical community. . . Low-dose dilantin works very well for the pain. . . Preliminary studies seem to show a reduction in the accumulation of glycosphingolipids. . . Interestingly, some transplanted patients show improvement in their pain. . . Group B blood groups tend to do worse. . . Of all X-linked recessive diseases, this one has the largest number of symptomatic female carriers. . . Enzyme replacement therapy is now available.   *KH, JW*

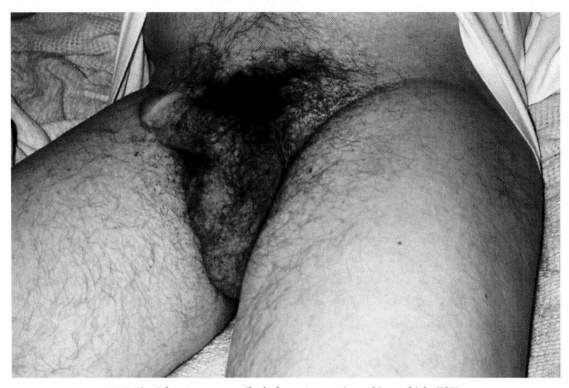

11.3. *Angiokeratomas on penile shaft, scrotum, groin, and inner thigh. (121)*

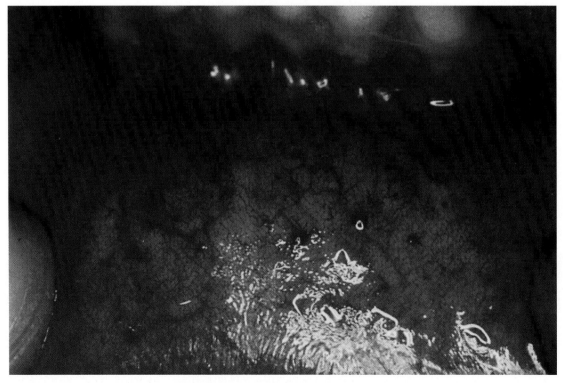

11.4. *Angiokeratomas studding the labial mucosa. (122)*

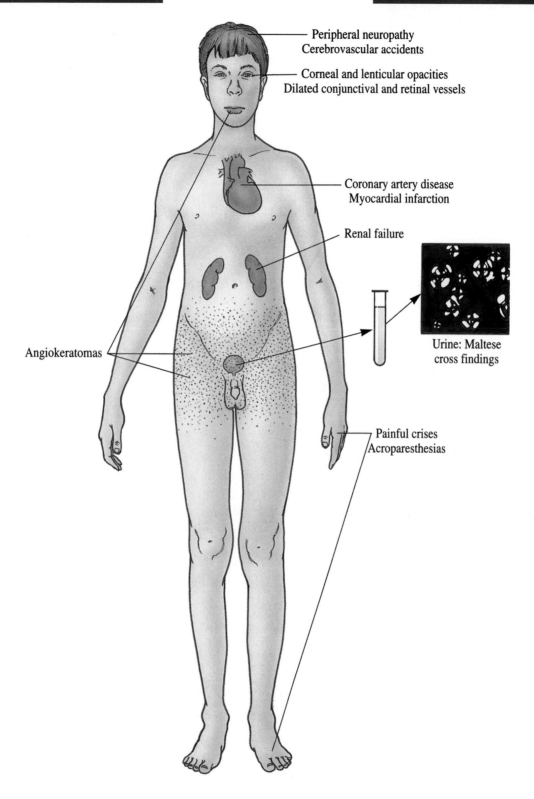

Peripheral neuropathy
Cerebrovascular accidents

Corneal and lenticular opacities
Dilated conjunctival and retinal vessels

Coronary artery disease
Myocardial infarction

Renal failure

Urine: Maltese
cross findings

Angiokeratomas

Painful crises
Acroparesthesias

Gaucher Disease

Inheritance	Autosomal recessive; acid-β-glucocidase (*GBA*) gene locus 1q21
Prenatal Diagnosis	CVS/amniocentesis—glucocerebrosidase enzyme assay Ultrasound: hydrops fetalis, hepatosplenomegaly may be seen in type II disease DNA analysis
Incidence	Over 350 patients reported; type I is 20 times more common than type II and increased in Ashkenazi Jewish population; M=F
Age at Presentation	Type II (infantile)—2 to 3 months of life Type I (adult)—may begin within first decade of life; usually begins later in adulthood
Pathogenesis	Mutation in *GBA* gene leads to decreased glucocerebrosidase activity resulting in accumulation of glucocerebroside in histiocytes (Gaucher's cells) in spleen, liver, bone marrow, lymph nodes, and brain (infantile only); adult form without CNS accumulation secondary to adequate neuronal glucocerebrosidase activity

Key Features

Type I (Adult)

Skin
May have diffuse hyperpigmentation on face, neck, hands; petechiae, ecchymoses

Musculoskeletal
Bone pain, fractures with thinned cortex, vertebral collapse, aseptic necrosis of femoral head

Gastrointestinal
Hepatomegaly, hypersplenism with secondary pancytopenia, hemorrhage

Lymphatics
Enlarged lymph nodes

Eyes
Pingueculae

Type II (Infantile)

Central Nervous System
Hypertonicity, neck rigidity, laryngeal spasm, difficulty swallowing, catatonia, developmental retardation

Gastrointestinal
Hepatosplenomegaly

Lungs
Chronic aspiration, fatal bronchopneumonia

Type III
Rarest, rapidly deteriorates like type II; hepatosplenomegaly, bone involvement, strabismus, slow neurodegeneration

Differential Diagnosis	Niemann-Pick disease (p. 314) Other lysosomal storage diseases

Laboratory Data

Serum glucocerebrosidase enzyme assay
Bone marrow biopsy—Gaucher cells
Bone x-rays
Serum acid phosphatase elevated

Management

Type II—supportive care, antibiotics
Type I—enzyme replacement, bone marrow transplant, splenectomy, referral to orthopedic surgeons for conservative management, referral to hematologist-oncologist

Prognosis

Type II—fatal by 1 to 2 years of age secondary to aspiration pneumonia
Type I—variable life span, potential premature death secondary to infection, anemia, hemorrhage without treatment; many may achieve a normal life span

Clinical Pearls

Infantile and adult forms may share mutation. . . Type II's are kids with big spleens and livers who neurologically deteriorate rapidly. . . There's essentially no residual enzyme in the infants. . . Type I's always have some residual enzyme. . . The brain probably doesn't need as much enzyme to dispose of the lipid. . . We are screening Ashkenazi Jews before pregnancy for both enzyme and DNA. . . Now we can treat symptomatic patients with enzyme. . . Livers and spleens shrink right up with the enzyme. . . There's a joke that we have to provide the kids with suspenders along with their Ceredase because their pants start falling down. . . The enzyme can't help the neuropathic forms (types II and III) because it doesn't cross the blood-brain barrier. . . Bony problems improve with enzyme if one intervenes early on. . . All kids who present with hepatosplenomegaly are initially worked up with an enzyme assay.   *KH, JW*

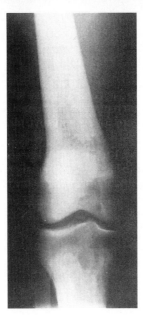

11.5. *X-ray depicting tapered femoral midshaft with widening of the distal femur-characteristic "Ehrlenmeyer flask" deformity.* (123)

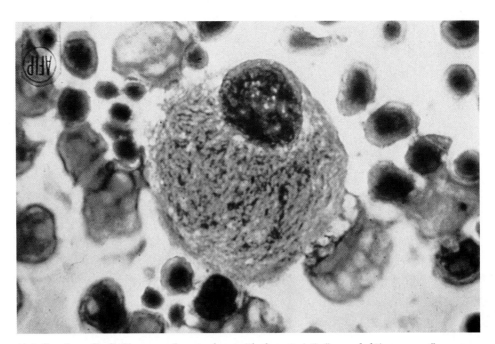

11.6. *Gaucher cell—lipid–engorged macrophage with characteristic "crumpled tissue paper" appearance obtained from bone marrow.* (48)

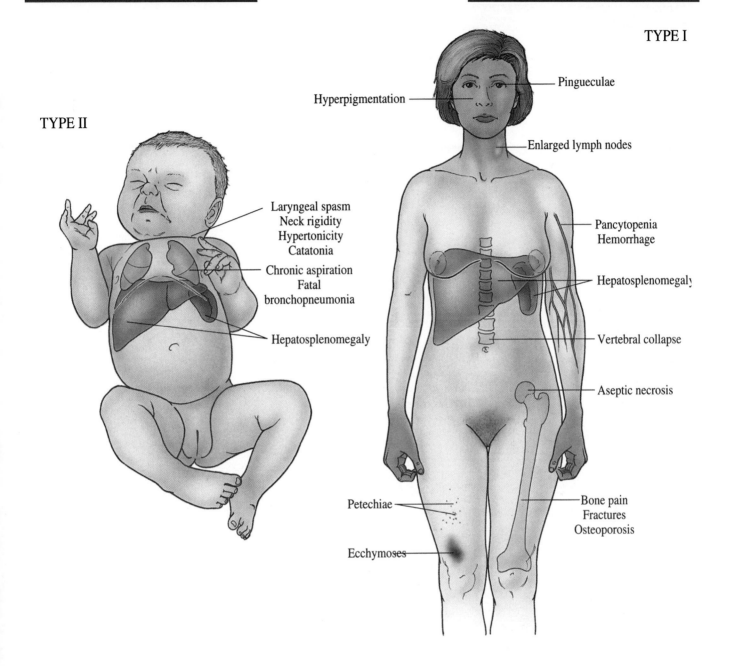

TYPE I

TYPE II

Hyperpigmentation

Pingueculae

Enlarged lymph nodes

Laryngeal spasm
Neck rigidity
Hypertonicity
Catatonia

Chronic aspiration
Fatal
bronchopneumonia

Hepatosplenomegaly

Pancytopenia
Hemorrhage

Hepatosplenomegaly

Vertebral collapse

Aseptic necrosis

Petechiae

Ecchymoses

Bone pain
Fractures
Osteoporosis

Niemann-Pick Disease

Inheritance

Autosomal recessive; sphingomyelin phosphodiesterase-1 (*SMPD-1*) gene locus 11p15.4–15.1 (types A, B)
Type C—gene locus 18p

Prenatal Diagnosis

CVS/amniocentesis—sphingomyelinase enzyme assay from cultured chorionic villus tissue/amniotic fluid cells
DNA analysis

Incidence

Type A most common—over 50% are Ashkenazi Jews; a few hundred cases reported; M=F

Age at Presentation

Type A—infancy
Type B—infancy to childhood
Type C—childhood

Pathogenesis

Mutations in *SMPD-1* results in acid sphingomyelinase deficiency in types A and B with subsequent accumulation of sphingomyelin in characteristic foam cells within all organs, increased in brain (except type B), liver, spleen, lymph nodes, and lungs; cholesterol esterification defect in type C with normal sphingomyelinase

Key Features

Type A
  Skin
    Xanthomas; yellow-brown, waxy induration on exposed surfaces
  Central Nervous System
    Progressive psychomotor deterioration, hypotonicity, muscle weakness
  Gastrointestinal
    Hepatosplenomegaly, emaciated appearance—failure to thrive, vomiting
  Lymphatics
    Generalized enlarged lymph nodes
  Eyes
    Blindness, cherry red spots
  Ear-Nose-Throat
    Deafness
  Lungs
    Bronchopneumonia, infiltration of foam cells
Type B
  CNS spared, otherwise similar to type A
Type C
  Developmental delay, hepatosplenomegaly, progressive psychomotor deterioration

Differential Diagnosis   Gaucher disease (p. 310)
Tay-Sachs disease

Laboratory Data   Serum sphingomyelinase assay
Bone marrow biopsy

Management   Supportive care—parenteral nutrition, antibiotics, transfusions, splenectomy
Bone marrow transplant—type B

Prognosis   Type A—death by 2 to 3 years of age secondary to progressive deterioration, fatal pulmonary infection
Type B—death in adolescence; may survive into adulthood
Type C—death in adolescence

Clinical Pearls

The gene has been cloned and most mutations in Ashkenazi Jews are pretty well known. . . We screen Ashkenazi Jewish couples preconceptually for carrier status. . . Same gene for types A and B, different mutations. . . Type B's have higher residual enzyme and thus don't get neurologic sequelae. . . B's can get terrible lung disease. . . We have an ongoing study looking at replacement therapy in type B. . . Type C is a different gene seen in French-Canadians. . . The defect in C secondarily affects sphingomyelin. . . As in all babies with vomiting, their formulae are changed five times prior to diagnosis. . . Cherry red spots are also seen in Tay-Sachs, generalized sialidosis, and Sandhoff's disease.   *KH, JW*

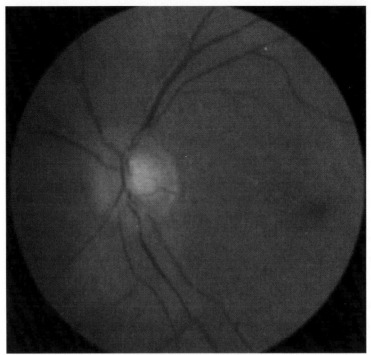

11.7. Cherry red spot in fovea. (124)

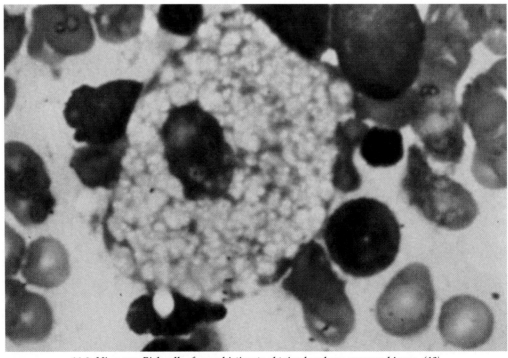

11.8. Niemann-Pick cell—foamy histiocyte obtained on bone marrow biopsy. (48)

TYPE A

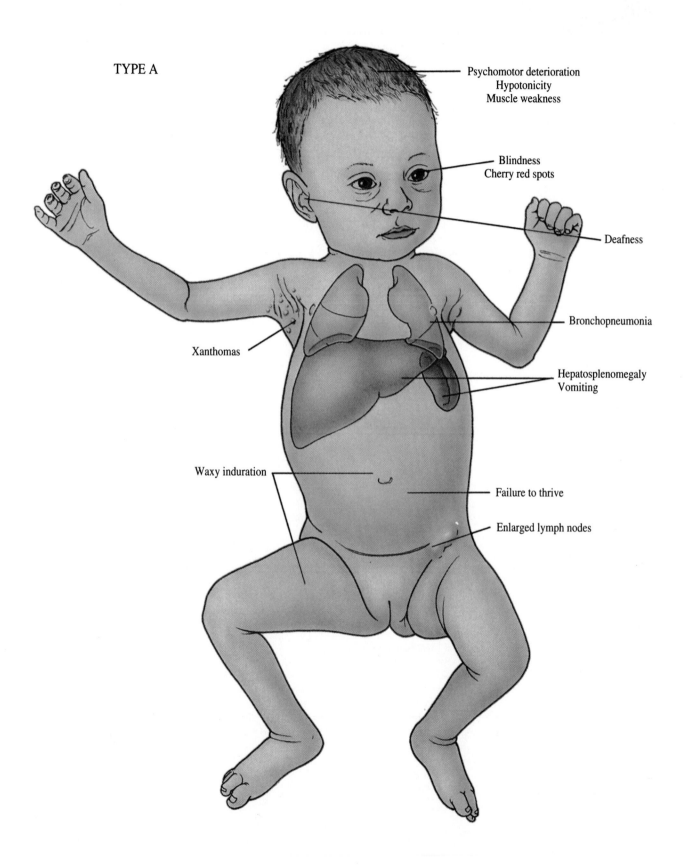

Psychomotor deterioration
Hypotonicity
Muscle weakness

Blindness
Cherry red spots

Deafness

Bronchopneumonia

Xanthomas

Hepatosplenomegaly
Vomiting

Waxy induration

Failure to thrive

Enlarged lymph nodes

Mucopolysaccharidoses

Inheritance Autosomal recessive except X-linked recessive in Hunter's syndrome
Gene loci
Hurler, Scheie syndrome—4p16.3
Hunter's syndrome—Xq27.3–q28
Sanfilippo syndrome—several loci reported
Morquio syndrome (A)—16q24.3
Maroteaux-Lamy syndrome—5q11–q13

Prenatal Diagnosis CVS/amniocentesis—enzyme assay from cultured chorionic villus tissue/amniotic fluid cells
DNA analysis

Incidence Hurler's—approximately 1:100,000; M=F
Scheie's—rare; M=F
Hunter's—approximately 1:100,000; all males
Sanfilippo's—approximately 1:25,000; M=F
Morquio's—<1:100,000; M=F
Maroteaux-Lamy's—rare; M=F

Age at Presentation Hurler's, Hunter's, Sanfilippo's, Morquio's, Maroteaux-Lamy—normal at birth, within first 2 years of life
Scheie's—birth (corneal clouding, herniae); childhood (stiff joints)

Pathogenesis Lysosomal enzymes responsible for breakdown of mucopolysaccharides are deficient; increased mucopolysaccharides throughout system
Syndrome: Enzyme; Mucopolysaccharides
Hurler's, Scheie: α-L-iduronidase; dermatan, heparan sulfate
Hunter's: iduronate sulfatase; dermatan, heparan sulfate
Sanfilippo's: (A) heparan-N-sulfatase, (B) α-N acetylglucosaminidase, (C) acetyl-CoA: α-glucosaminide acetyltransferase, (D) N-acetylglucosamine 6-sulfatase; heparan sulfate
Morquio's: (A) hexosamine 6-sulfatase, (B) beta-galactosidase; keratan sulfate
Maroteaux-Lamy's: arylsulfatase B; dermatan sulfate

Key Features **Skin**
Firm, ivory-colored papules symmetrically distributed between angles of the scapulae and posterior axillary line (Hunter)
Thick, coarse (all)
Hair
Generalized hirsutism (all)
Craniofacial
Coarse facies with thick nose and depressed nasal bridge, thick lips and tongue, short neck, macrocephaly (Hurler's, Hunter's, Sanfilippo's—mild, Maroteaux-Lamy's)
Central Nervous System
Mental retardation (Hurler's, Hunter's—severe form, Sanfilippo's), progressive neurologic impairment (Hunter's—severe form, Sanfilippo's), deafness (Hurler's, Hunter's), hyperactivity/behavioral problems (Sanfilippo's), hydrocephalus (Hurler's, Hunter's—severe form)
Musculoskeletal
Short stature (all except Scheie's), broad hands with short fingers (all), "dysostosis multiplex"—stiff joints, contractures, kyphoscoliosis, claw deformity of hand (Hurler's, Scheie's, Hunter's, Maroteaux-Lamy's), odontoid hypoplasia (Morquio's, Hurler's), joint laxity (Morquio's), lumbar lordosis (Morquio's), umbilical/inguinal hernia (Hurler's, Scheie's, Hunter's, Maroteaux-Lamy's)

Mucopolysaccharidoses *(continued)*

Eyes
Corneal clouding (all except Hunter's, Sanfilippo's)

Cardiovascular
Deposition of mucopolysaccharides with valvular and coronary heart disease (Hurler's, Scheie's, Hunter's, Morquio's, Maroteaux-Lamy's), aortic valve disease (Scheie's)

Gastrointestinal
Hepatosplenomegaly (Hurler's, Hunter's, Maroteaux-Lamy's)

Lungs
Bronchopneumonia—often end-stage, sleep apnea with narrow upper airway (Hurler's, Scheie's, Hunter's, Maroteaux-Lamy's)

Differential Diagnosis

Mucolipidoses

Laboratory Data

Mucopolysaccharide detection in urine
Enzyme assay: fibroblasts, leukocytes, serum
Spine films
Echocardiogram

Management

Supportive care with physical therapy, special education, hearing aids
Surgical correction of cornea, cardiac valve, cervical spine, joint contractures, hernia may help
Bone marrow transplantation—some success

Prognosis

Progressive worsening with no cure; death usually within second decade because of respiratory/cardiac decompensation; milder forms may survive into adulthood
Scheie's—normal life span

Clinical Pearls

The coarse facies may not be apparent when they're very young. . . The early tip off to the pediatrician is hepatosplenomegaly and a gibbous deformity of the lower spine. . . Early on, get a lateral lumbar spine and/or lateral skull seeing the j-shaped deformity of the sella turcica. . . Kids with Sanfilippo's are physically very mild, but mentally can be difficult with hyperactivity, aggressive behavior. . . Four or five different enzyme defects can lead to Sanfilippo's. . . As opposed to Hurler's where different mutations in the same gene gives different disease. . . Most kids with storage disease seem to begin life reaching their early milestones and then drop off. . . If the mother tells you the kid isn't doing what he's supposed to be doing at 6 months or so, you really need to start looking. . . To obtain skin for fibroblast cultures, I (*KH*) take a tuberculin syringe, raise a bleb in the skin with lidocaine, and then come out the other end of the bleb. . . I lift it and shear off the base with a scalpel. . . Fibroblasts grow beautifully. . . We do echoes and spine films on all of them. . . As with Down's, patients with Hurler's and Morquio's lack their occipito-atlantic prominence that anchors the cervical spine to the skull. . . They can split and become quadriplegic. . . You must fuse this area. . . We keep them in physical therapy to prevent contractures. . . The group in Minnesota has studied bone marrow transplants in all patients with mucopolysaccharidoses (MPS). . . They believe it may mitigate the retardation. . . They've transplanted a kid with Hurler's in utero. . . They may be slowing things down some but those cells are not going to correct the brain. . . You're going to have to wait for gene therapy. . . Corneal transplants stay clear because they produce their own enzyme. . . The MPS society is very active. . . Gene replacement is being done on animal models like the Siamese cat for Maroteaux-Lamy's.   *KH, JW*

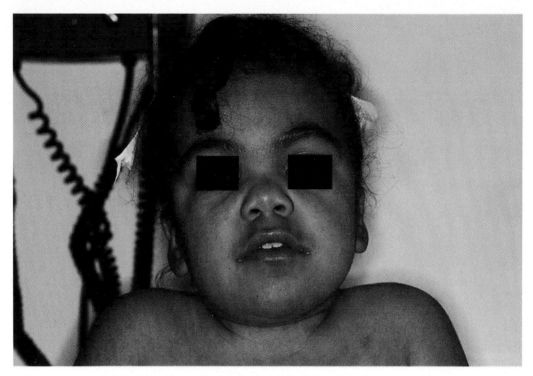

11.9. *Typical coarse facies in a girl with Hurler syndrome.*

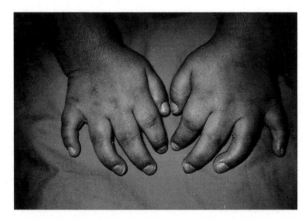

11.10. *Broad hands with short fingers, thick coarse skin. (1)*

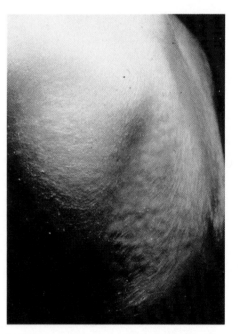

11.11. *Ivory-colored papules in "cobblestone" pattern between scapula and posterior axillary line in patient with Hunter's syndrome. (125)*

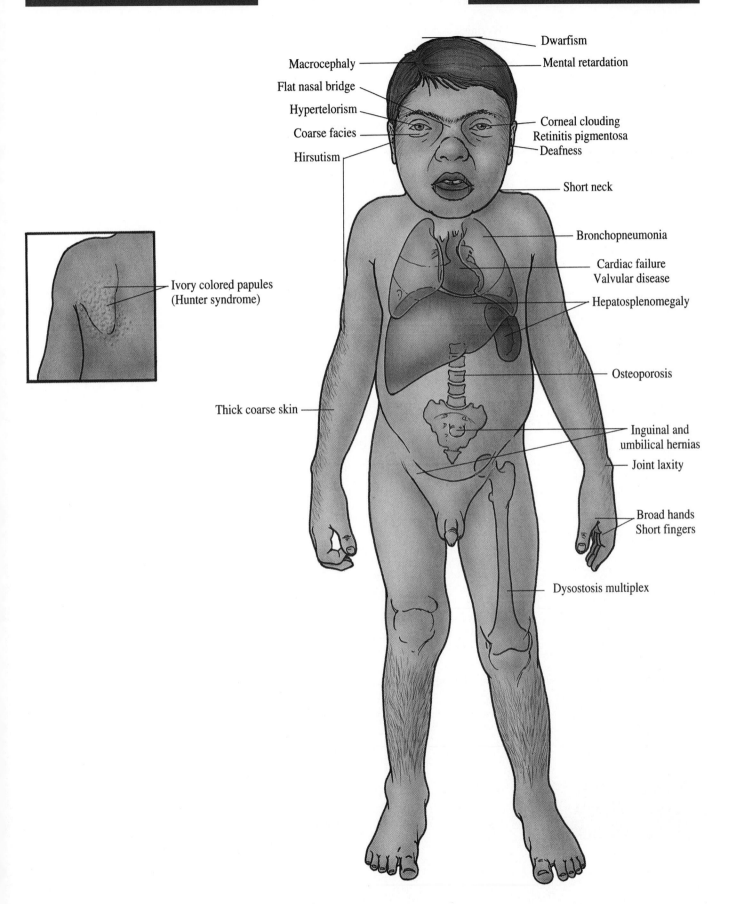

Dwarfism

Macrocephaly

Mental retardation

Flat nasal bridge

Hypertelorism

Corneal clouding
Retinitis pigmentosa
Deafness

Coarse facies

Hirsutism

Short neck

Ivory colored papules
(Hunter syndrome)

Bronchopneumonia

Cardiac failure
Valvular disease

Hepatosplenomegaly

Osteoporosis

Thick coarse skin

Inguinal and
umbilical hernias

Joint laxity

Broad hands
Short fingers

Dysostosis multiplex

Multiple Carboxylase Deficiency

Synonym	Biotinidase deficiency Holocarboxylase synthetase deficiency
Inheritance	Both autosomal recessive; holocarboxylase synthetase (*HLCS*) gene on 21q22; biotinidase (*BTD*) gene on 3p25
Prenatal Diagnosis	CVS/amniocentesis: biotinidase or holocarboxylase synthetase assay
Incidence	Biotinidase deficiency: 1:70,000 to 80,000; M=F Holocarboxylase synthetase deficiency: unknown, rare: M=F
Age at Presentation	Biotinidase deficiency: approximately 6 months old Holocarboxylase synthetase deficiency: first few days to months of life
Pathogenesis	Mutations in *HLCS* or *BTD* render the patient deficient in holocarboxylase synthetase or biotinidase respectively, resulting in decreased free serum biotin and metabolic acidosis with resultant phenotype
Key Features	**Skin** Periorificial/generalized dermatitis with/without candida infection **Hair** Sparse to total alopecia **Central Nervous System** Hypotonia, seizures, ataxia, coma **Gastrointestinal** Vomiting (holocarboxylase synthetase deficiency) **Eyes** Optic atrophy (biotinidase deficiency) **Ear-Nose-Throat** High-frequency hearing loss (biotinidase deficiency) **Metabolism** Metabolic acidosis, hyperammonemia, organic aciduria
Differential Diagnosis	Atopic dermatitis Seborrheic dermatitis Acrodermatitis enteropathica (p. 328) Mucocutaneous candidiasis Essential fatty acid deficiency
Laboratory Data	Screen urine for organic aciduria Serum biotinidase/holocarboxylase synthetase assay Screen blood—metabolic acidosis, hyperammonemia
Management	Biotin 10 mg per day for life
Prognosis	If biotin instituted prior to neurologic sequelae, normal life span with normal growth and development

Clinical Pearls

Clearly, we look for it in a kid who is acidotic in a precomatose state. . . We also look for all the other inborn errors that can do this. . . Any child who presents with failure to thrive and skin manifestations should to have their urine screened for organic acids.   *KH, JW*

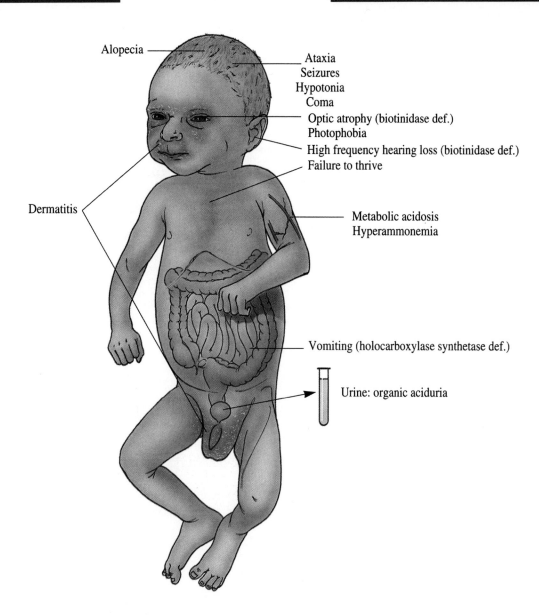

Alopecia

Dermatitis

Ataxia
Seizures
Hypotonia
Coma

Optic atrophy (biotinidase def.)
Photophobia
High frequency hearing loss (biotinidase def.)
Failure to thrive

Metabolic acidosis
Hyperammonemia

Vomiting (holocarboxylase synthetase def.)

Urine: organic aciduria

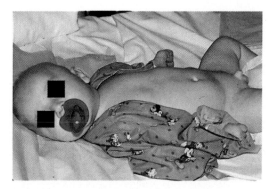

11.12. *Infant with alopecia, hypotonia, and groin dermatitis. (5)*

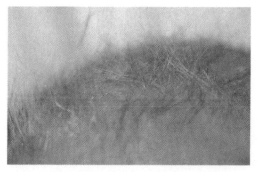

11.13. *Sparse, lusterless, brittle scalp hair on close-up view. (5)*

323

Phenylketonuria

Inheritance	Autosomal recessive; phenylalanine hydroxylase (*PAH*) gene locus 12q24.1
Prenatal Diagnosis	CVS/amniocentesis—enzyme assay, metabolite levels, DNA analysis
Incidence	1:10,000 caucasian births; M=F
Age at Presentation	Birth
Pathogenesis	Mutation in *PAH* leads to a deficiency of phenylalanine hydroxylase with subsequent accumulation of phenylalanine and its metabolites; increased phenylalanine competitively inhibits tyrosine in melanogenesis and has toxic affects on the CNS
Key Features	**Skin**
	Generalized hypopigmentation, eczematous dermatitis, sclerodermoid changes
	Hair
	Blonde
	Eyes
	Blue
	Central Nervous System
	Mental retardation, seizures, hyperreflexia, psychomotor delay
Differential Diagnosis	Albinism
	Chédiak-Higashi syndrome (p. 62)
	Scleroderma/morphea
Laboratory Data	Urine (mousy odor), blood screen for phenylalanine and its metabolites
Management	Routine neonatal screening
	Low-phenylalanine diet instituted early on will prevent CNS and skin changes
Prognosis	Normal life span with normal intelligence with treatment; without treatment shortened life span with chronic seizures and mental retardation

Clinical Pearls

We don't see it anymore. . . We're screening them all at birth. . . I (*KH*) remember seeing a kid with phenylketonuria (PKU) who came from blonde-haired parents. . . He looked like an albino. . . Pregnant women with PKU must be on strict diet control to protect heterozygote fetus from malformations and severe retardation. . . Patients need to be on formula diet for rest of their lives. . . Tastes terrible. . . If the patient's not under control, the mousy odor will be present. . . The enzyme is not expressed in cultured amniocytes. . . Prenatal diagnosis by molecular techniques if the mutation is known. . . People are using polymerase chain reaction (PCR) in situations where fibroblast or lymphocyte cultures don't express enough enzyme to make the diagnosis.   *KH, JW*

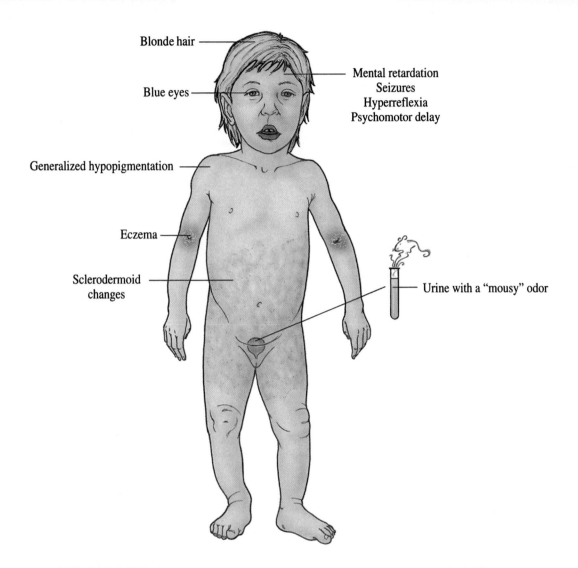

Blonde hair

Blue eyes

Generalized hypopigmentation

Eczema

Sclerodermoid
changes

Mental retardation
Seizures
Hyperreflexia
Psychomotor delay

Urine with a "mousy" odor

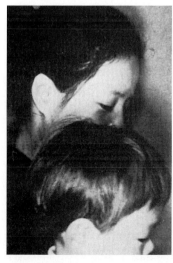

11.14. *Lighter hair color in affected Japanese child compared to unaffected mother. (126)*

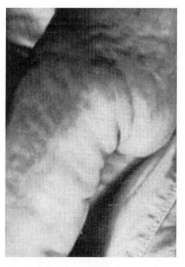

11.15. *Sclerodermoid changes on buttocks and thigh of 1-year-old. (127)*

Wilson's Disease

Synonym	Hepatolenticular degeneration
Inheritance	Autosomal recessive; *ATB7B* gene on 13q14.2–q21
Prenatal Diagnosis	DNA analysis
Incidence	1:50 to 100,000: M=F
Age at Presentation	Childhood to adulthood
Pathogenesis	Mutation in *ATB7B*, a gene encoding an adenosine triphosphatase (ATPase) CU^{2+}-transporting polypeptide results in a defect in biliary excretion of copper/copper transport and leads to accumulation of copper in liver, brain, cornea
Key Features	**Gastrointestinal** Hepatomegaly, cirrhosis/liver failure **Central Nervous System** Dysarthria, decreased voluntary motor coordination, ataxia, dementia **Eyes** **Kayser-Fleischer ring**—yellow-brown copper deposition in Descemet's membrane of the cornea **Skin** Pretibial hyperpigmentation **Nails** Blue lunulae (rare)
Differential Diagnosis	Gaucher disease (p. 310) Argyria Other causes of chronic liver disease Other causes of dementia and ataxia
Laboratory Data	Decreased incorporation of copper into ceruloplasmin after intravenous copper-64 isotope administration over 48 hours Decreased serum ceruloplasmin levels Increased urinary/serum copper levels
Management	Slit-lamp eye examination Oral penicillamine, trientine-copper chelators Liver transplantation Decrease copper intake, increased zinc
Prognosis	Shortened life span if untreated; if treatment instituted early on, most symptoms will reverse itself (except CNS) and life span is normal

Clinical Pearls

Patients can present at any age, even with fulminant hepatic failure in childhood. . . I've (*KH*) seen a 2-year-old with ataxia. . . Need to do a copper excretion study and slit-lamp to rule out Wilson's in kids with unexplained liver disease. . . Most interesting recent finding is that when they found the Menkes gene, a copper transport gene, they looked for and located homologous DNA on chromosome 13 in region of Wilson's disease. . . Penicillamine most commonly used but has nasty side effects. . . The first liver transplant for genetic disease was a patient with Wilson's. . . The new liver will make the transport protein and properly process all the copper. . . All of them are being transplanted now. . . This is a good disease for hepatic gene therapy in future.   *KH, JW*

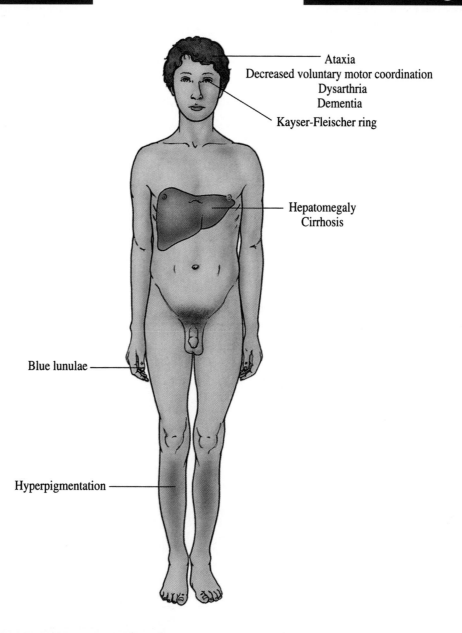

Ataxia
Decreased voluntary motor coordination
Dysarthria
Dementia
Kayser-Fleischer ring

Hepatomegaly
Cirrhosis

Blue lunulae

Hyperpigmentation

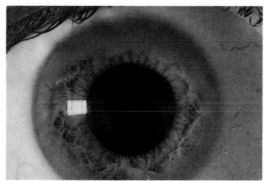

11.16. *Kayser-Fleischer ring. (1)*

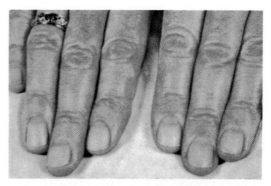

11.17. *Blue lunulae. (128)*

Acrodermatitis Enteropathica

Inheritance	Autosomal recessive; *SLC39A4* on 8q24.3
Prenatal Diagnosis	DNA mutation analysis if known
Incidence	Rare; approximately 1:500,000 in Denmark; M=F
Age at Presentation	Days to weeks after birth in bottle-fed infants; after weaning breast-fed older infants
Pathogenesis	Mutation in *SLC39A4*, a gene encoding an intestinal zinc-specific transporter protein, results in defective zinc absorption from the gut, low serum zinc levels, and characteristic phenotype; human milk has zinc-binding ligands that facilitates transport of zinc into epithelial cells
Key Features	**Skin** Periorificial, scalp, and acral dermatitis with erythema, scaling, vescicles/bullae, erosions; bacterial or candidal superinfection **Hair** Alopecia **Gastrointestinal** Diarrhea, failure to thrive, stomatitis, glossitis **Central Nervous System** Irritability **Eyes** Photophobia
Differential Diagnosis	Atopic dermatitis Seborrheic dermatitis Multiple carboxylase deficiency (p. 322) Other causes of zinc deficiency
Laboratory Data	Serum zinc level
Management	Lifelong oral zinc supplementation
Prognosis	All symptoms clear within 1 to 2 days of zinc supplementation

Clinical Pearls

Very rare genetic entity. . . I have seen it only in the setting of long-term total parenteral nutrition (TPN). . . Only a few years ago, TPN lacked zinc. . . Zinc perks these kids right up. *KH, JW*

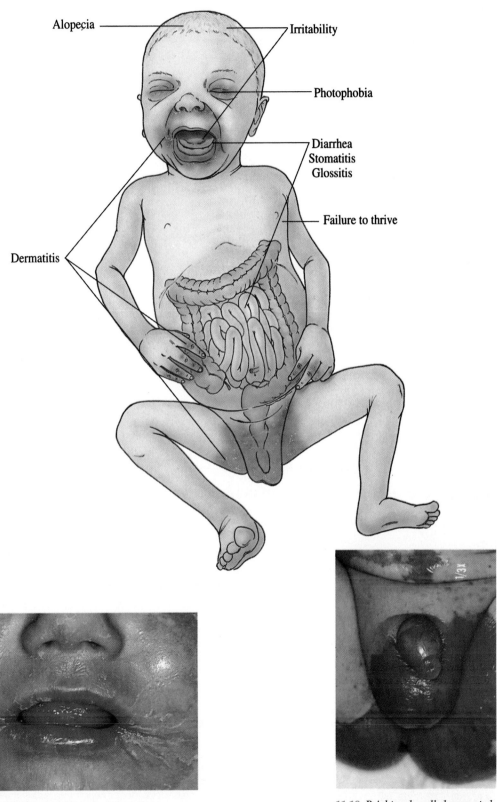

Alopecia

Irritability

Photophobia

Diarrhea
Stomatitis
Glossitis

Failure to thrive

Dermatitis

11.18. *Marked perioral erythema, scale, and erosions. (129)*

11.19. *Bright-red, well-demarcated perianal and scrotal erosion. (129)*

Hemochromatosis

Inheritance
Autosomal recessive; classic hemochromatosis-*HFE* gene on locus 6p21.3

Prenatal Diagnosis
DNA analysis available

Incidence
Approximately 1:333; 8% to 10% of population are heterozygotes; M>F

Age at Presentation
Usually around fifth decade of life

Pathogenesis
A mutation in *HFE* leads to increased intestinal iron absorption, iron overload and deposition in a variety of organs; presumably, females are less likely to be affected given natural iron loss with menstruation

Key Features
Skin
Generalized metallic-grey hyperpigmentation
Nails
Koilonychia
Hair
Generalized sparse to absent
Gastrointestinal
Hepatomegaly, abdominal pain, weight loss
Cardiovascular
Cardiac failure, arrhythmias, heart block
Endocrine
Insulin-dependent diabetes mellitus, hypogonadism, loss of libido
Musculoskeletal
Polyarthritis

Differential Diagnosis
Addison's disease
Wilson disease (p. 326)
Argyria
Chrysiasis
Gaucher disease (p. 310)
Niemann-Pick disease (p. 314)

Laboratory Data
Plasma ferritin, iron, total iron-binding capacity levels

Management
Phlebotomy
Deferoxamine—iron chelator
Supportive care—insulin, testosterone, anti-arrhythmic agents
Screen first-degree relatives by DNA

Prognosis
Early diagnosis and treatment will decrease symptomatology and extend life span; premature death may occur secondary to cardiac failure, hepatocellular carcinoma, hepatic coma

Clinical Pearls

Fascinating disease. . . Far more common than people are led to believe. . . Significantly more common than Wilson's. . . Think of the diagnosis if you have a 40-year-old with unexplained liver disease. . . Almost always expresses itself in the context of a specific human leukocyte antigen (HLA) type. . . You have to identify patients early enough to prevent liver damage. . . Skin pigmentation is diffuse. . . Alcoholics who destroy their livers more rapidly than one would expect should be screened for hemochromatosis. . . Population screening is controversial, because many homozygotes for the common mutation will never develop disease.   *KH, JW*

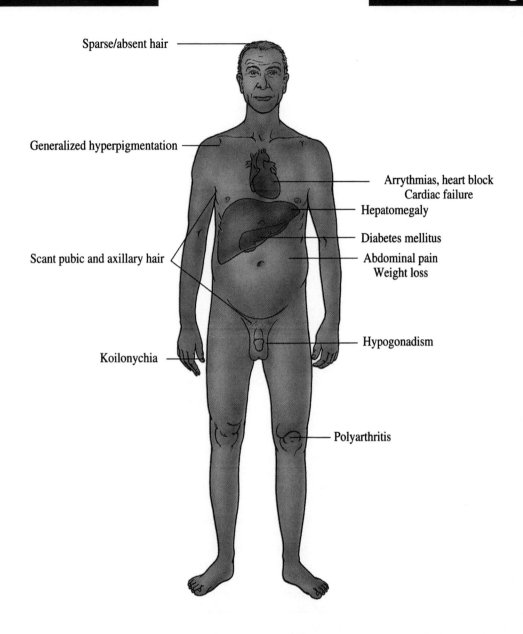

Sparse/absent hair

Generalized hyperpigmentation

Arrythmias, heart block
Cardiac failure

Hepatomegaly

Diabetes mellitus

Scant pubic and axillary hair

Abdominal pain
Weight loss

Hypogonadism

Koilonychia

Polyarthritis

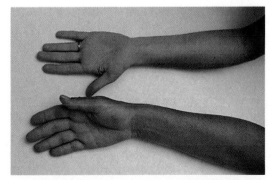

11.20. *Top arm. Normal pigment in patient's sibling. Bottom arm. Metallic-gray hyperpigmentation in affected patient. (130)*

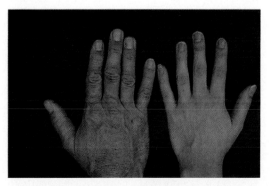

11.21. *Left. Hyperpigmentation on patient's hand. Right. Normal sibling's hand. (130)*

Homocystinuria

Inheritance
Autosomal recessive; cystathionine β-synthase (*CBS*) gene on 21q22.3

Prenatal Diagnosis
CVS/amniocentesis—cystathionine β-synthase assay with chorionic villus tissue/amniotic fluid cell culture
DNA analysis

Incidence
Approximately 1:200,000; increased incidence in Ireland; M=F

Age at Presentation
Early childhood

Pathogenesis
Mutations in the *CBS* gene leads to cystathionine beta-synthase deficiency with accumulation of homocystine

Key Features
Skin
Malar flush, deep venous thromboses, livedo reticularis, leg ulcers
Hair
Fine, sparse
Eyes
Downward lens dislocation, myopia, glaucoma
Musculoskeletal
Marfanoid habitus with dolichostenomelia, arachnodactyly, osteoporosis, kyphoscoliosis, pectus excavatum/carinatum, genu valgum, pes cavus
Cardiovascular
Arterial and venous thromboses with emobolic phenomenon to heart, lungs, brain, kidney
Central Nervous System
Mental retardation, seizures, psychiatric disorders

Differential Diagnosis
Marfan syndrome (p. 140)
Congenital contractural arachnodactyly
Multiple endocrine neoplasia (MEN) IIB (p. 190)

Laboratory Data
Increased homocystine and methionine levels in blood and urine
Newborn screening is based on elevated plasma methionine

Management
Vitamin B$_6$ (pyridoxine)—response in patients with residual cystathionine β-synthase activity
Low-methionine, high-cystine diet
Referral to symptom-specific specialist

Prognosis
Vitamin B$_6$ responders may have normal life span with early intervention; early diet control in non-responders may improve outcome; otherwise premature death secondary to thrombotic events

Clinical Pearls

Usually not as tall as patients with Marfan's. . . Patients with Marfan's don't have the neuropsychiatric changes we see here. . . Mental retardation can be quite variable. . . In general, patients' IQs are significantly lower than their siblings'. . . However, I (*KH*) know a homocystinuric who's in college. . . Of course, their skin findings, namely the malar rash and chronic leg ulcers, are also distinguishing features. . . Death usually in third to fourth decade from vascular event.   *KH, JW*

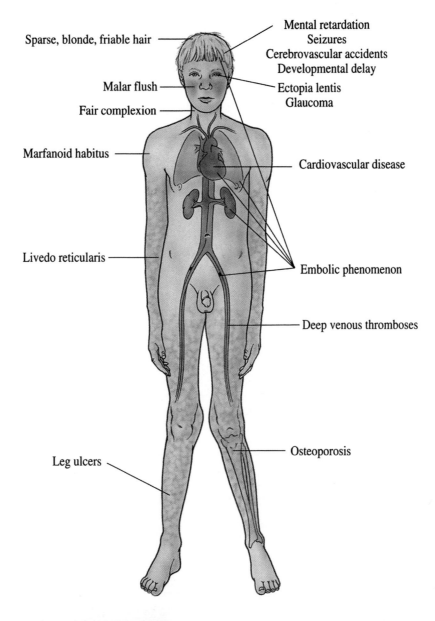

Sparse, blonde, friable hair

Malar flush

Fair complexion

Marfanoid habitus

Livedo reticularis

Leg ulcers

Mental retardation
Seizures
Cerebrovascular accidents
Developmental delay

Ectopia lentis
Glaucoma

Cardiovascular disease

Embolic phenomenon

Deep venous thromboses

Osteoporosis

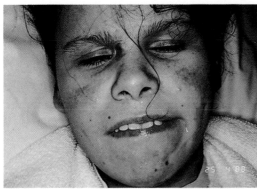

11.22. Typical malar flush in mentally retarded female. (20)

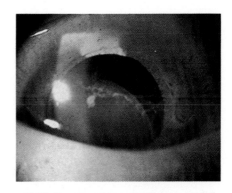

11.23. Downward lens displacement. (131)

Hyperlipoproteinemias

Synonym

Type I hyperlipoproteinemia (I)—familial lipoprotein lipase deficiency
Type II hyperlipoproteinemia (II)—familial hypercholesterolemia
Type III hyperlipoproteinemia (III)—familial dysbetalipoproteinemia
Type IV hyperlipoproteinemia (IV)—familial hypertriglyceridemia
Type V hyperlipoproteinemia (V)

Inheritance

I—autosomal recessive; lipoprotein lipase gene (*LPL*) on 8p22; 19 (apoC-II)
II—autosomal dominant; gene locus 19p13
III—autosomal recessive; apolipoprotein E (*APOE*) gene on 19q13
IV—autosomal dominant; gene locus 15q11.2–13.1
V—autosomal dominant; gene locus unknown

Prenatal Diagnosis

I—CVS/amniocentesis—lipoprotein lipase activity in cultured chorionic villus tissue/amniotic fluid cells; DNA analysis
II—DNA analysis
III—DNA analysis
IV—DNA analysis
V—unknown

Incidence

I—rare; M=F
II—1:500 heterozygotes; M=F
III—1:2,000 to 10,000; M > F
IV—unknown; likely 1 to 10:1,000; M=F
V—1:1,000; M=F

Age at Presentation

I—childhood
II—heterozygotes: third to fourth decade
II—homozygotes: first decade
III—fourth to fifth decade
IV—early adulthood
V—usually in adulthood

Pathogenesis

I—mutation in the *LPL* gene leads to decreased lipoprotein lipase activity with secondary defective lipolysis and increased chylomicronemia; apoC-II cofactor deficiency will secondarily decrease lipoprotein lipase activity and produce similar phenotype
II—structural and functional defect of LDL receptor on cell membrane with marked increase in LDL and cholesterol levels
III—mutation in *APOE* gene leads to an apolipoprotein E defect with defective clearing of intermediate density lipoproteins and chylomicrons by the liver
IV—multiple causative factors
V—multiple causes including insulin-dependent diabetes mellitus, alcohol abuse, contraceptive steroids, and glycogen storage disease I

Key Features

Skin
Eruptive xanthomas (I, III, V); xanthelasma (II, III); xanthoma striata palmaris (III); tendinous xanthoma (II); tuberous xanthomas at pressure points (II,III); planar xanthoma (II)
Eyes
Lipemia retinalis (I, V); arcus juvenilis (II)
Cardiovascular
Premature atherosclerosis (II, III, and less common in IV)
Gastrointestinal
Pancreatitis (I, V, may occur in IV), hepatosplenomegaly (I, V) abdominal pain (I, V)
Central Nervous System
Neuropsychiatric symptoms (I, V)
Endocrine
Glucose intolerance (III, IV, V), hypothyroidism (III), obesity (III, IV, V), hyperuricemia (III, IV, V)

Differential Diagnosis

Secondary causes of hyperlipoproteinemia: diabetes mellitus, primary biliary cirrhosis, hypothyroidism, chronic pancreatitis, nephrotic syndrome, multiple myeloma, oral contraceptives
Pseudoxanthoma elasticum (p. 144)

Laboratory Data

I—plasma chylomicrons, triglycerides markedly increased; cholesterol normal; very low-density lipoprotein (VLDL), high-density lipoprotein (HDL), low-density lipoprotein (LDL) normal or decreased; enzyme assay for lipoprotein lipase/apoCII activity; cream top layer on standing at 4°C for 18 hours
II—plasma LDL, cholesterol markedly increased; LDL receptor assay; turbid plasma
III—plasma cholesterol, triglycerides increased; presence of β-VLDL on lipoprotein electrophoresis; apoE phenotyping; turbid plasma
IV—plasma VLDL, triglycerides markedly increased; turbid plasma
V—plasma chylomicrons, triglycerides, VLDL markedly increased; cholesterol increased; cream top layer

Management

Close routine care by primary physician—screen children with family history of early infarcts, hyperlipoproteinemia
Referral to nutritionist:
    I,V—restriction of fat intake/medium-chain triglyceride diet
    II—low-fat, low-cholesterol diet with reduction of saturated fats, increase in polyunsaturated and monounsaturated fats
    III—low-calorie/cholesterol/saturated-fat diet
    IV—low-calorie, low-carbohydrate diet
Plasmapheresis, liver transplantation (II)
Lipid lowering agents including HMG-CoA reductase inhibitors, nicotinic acid, gemfibrozil, cholestyramine (II, III, IV, V)
Treatment of diabetes, hypothyroidism, obesity (III, IV, V)
Referral to symptom-specific subspecialist
Avoidance of alcohol, oral contraceptives

Prognosis

I, V—may succumb prematurely to pancreatitis; otherwise normal life span
II—premature myocardial infarction/death secondary to atherosclerotic event in first few decades of life; may improve with early intervention (medication, diet modification, plasmapheresis, transplantation)
III—lipid changes very responsive to diet modification/caloric restriction and medication; may decrease cardiovascular events
IV—lipid changes respond to weight loss, caloric restriction, medication; unknown decrease in cardiovascular events

Clinical Pearls

First thing to do is determine what kind of xanthoma you're dealing with. . . Type II's "xanthelasmas" are really tuberous xanthomas and can occur where eyeglasses apply pressure on nasal bridge. . . Although xanthelasma is common as a normal variant, check lipid status on all patients. . . Arcus juvenilis is a specific sign for hyperlipoproteinemia. . . Lipemia retinalis is an interesting phenomenon—if you have somebody with high triglycerides from any cause, look for sludging of red blood cells in conjunctival or retinal vessels. . . One of the allelic types of apoE has been associated with Alzheimer's. . . Type I's present with horrible, "screaming" abdominal pain. . . Could be their liver or pancreas. . . Initially, little kids need some fat to grow. . . Must balance belly aches with growth when managing diet in type I's. . . After 2 to 3 years old, essentially need fat-free diets. . . Homozygous II's need liver transplantation to survive. . . Gene therapy is next step. . . Easy to misdiagnose chest pain in a young kid. . . Especially if xanthomas not present yet. . . After you listen to a normal chest, look at a normal x-ray, then do an ECG. . . You'll pick up angina, myocardial infarctions. . . Only other kids to get heart attacks are those with vasculitis, sickle cell disease, and occasionally homocystinurics. . . Some places are screening for genes. . . Nutritionist is critical.   *KH, JW*

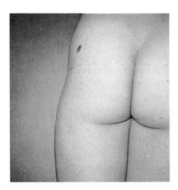

11.24. *Eruptive xanthomas on buttocks and thigh. (132)*

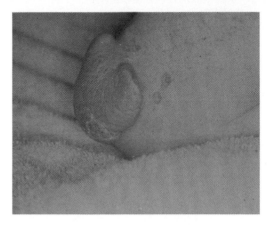

11.25. *Tuberous xanthoma on elbow. (132)*

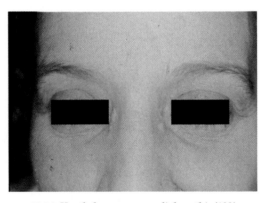

11.26. *Xanthelasma near medial canthi. (132)*

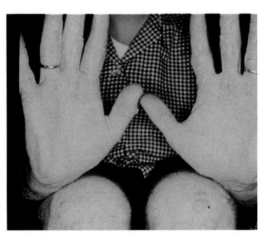

11.27. *Xanthoma striata palmaris with tuberous xanthomas of knees. (132)*

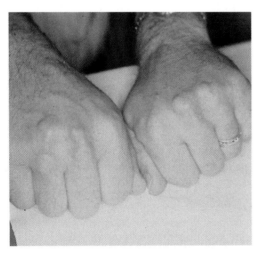

11.28. *Tendinous xanthomas on hands. (132)*

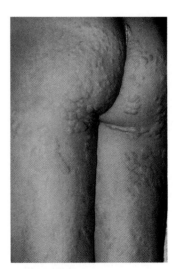

11.29. *Diffuse planar xanthoma on buttocks and lower extremities. (102)*

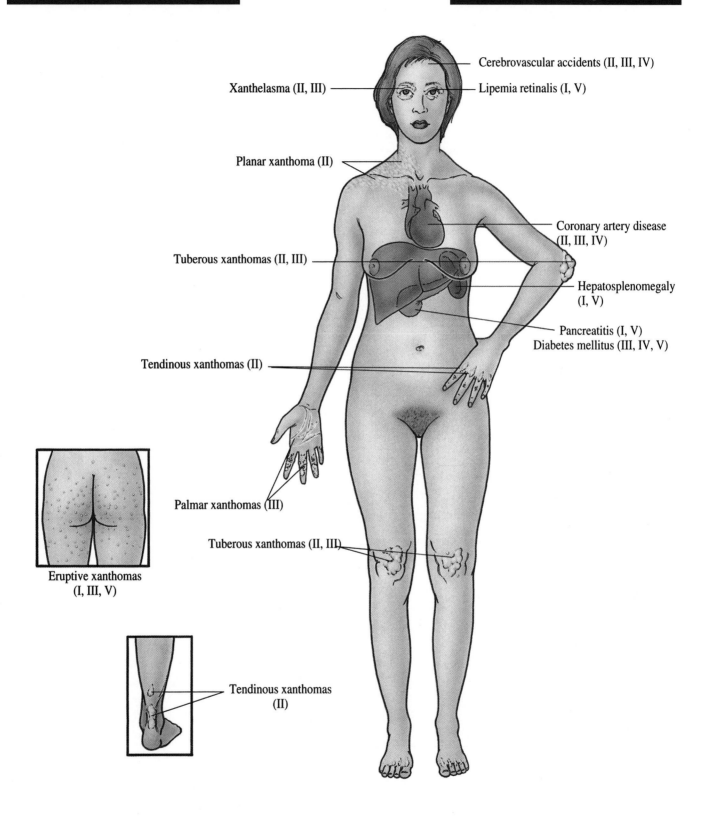

Cerebrovascular accidents (II, III, IV)

Xanthelasma (II, III)

Lipemia retinalis (I, V)

Planar xanthoma (II)

Coronary artery disease (II, III, IV)

Tuberous xanthomas (II, III)

Hepatosplenomegaly (I, V)

Pancreatitis (I, V)
Diabetes mellitus (III, IV, V)

Tendinous xanthomas (II)

Eruptive xanthomas (I, III, V)

Palmar xanthomas (III)

Tuberous xanthomas (II, III)

Tendinous xanthomas (II)

Suggested Reading

Alkaptonuria

Albers SE, Brozena SJ, Glass LF, et al. Alkaptonuria and ochronosis: case report and review. *J Am Acad Dermatol* 1992;27:609–614.

Beltran-Valero de Bernabe D, Peterson P, Luopajarvi K, et al. Mutational analysis of the HGO gene in Finnish alkaptonuria patients. *J Med Genet* 1999;36:922–923.

Beltran-Valero de Bernabe D, Jimenez FJ, Aquaron R, et al. Analysis of alkaptonuria (AKU) mutations and polymorphisms reveals that the CCC sequence motif is a mutational hot spot in the homogentisate 1,2-dioxygenase gene (HGO). *Am J Hum Genet* 1999;64:1316–1322.

Brenton OF, Krywawych S. Alkaptonuria. *Clin Rheum Dis* 1986;12:755–769.

Carrier DA, Harris CM. Bilateral hip and bilateral knee arthroplasties in a patient with ochronotic arthropathy. *Orthop Rev* 1990;19:1005–1009.

Garrod AE. The incidence of alkaptonuria: a study in chemical individuality. *Lancet* 1902;11:1616–1620.

Janocha S, Wolz W, Srsen S, et al. The human gene for alkaptonuria (AKU) maps to chromosome 3q. *Genomics* 1994;19:5–8.

La Du BN. Alkaptonuria. In: Scriver CR, Beaudet A, Sly W, Valle D, eds. *The Metabolic and Molecular Bases of Inherited Disease.* 7th ed. New York: McGraw-Hill, 2001:1371.

Lorenzini S, Mannoni A, Selvi E. Alkaptonuria. *N Engl J Med* 2003;348:1408; author reply 1408.

Mannoni A, Selvi E, Lorenzini M, et al. Alkaptonuria, ochronosis, and ochronotic arthropathy. *Semin Arthritis Rheum* 2004;33:239–248.

O'Brien WM, La Du BN, Bunim JJ. Biochemical, pathologic and clinic aspects of alcaptonuria, ochronosis and ochronotic arthropathy: review of world literature (1584–1962). *Am J Med* 1963;34:813–838.

Phornphutkul C, Introne WJ, Perry MB, et al. Natural history of alkaptonuria. *N Engl J Med* 2002;349:2111–2121.

Rodriguez JM, Timm DE, Titus GP, et al. Structural and functional analysis of mutations in alkaptonuria. *Hum Mol Genet* 2000;9:2341–2350.

Suzuki Y, Oda K, Yoshikawa Y, et al. A novel therapeutic trial of homogentistic aciduria in a murine model of alkaptonuria. *J Hum Genet* 1999;44:79–84.

Toth K, Lenart E, Janositz G, et al. Ochronotic arthropathy. *Scand J Rheumatol* 2003;32:315–317.

Uyguner O, Goicoechea de Jorge E, Cefle A, et al. Molecular analyses of the HGO gene mutations in Turkish alkaptonuria patients suggest that the R58fs mutation originated from central Asia and was spread throughout Europe and Anatolia by human migrations. *J Inherit Metab Dis* 2003;26:17–23.

Zatkova A, de Bernabe DB, Polakova H, et al. High frequency of alkaptonuria in Slovakia: evidence for the appearance of multiple mutations in HGO involving different mutational hot spots. *Am J Hum Genet* 2000;67:1333–1339.

Zatkova A, Chmelikova A, Polakova H, et al. Rapid detection methods for five HGO gene mutations causing alkaptonuria. *Clin Genet* 2003;63:145–149.

Fabry Disease

Ashley GA, Shabbeer J, Yasuda M, et al. Fabry disease: twenty novel a-galactosidase A mutations causing the classical phenotype. *J Hum Genet* 2001;46:192–196.

Chesser RS, Gentry RH, Fitzpatrick JE, et al. Perioral telangiectases: a new cutaneous finding in Fabry's disease. *Arch Dermatol* 1990;126:1655–1656.

Cho ME, Kopp JB. Fabry disease in the era of enzyme replacement therapy: a renal perspective. *Pediatr Nephrol* 2004;19:583–593.

Clement M, McGonigle RJS, Monkhouse PM, et al. Renal transplantation in Anderson-Fabry disease. *J R Soc Med* 1982;75:557–560.

Desnick RJ. a-Galactosidase A deficiency: Fabry disease. In: Scriver CR, Beaudet AL, Sly WS, Valle D, eds. *The Metabolic and Molecular Bases of Inherited Disease.* 8th ed. New York: McGraw-Hill, 2001:3733.

Eng CM, Guffon N, Wilcox WR, et al. Safety and efficacy of recombinant human a-galactosidase A—replacement therapy in Fabry's disease. *N Engl J Med* 2001;345:9–16.

Eng CM, Resnick-Silverman LA, Niehaus DJ, et al. Nature and frequency of mutations in the alpha galactosidase A gene causing Fabry disease. *Am J Hum Genet* 1993;53:1186–1197.

Fisher EA, Desnick RJ, Gordon RE, et al. Fabry disease: an unusual cause of severe coronary disease in a young man. *Ann Intern Med* 1992;117:221–223.

Hilz MJ, Brys M, Marthol H, et al. Enzyme replacement therapy improves function of C-, Adelta-, and Abeta-nerve fibers in Fabry neuropathy. *Neurology* 2004;62:1066–1072.

Kotanko P, Kramar R, Devrnja D, et al. Results of a nationwide screening for Anderson-Fabry disease among dialysis patients. *J Am Soc Nephrol* 2004;15:1323–1329.

Linhart A, Palecek T, Bultas J, et al. New insights in cardiac structural changes in patients with Fabry's disease. *Am Heart J* 2000;139:1101–1108.

Linthorst GE, De Rie MA, Tjiam KH, et al. Misdiagnosis of Fabry disease: importance of biochemical confirmation of clinical or pathological suspicion. *Br J Dermatol* 2004;150:575–577.

Mitsias P, Levine SR. Cerebrovascular complications of Fabry's disease. *Ann Neural* 1996;40:8–17.

Morgan SH, Rudge P, Smith SJ, et al. The neurological complications of Anderson-Fabry disease (alphagalactosidase A deficiency)—investigation of symptomatic and presymptomatic patients. *Q J Med* 1990;75:491–507.

Nguyen J, Egbert BM, Swetter SM. Diffuse verrucous, vascular nodules on the extremities and trunk. *Arch Dermatol* 2004;140:353–358.

Ojo A, Meier-Kriesche HU, Friedman G, et al. Excellent outcome of renal transplantation in patients with Fabry's disease. *Transplantation* 2000;69:2337–2339.

Pastores GM, Thadani R. Enzyme-replacement therapy for Anderson-Fabry disease. *Lancet* 2001;358:601–603.

Schiffmann R, Murray GJ, Treco D, et al. Infusion of a-galactosidase A reduces tissue globo-triaosylceramide storage in patients with Fabry disease. *Proc Natl Acad Sci USA* 2000;97:365–370.

Schiffmann R, Kopp JB, Austin HA 3rd, et al. Enzyme replacement therapy in Fabry disease: a randomized controlled trial. *JAMA* 2001;285:2743–2749.

Thurberg BL, Randolph Byers H, Granter SR, et al. Monitoring the 3-year efficacy of enzyme replacement therapy in fabry disease by repeated skin biopsies. *J Invest Dermatol* 2004;122:900–908.

Gaucher Disease

Barton NW, Brady RO, Dambrosia JM, et al. Replacement therapy for inherited enzyme deficiency: macrophage-targeted glucocerebrosidase for Gaucher's disease. *N Engl J Med* 1991;324:1464–1470.

Beutler E. Gaucher disease as a paradigm of current issues regarding single gene mutations of humans. *Proc Nat Acad Sci* 1993;90:5384–5390.

Brady RO, Barton NW, Grabowski GA. The role of neurogenetics in Gaucher disease. *Arch Neurol* 1993;50:1212–1224.

Desnick RJ. Gaucher disease: a century of delineation and understanding. *Prog Clin Biol Res* 1982;95:1–30.

Frenkel EP. Gaucher disease: a heterogeneous clinical complex for which effective enzyme replacement has come of age. *Am J Med Sci* 1993;305:331–344.

Goldblatt J, Beighton P. Cutaneous manifestations of Gaucher disease. *Br J Dermatol* 1984;111:331–334.

Grabowski GA. Gaucher disease. Enzymology, genetics, and treatment. *Adv Hum Genet* 1993;21:377–441.

Filocamo M, Mazzotti R, Stroppiano M, et al. Analysis of the glucocerebrosidase gene and mutation profile in 144 Italian gaucher patients. *Hum Mutat* 2002;20:234–235.

Orvisky E, Park JK, Parker A, et al. The identification of eight novel glucocerebrosidase (GBA) mutations in patients with Gaucher disease. *Hum Mutat* 2002;19:458–459.

Zevin S, Abrahamov A, Hadas-Halpern I, et al. Adult-type Gaucher disease in children: genetics, clinical features and enzyme replacement therapy. *Q J Med* 1993;86:565–573.

Niemann-Pick Disease

Bayever E, August CS, Kamani N, et al. Allogeneic bone marrow transplantation for Niemann-Pick disease (type IA). *Bone Marrow Transplant* 1992;10:85–86.

Crocker AC, Farber S. Niemann-Pick disease: a review of 18 patients. *Medicine* 1958;37:1–95.

Fernandez-Burriel M, Pena L, Ramos JC, et al. The R608del mutation in the acid sphingomyelinase gene (SMPD1) is the most prevalent among patients from Gran Canaria Island with Niemann-Pick disease type B. *Clin Genet* 2003;63:235–236.

Filling-Katz MR, Fink JK, Gorin MB, et al. Ophthalmologic manifestations of type B Niemann-Pick diseases. *Metab Pediatr Syst Ophthalmol* 1992;15:16–20.

Harzer K, Rolfs A, Bauer P, et al. Niemann-Pick disease type A and B are clinically but also enzymatically heterogeneous: pitfall in the laboratory diagnosis of sphingomyelinase deficiency associated with the mutation Q292 K. *Neuropediatrics* 2003;34:301–306.

Jin HK, Schuchman EH. Ex vivo gene therapy using bone marrow-derived cells: combined effects of intracerebral and intravenous transplantation in a mouse model of Niemann-Pick disease. *Mol Ther* 2003;8:876–885.

Kivlin JD, Sanborn GE, Myers GG. The cherry-red spot in Tay-Sachs and other storage diseases. *Ann Neurol* 1985;17:356–360.

Lee CY, Krimbou L, Vincent J, et al. Compound heterozygosity at the sphingomyelin phosphodiesterase-1 (SMPD1) gene is associated with low HDL cholesterol. *Hum Genet* 2003;112:552–562.

Levade T, Salvayre R, Douste-Blazy L. Sphingomyelinases and Niemann-Pick disease. *J Clin Chem Clin Biochem* 1986;24:205–220.

Mardini MK, Gergen P, Akhtar M, et al. Niemann-Pick disease: report of a case with skin involvement. *Am J Dis Child* 1982;136:650–651.

Sikora J, Pavlu-Pereira H, Elleder M, et al. Seven novel acid sphingomyelinase gene mutations in Niemann-Pick type A and B patients. *Ann Hum Genet.* 2003;67:63–70.

Smanik EJ, Tavill AS, Jacobs GH, et al. Orthotopic liver transplantation in two adults with Niemann-Pick and Gaucher's diseases: implications for the treatment of inherited metabolic disease. *Hepatology* 1993;17:42–49.

Vanier MT, Pentchev P, Rodriguez-Lafrasse C, et al. Niemann-Pick disease type C: an update. *J Inherit Metab Dis* 1991;14:580–595.

Victor S, Coulter JB, Besley GT, et al. Niemann-Pick disease: sixteen-year follow-up of allogeneic bone marrow transplantation in a type B variant. *J Inherit Metab Dis* 2003;26:775–785.

Mucopolysaccharidoses

Baker E, Guo XH, Orsborn AM, et al. The Morquio A syndrome (mucopolysaccharidosis IVA) gene maps to 16q24. 3. *Am J Hum Genet* 1993;52:96–98.

Bredenkamp JK, Smith ME, Dudley JP, et al. Otolaryngologic manifestations of the mucopolysaccharidoses. *Ann Otol Rhinol Laryngol* 1992;101:472–478.

Brooks DA. Review: the immunochemical analysis of enzyme from mucopolysaccharidoses patients. *J Inherit Metab Dis* 1993;16:3–15.

Brusselbach S. Extracellular beta-glucuronidase for gene-directed enzyme-prodrug therapy. *Methods Mol Med* 2004;90:303–330.

Dembure PP, Drumbeller JE, Barr SM, et al. Selective urinary screening for mucopolysaccharidoses. *Clin Biochem* 1990;23:91–96.

Demitsu T, Kakurai M, Okubo Y, et al. Skin eruption as the presenting sign of Hunter syndrome IIB. *Clin Exp Dermatol* 1999;24:179–182.

Diaz JH, Belani KG. Perioperative management of children with mucopolysaccharidoses. *Anesth Analg* 1993;77:1261–1270.

Di Natale P, Annella T, Daniele A, et al. Biochemical diagnosis of mucopolysaccharidoses: experience of 297 diagnoses ina 15-year period (1977–1991). *J Inherit Metab Disease* 1993;16:473–483.

Finlayson LA. Hunter syndrome (mucopolysaccharidosis II). *Pediatr Dermatol* 1990;7:150–152.

Gabriella O, Polonara G, Regnicolo L, et al. Correlation between cerebral MRI abnormalities and mental retardation in patients with mucopolysaccharidoses. *Am J Med Genet* 2004;125A:224–231.

Gerich JE. Hunter's syndrome: beta-galactosidase deficiency in skin. *N Engl J Med* 1969;280:799–802.

Greaves MW, Inman PM. Cutaneous changes in the Morquio syndrome. *Br J Dermatol* 1969;81:2–36.

Hopwood JJ, Morris CP. The mucopolysaccharidoses. Diagnosis, molecular genetics and treatment. *Mol Biol Med* 1990;7:381–404.

Jin WD, Jackson CE, Desnick RJ. Mucopolysaccharidosis type VI: identification of three mutations in the arylsulfatase B gene of patients with the severe and mild phenotypes provides molecular evidence for genetic heterogeneity. *Am J Hum Genet* 1992;50:795–800.

Kakkis ED, Mucnzer J, Tiller GE, et al. Enzyme-replacement therapy in mucopolysaccharidosis I. *N Engl J Med* 2001;344:182–188.

Karageorgos L, Harmatz P, Simon J, et al. Mutational analysis of mucopolysaccharidosis type VI patients undergoing a trial of enzyme replacement therapy. *Hum Mutat* 2004;23:229–233.

Krivit W, Pierpont ME, Ayaz K, et al. Bone-marrow transplantation in the Maroteaux-Lamy syndrome (mucopolysaccharidosis type VI): biochemical and clinical status 24 months after transplantation. *N Eng J Med* 1984;311:1606–1611.

Lee C, Dineen TE, Brack M, et al. The mucopolysaccharidoses: characterization by cranial MR imaging. *Am J Neuroradiol* 1993;14:1285–1292.

McDowell GA, Cown TM, Blitzer MG, et al. Intrafamilial variability in Hurler syndrome and Sanfilippo syndrome type A: implications for evaluation of new therapies. *Am J Med Genet* 1993;47:1092–1095.

McKusick VA. Relative frequency of the Hunter and Hurler syndromes. *N Eng J Med* 1970;283:853–854.

Nelson J. Incidence of the mucopolysaccharidoses in Northern Ireland. *Hum Genet* 1997;101:355–358.

Nelson J, Shields MD, Mulholland HC. Cardiovascular studies in the mucopolysaccharidoses. *J Med Genet* 1990;27:94–100.

Schroder W, Petruschka L, Wehnert M, et al. Carrier detection of Hunter syndrome (MPS II) by biochemical and DNA techniques in families at risk. *J Med Genet* 1993;30:210–213.

Scott HS, Guo XH, Hopwood JJ, et al. Structure and sequence of the human alpha-L-iduronidase gene. *Genomics* 1992;13:1311–1313.

Steen-Bondeson ML, Dahl N, Tonnesen T, et al. Molecular analysis of patients with Hunter syndrome: implication of a region prone to structural alterations within the IDS gene. *Hum Mol Genet* 1992;1:195–198.

Tan CTT, Schaff HV, Miller FA Jr, et al. Valvular heart disease in four patients with Maroteaux-Lamy syndrome. *Circulation* 1992;85:188–195.

Thappa DM, Singh A, Jaisankar TJ, et al. Pebbling of the skin: a marker of Hunter's syndrome. *Pediatr Dermatol* 1998;15:370–373.

Shinhar SY, Zablocki H, Madgy DN. Airway management in mucopolysaccharide storage disorders. *Arch Otolaryngol Head Neck Surg* 2004;130:233–237.

Weisstein JS, Delgado E, Steinbach LS, et al. Musculoskeletal manifestations of Hurler syndrome: long-term follow-up after bone marrow transplantation. *J Pediatr Orthop* 2004;24:97–101.

Yogalingam G, Hopwood JJ. Molecular genetics of mucopolysaccharidosis type IIIA and IIIB: diagnostic, clinical, and biological implications. *Hum Mutat* 2001;18:264–281.

Zlotogora J, Schaap T, Zeigler M, et al. Hunter syndrome in Jews in Israel: further evidence for prenatal selection favoring the Hunter allele. *Hum Genet* 1991;86:531–533.

Multiple Carboxylase Deficiency

Burri BJ, Sweetman L, Nyhan WL. Heterogeneity of holocarboxylase synthetase in patients with biotin-responsive multiple carboxylase deficiency. *Am J Hum Genet* 1985;37:326–337.

Forman DT, Bankson DD, Highsmith WE Jr. Neonatal screening for biotinidase deficiency. *Ann Clin Lab Sci* 1992;22:144–154.

Fuchshuber A, Suormala T, Roth B, et al. Holocarboxylase synthetase deficiency: early diagnosis and management of a new case. *Eur J Pediatr* 1993;152:446–449.

Levy HL. Nutritional therapy for selected inborn errors of metabolism. *J Am Coll Nutr* 1989;8:54S–60S.

Navarro PC, Guerra A, Alvarez JG. Cutaneous and neurologic manifestations of biotinidase deficiency. *Int J Dermatol* 2000;39:363–365.

Norrgard KJ, Pomponio RJ, Hymes J, et al. Mutations causing profound biotinidase deficiency in children ascertained by newborn screening in the United States occur at different frequencies than in symptomatic children. *Pediatr Res* 1999;46:20–27.

Nyhan WL. Multiple carboxylase deficiency. *Int J Biochem* 1988;20:363–370.

Roth KS. Prenatal treatment of multiple carboxylase deficiency. *Ann NY Acad Sci* 1985;447:263–271.

Solorzano-Vargas RS, Pacheco-Alvarez D, Leon-Del-Rio A. Holocarboxylase synthetase is an obligate participant in biotin-mediated regulation of its own expression and of biotin-dependent carboxylases mRNA levels in human cells. *Proc Natl Acad Sci USA* 2002;99:5325–5330.

Thuy LP, Jurecki E, Nemzer L, et al. Prenatal diagnosis of holocarboxylase synthetase deficiency by assay of the enzyme in chorionic villus material followed by prenatal treatment. *Clin Chim Acta* 1999;284:59–68.

Williams ML. Biotin-responsive multiple carboxylase deficiency and immunodeficiency. *Curr Probl Dermatol* 1989;18:89–92.

Wolf B. Biotinidase deficiency: new directions and practical concerns. *Curr Treat Options Neurol* 2003;5:321–328.

Wolf B. Disorders of biotin metabolism. In: Scriver CR, Beaudet AL, Sly WS, Valle D, eds. *The Metabolic and Molecular Basis of Inherited Disease.* 8th ed. New York: McGraw-Hill, 2001:3935.

Wolf B, Feldman GL. The biotin-dependent carboxylase deficiencies. *Am J Hum Genet* 1982;34:699–716.

Wolf B, Grier RE, Parker WD, et al. Deficient biotinidase activity in late-onset multiple carboxylase deficiency. *N Engl J Med* 1983;308:161.

Wolf B, Heard GS, Jefferson LG, et al. Clinical findings in four children with biotinidase deficiency detected through a statewide neonatal screening program. *N Engl J Med* 1985;313:16–19.

Wolf B, Heard GS, Weissbecker KA, et al. Biotinidase deficiency: initial clinical features and rapid diagnosis. *Ann Neurol* 1985;18:614–617.

Wolf B, Jensen K, Huner G, et al. Seventeen novel mutations that cause profound biotinidase deficiency. *Mol Genet Metab* 2002;77:108–111.

Yang X, Aoki Y, Li X, et al. Structure of human holocarboxylase synthetase gene and mutation spectrum of holocarboxylase synthetase deficiency. *Hum Genet* 2001;109:526–534.

Phenylketonuria

Abadie V, Berthelot J, Feillet F, et al. Neonatal screening and long-term follow-up of phenylketonuria: the French database. *Early Hum Dev* 2002;65:149–158.

Aulehla-Scholz C, Heilbronner H. Mutational spectrum in German patients with phenylalanine hydroxylase deficiency. *Hum Mutat* 2003;21:399–400.

Coskun T, Ozalp I, Kale G, et al. Scleroderma-like skin lesions in two patients with phenylketonuria. *Eur J Pediatr* 1990;150:109–110.

Dashman T, Sansaricq C. Nutrition in the management of inborn errors of metabolism. *Clin Lab Med* 1993;13:407–432.

Ding Z, Harding CO, Thony B. State-of-the-art 2003 on PKU gene therapy. *Mol Genet Metab* 2004;81:3–8.

Eisensmith RC, Woo SI. Molecular basis of phenylketonuria and related hyperphenylalaninemias: mutations and polymorphisms in the human phenylalanine hydroxylase gene. *Hum Mutat* 1992;1:13–23.

Erlandsen H, Patch MG, Gamez A, et al. Structural studies on phenylalanine hydroxylase and implications toward understanding and treating phenylketonuria. *Pediatrics* 2003;112:1557–1565.

Farishian P, Shittaker J. Phenylalanine lowers melanin synthesis in mammalian melanocytes by reducing tyrosine uptake: implications for pigment reduction in phenylketonuria. *J Invest Dermatol* 1980;74:85–89.

Fisch RO, Tsai MY, Gentry WC Jr. Studies of phenylketonurics with dermatitis. *J Am Acad Dermatol* 1981;4:284–290.

Gamez A, Wang L, Straub M, et al. Toward PKU enzyme replacement therapy: PEGylation with activity retention for three forms of recombinant phenylalanine hydroxylase. *Mol Ther* 2004;9:124–129.

Holtzman NA, Kronmal RA, van Doornick W, et al. Effect of age at loss of dietary control on intellectual performance and behavior of children with phenylketonuria. *N Eng J Med* 1986;314:593–598.

Irons M. Screening for metabolic disorders. How are we doing? *Pediatr Clin North Am* 1993;40:1073–1085.

Lenke RR, Levy HL. Maternal phenylketonuria and hyperphenylalaninemia: an international survey of the outcome of untreated and treated pregnancies. *N Engl J Med* 1980;303:1202–1208.

Lundstedt G, Johansson A, Melin L, et al. Adjustment and intelligence among children with phenylketonuria in Sweden. *Acta Pediatr* 2001;90:1147–1152.

Mocbizuki S, Mizukami H, Ogura T, et al. Long-term correction of hyperphenylalaninemia by AAV-mediated gene transfer leads to behavioral recovery in phenylketonuria mice. *Gene Ther* 2004;11:1081–1086.

Nagasaki Y, Matsubara Y, Takano H, et al. Reversal of hypopigmentation in phenylketonuria mice by adenovirus-mediated gene transfer. *Pediatr Res* 1999;45:465–473.

National Institutes of Health Consensus Development Panel. National Institutes of Health Consensus Conference Statement: phenylketonuria: screening and management. *Pediatrics* 2001;108:972–982.

Nova MP, Kaufman M, Halperin A. Scleroderma-like skin indurations in a child with phenylketonuria: a clinicopathologic correlation and review of the literature. *J Am Acad Dermatol* 1992;26:329–333.

Scriver CR, Kaufman S. Hyperphenylalaninemia phenylalanine hydroxylase deficiency. In: Scriver CR, Beaudet A, Sly W, Valle D, eds. *The Metabolic and Molecular Bases of Inherited Disease.* 8th ed. New York: McGraw-Hill, 2001:1667

Verlinsky Y, Rechitsky S, Verlinsky O, et al. Preimplantation testing for phenylketonuria. *Fertil Steril* 2001;76:346–349.

Weglage J, Wiedermann D, Denecke J, et al. Individual blood-brain barrier phenylalanine transport determines clinical outcome in phenylketonuria. *Ann Neurol* 2001;50:463–467.

Wilson's Disease

Bearn AG, McKusick VA. Azure lunulae: an unusual change in the fingernails in two patients with hepatolenticular degeneration (Wilson's disease). *JAMA* 1958;166:904–906.

Bull PC, Thomas GR, Rommens JM, et al. The Wilson disease gene is a putative copper transporting P-type ATPase similar to the Menkes gene. *Nat Genet* 1993;5:327–337.

Cossu P, Pirastu M, Nucaro A, et al. Prenatal diagnosis of Wilson's disease by analysis of DNA polymorphism. *N Engl J Med* 1992;327:57.

Cullen LM, Prat L, Cox DW. Genetic variation in the promoter and 5' UTR of the copper transporter, ATP7B, in patients with Wilson disease. *Clin Genet* 2003;64:429–432.

Culotta VC, Gitlin JD. Disorders of copper transport. In: Scriver CR, Beaudet A, Sly W, Valle D, eds. *The Metabolic and Molecular Basis of Inherited Disease*. 8th ed. New York: McGraw Hill, 2001:3105–3118.

Deguti MM, Genschel J, Cancado EL, et al. Wilson disease: novel mutations in the ATP7B gene and clinical correlation in Brazilian patients. *Hum Mutat* 2004;23:398.

Dening TR. The neuropsychiatry of Wilson's disease: a review. *Int Psychiatry Med* 1991;21:135–148.

Lutsenko S, Efremov RG, Tsivkovskii R, et al. Human copper-transporting ATPase ATP7B (the Wilson's disease protein): biochemical properties and regulation. *J Bioenerg Biomembr* 2002;34:351–362.

Menkes JH. Menkes disease and Wilson disease: two sides of the same copper coin. Part II: Wilson disease. *Eur J Paediatr Neurol* 1999;3:245–253.

Petrukhin K, Fischer SG, Pirastu M, et al. Mapping, cloning and genetic characterization of the region containing the Wilson disease gene. *Nat Genet* 1993;5:338–343.

Polio J, Enriquez RE, Chow A, et al. Hepatocellular carcinoma in Wilson's disease. Case report and review of the literature. *J Clin Gastroeneterol* 1989;11:220–224.

Schafer DF, Shaw BW Jr. Fulminant hepatic failure and orthotopic liver transplantation. *Semin Liver Dis* 1989;9:189–194.

Suzuki M, Gitlin JD. Intracellular localization of the Menkes and Wilson's disease proteins and their role in intracellular copper transport. *Pediatr Int* 1999;41:436–442.

Acrodermatitis Enteropathica

Ford D. Intestinal and placental zinc transport pathways. *Proc Nutr Soc* 2004;63:21–29.

Fraker PJ, King LE, Laakko T, et al. The dynamic link between the integrity of the immune system and zinc status. *J Nutr* 2000;130:1399–1406.

Goskowicz M, Eichenfield LF. Cutaneous findings of nutritional deficiencies in children. *Curr Opin Pediatr* 1993;5:441–445.

Gunshin H, Mackenzie B, Berger UV, et al. Cloning and characterization of a mammalian proton-coupled metal-ion transporter. *Nature* 1997;388:482–488.

Kenny F, Sriram K, Hammond JB. Clinical zinc deficiency during adequate enteral nutrition. *J Am Coll Nutr* 1989;8:83–85.

Kury S, Dreno B, Bezieau S, et al. Identification of SLC39A4, a gene involved acrodermatitis enteropathica. *Nat Genet* 2002;31:239–240.

Kury S, Kharfi M, Kamonn R, et al. Mutation spectrum of human SLC39A4 in a panel of patients with acrodermatitis enteropathica. *Hum Mutat* 2003;22:337–338.

Lee MG, Hong KT, Kim JJ. Transient symptomatic zinc deficiency in a full-term breast-fed infant. *J Am Acad Dermatol* 1990;23:375–379.

McMahon RJ, Cousins RJ. Mammalian zinc transporters. *J Nutr* 1998;128:667–670.

Neldner KH, Hambidge KM. Zinc therapy of acrodermatitis enteropathica. *N Engl J Med* 1975;292:879–882.

Perafan-Rivero C, Franca LF, Alves AC, et al. Acrodermatitis enteropathica: case report and review of the literature. *Pediatr Dermatol* 2002;19:426–431.

Prasad AS. Clinical, endocrinological and biochemical effects of zinc deficiency. *Clin Endocrinol Metab* 1985;14:567–589.

Sehgal VN, Jain S. Acrodermatitis enteropathica. *Clin Dermatol* 2000;18:745–748.

Stevens J, Lubitz C. Symptomatic zinc deficiency in infants. *J Paediatr Child Health* 1998;34:97–100.

Van Wouwe JP. Clinical and laboratory diagnosis of acrodermatitis enteropathica. *Eur J Pediatr* 1989;149:2–8.

Wang K, Pugh EW, Griffen S, et al. Homozygosity mapping places the acrodermatitis entero-pathica gene on chromosomal region 8q24.3. *Am J Hum Genet* 2001;68:1055–1060.

Wang K, Zhou B, Kuo YM, et al. A novel member of a zinc transporter family is defective in acrodermatitis enteropathical. *Am J Hum Genet* 2002;71:66–73.

Wang F, Kim BE, Dufner-Beattie J, et al. Acrodermatitis enteropathica mutations affect transport activity, localization and zinc-responsive trafficking of the mouse ZIP4 zinc transporter. *Hum Mol Genet* 2004;13:563–571.

Hemochromatosis

Andersen RV, Tybjaerg-Hansen A, Appleyard M, et al. Hemochromatosis mutations in the general population: iron overload progression rate. *Blood* 2004;103:2914–2919.

Bento MC, Ribeiro ML, Relvas L. Gene symbol: HFE. Disease: haemochromatosis. *Hum Genet* 2004;114:405.

Chevrant-Breton J, Simon M, Bourel M, et al. Cutaneous manifestations of idiopathic hemochromatosis. *Arch Dermatol* 1977;113:161–165.

Deugnier YM, Guyader D, Crantock L, et al. Primary liver cancer in genetic hemochromatosis: a clinical, pathological, and pathogenetic study of 54 cases. *Gastroeneterology* 1993;104:228–234.

Edwards CQ, Griffen LM, Dadone MM, et al. Mapping the locus for hereditary hemochromatosis: localization between HLA-B and HLA-A. *Am J Hum Genet* 1986;805–811.

Edwards CQ, Griffen LM, Godlgar D, et al. Prevalence of hemochromatosis among 11,065 presumably healthy blood donors. *N Engl J Med* 1988;318:1355–1362.

Edwards CQ, Kushner JP. Screening for hemochromatosis. *N Engl J Med* 1993;328:1616–1620.

Flexner JM. Hemochromatosis: diagnosis and treatment. *Compr Ther* 1991;17:7–9.

Gasparini P, Camaschella C. Hereditary hemochromatosis: is the gene race over? *Eur J Hum Genet* 2004;12:341–342.

Holland HK, Spivak JL. Hemochromatosis. *Med Clin North Am* 1989;73:831–845.

Haynes H, Farroni J. Successful combined heart-liver transplantation in a patient with hemochromatosis. *Prog Transplant* 2004;14:39–40.

Nisselle A, Delatycki M, Collins V, et al. Implementation of HaemScreen, a workplace-based genetic screening program for hemochromatosis. *Clin Genet* 2004;65:358–367.

Powell LW. Does transplantation of the liver cure genetic hemochromatosis? *J Hepatol* 1992;16:259–261.

Schumacher HR, Straka PC, Krikker MA, et al. The arthropathy of hemochromatosis. Recent studies. *Ann NY Acad Sci* 1988;526:224–233.

Senden IP, De Groot CJ, Steegers EA, et al. Preeclampsia and the C282Y Mutation in the Hemochromatosis (FIFE) Gene. *Clin Chem* 2004;50:973–974.

Homocystinuria

Abbott MH, Foistein SE, Abbey H, et al. Psychiatric manifestations of homocystinuria due to cystathionine beta-synthase deficiency: prevalence, natural history, and relationship to neurologic impairment and vitamin B(6)-responsiveness. *Am J Med Genet* 1987;26:959–969.

Ambrosi P. Homocysteine and post-angioplasty restenosis. *Nutr Metab Cardiovasc Dis* 2003;13:391–397.

Boers GH, Fowler B, Smals AG, et al. improved identification of heterozygotes for homocystinuria due to cystathionine synthetase deficiency by the combination of methionine loading and enzyme determination in cultured fibroblasts. *Hum Genet* 1985;69:164–169.

Carey MC, Donovan DE, FitzGerald O, et al. Homocystinuria: a clinical and pathological study of nine subjects in six families. *Am J Med* 1968;45:7–25.

Clarke R, Daly L, Robinson K, et al. Hyperhomocysteinemia: an independent risk factor for vascular disease. *N Engl J Med* 1991;324:1149–1155.

Kraus JP. Molecular basis of phenotype expression in homocystinuria. *J Inherit Metab Dis* 1994;17:383.

Lieberman ER, Gomperts ED, Shaw KN, et al. Homocystinuria: clinical and pathologic review, with emphasis on thrombotic features, including pulmonary artery thrombosis. *Perspect Pediatr Pathol* 1993:17:125–147.

Miles EW, Kraus JP. Cystathionine β-synthase: structure, function, regulation and location of homocystinuria-causing mutations. *J Biol Chem* 2004;279:29871–29874.

Moat SJ, Bao L, Fowler B, et al. The molecular basis of cystathionine beta-synthase (CBS) deficiency in UK and US patients with homocystinuria. *Hum Mutat* 2004;23:206.

Munke M, Kraus JP, Ohura T, et al. The gene for cystathionine beta-synthase (CBS) maps to the subtelomeric region on human chromosome 2lq and to proximal mouse chromosome 17. *Am J Hunt Genet* 1988;42:550–559.

Orendac M, Zeman J, Stabler SP, et al. Homocystinuria due to cystathionine beta-synthase deficiency: novel biochemical findings and treatment efficacy. *J Inherit Metab Dis* 2003;26:761–773.

Sokolova J, Janosikova B, Terwilliger JD. Cystathionine beta-synthase deficiency in Central Europe: discrepancy between biochemical and molecular genetic screening for homocystinuric alleles. *Hum Mutat* 2001;18:548–549.

Yap S, Rushe H, Howard PM, et al. The intellectual abilities of early-treated individuals with pyridoxine-nonresponsive homocystinuria due to cystathione beta-synthase deficiency. *J Inherit Metab Dis* 2001;24:437–447.

Hyperlipoproteinemias

Agheli N, Cloarec M, Jacotot B. Effect of dietary treatment on the lipid, lipoprotein and fatty acid compositions in type IV familial hypertriglyceridemia. *Ann Nutr Metab* 1991;35:261–273.

Auwerx J, Leroy P, Schoonjans K. Lipoprotein lipase: recent contributions from molecular biology. *Crit Rev Clin Lab Sci* 1992;29:243–268.

Black DM, Sprecher DL. Dietary treatment and growth of hyperchylomicronemic children severely restricted in dietary fat. *Am J Dis Child* 1993;147:60–62.

Boerwinkle E, Utermann G. Simultaneous effects of the apolipoprotein E polymorphism on apolipoprotein E, apolipoprotein B, and cholesterol metabolism. *Am J Hum Genet* 1988;42:104–112.

Borgaonkar DS, Schmidt LC, Martin SE, et al. Linkage of late-onset Alzheimer's disease with apolipoprotein E type 4 on chromosome 19. *Lancet* 1993;342:625.

Boulton J, Henry R, Roddick LG, et al. Survival after neonatal myocardial infarction. *Pediatrics* 1991;88:145–150.

Brunzell JD, Deeb SS. Familial lipoprotein lipase deficiency, Apo C-II deficiency, and hepatic lipase deficiency. In: Scriver CR, Beaudet A, Sly W, Valle D, eds. *The Metabolic and Molecular Basis of Inherited Disease.* 8th ed. New York: McGraw Hill, 2001:2789.

Connor WE, Connor SL. Importance of diet in the treatment of familial hypercholesterolemia. *Am J Cardiol* 1993;72:42D–53D.

Cortner JA, Coates PM, Gallagher PR. Prevalence and expression of familial combined hyperlipidemia in childhood. *J Pediatr* 1990;116:514–519.

Cruz PD, East C, Bergstresser PR. Dermal, subcutaneous, and tendon xanthomas: diagnostic markers for specific lipoprotein disorders. *J Am Acad Dermatol* 1988;19:95–111.

Cuthbert JA, East CA, Bilheimer DW, et al. Detection of familial hypercholesterolemia by assaying functional low-density-lipoprotein receptors on lymphocytes. *N Engl J Med* 1986;314:879–883.

de Jongh S, Kerckhoffs MC, Grootenhuis MA, et al. Quality of life, anxiety and concerns among statin-treated children with familial hypercholesterolaemia and their parents. *Acta Paediatr* 2003;92:1096–1101.

Eichenbaum-Voline S, Olivier M, Jones EL, et al. Linkage and association between distinct variants of the APOA1/C3/A4/A5 gene cluster and familial combined hyperlipidemia. *Arterioscler Thromb Vase Biol* 2004;24:167–174.

Eichner JE, Dunn ST, Perveen G, et al. Apolipoprotein E polymorphism and cardiovascular disease: a HuGE review. *Am J Epidemiol* 2002;155:487–495.

Feussner G, Wagner A, Kohl B, et al. Clinical features of type III hyperlipoproteinemia: analysis of 64 patients. *Clin Invest* 1993;71:362–366.

Fojo SS, Brewer HB. Hypertriglyceridaemia due to genetic defects in lipoprotein lipase and apolipoprotein C-II. *J Intern Med* 1992;231:669–677.

Goldstein JL, et al. Familial hypercholesterolemia. In: Scriver CR, Beaudet A, Sly W, Valle D, eds. *The Metabolic and Molecular Basis of Inherited Disease.* 8th ed. New York: McGraw Hill, 2001:2863

Heaney AP, Sharer N, Ramch B, et al. Prevention of recurrent pancreatitis in familial lipoprotein lipase deficiency with high-dose antioxidant therapy. *J Clin Endocrinol Metab* 1999;84:1203–1205.

Hobbs HH, Brown MS, Goldstein JL. Molecular genetics of the LDL receptor gene in familial hypercholesterolemia. *Hum Mutat* 1992;1:445–466.

Illingworth DR. How effective is drug therapy in heterozygous familial hypercholesterolemia? *Am J Cardiol* 1993;72:54D–58D.

Kroger K. Dyslipoproteinemia and peripheral arterial occlusive disease. *Angiology* 2004;55:135–138.

Kypreos KE, Li X, van Dijk KW, et al. Molecular mechanisms of type III hyperlipoproteinemia: The contribution of the carboxy-terminal domain of ApoE can account for the dyslipidemia that is associated with the E2/E2 phenotype. *Biochemistry* 2003;42:9841–9853.

Lenaerts J, Verresen L, Van Steenbergen W, et al. Fatty liver hepatitis and type 5 hyperlipoproteinemia in juvenile diabetes mellitus. Case report and review of the literature. *J Clin Gastroenterol* 1990;12:93–97.

Liao JK. Isoprenoids as mediators of the biological effects of statins. *J Clin Invest* 2002;110:285.

Lloyd JK. Cholesterol: should we screen all children or change the diet of all children? *Acta Paediatr Scand Suppl* 1991;373:66–72.

Ma Y, Henderson HE, Ven Murthy MR, et al. A mutation in the human lipoprotein lipase gene as the most common cause of familial chylomicronemia in French-Canadians. *N Engl J Med* 1991;324:1761–1766.

Mahley RW, Huang Y, Rail SC Jr. Pathogenesis of type III hyperlipoproteinemia (dysbetalipoproteinemia): questions, quandaries, and paradoxes. *J Lipid Res* 1999;40:1933–1949.

Mahley RW, Rail SC Jr. Type III hyperlipoprotein (dysbetalipoproteinemia): the role of apolipoprotein E in normal and abnormal lipoprotein metabolism. In: Scriver CR, Beaudet A, Sly W, Valle D, eds. *The Metabolic and Molecular Basis of Inherited Disease.* 8th ed. New York: McGraw Hill, 2001:2835.

Marcoval J, Moreno A, Bordas X, et al. Diffuse plane xanthoma: clinicopathologic study of 8 cases. *J Am Acad Dermatol* 1998;39:439–442.

Milionis HJ, Miltiadous GA, Cariolou M, et al. Pinpoint skin lesions in a familial hypercholesterolaemia homozygote. *Acta Paediatr* 2003;92:1109–1110.

Molgaard J, von Schenck H, Lassvik C, et al. Effect of fish oil treatment on plasma lipoproteins in type Ill hyperlipoproteinaemia. *Atherosclerosis* 1990;81:1–9.

Neil HA, Hammond T, Mant D, et al. Effect of statin treatment for familial hypercholesterolaemia on life assurance: results of consecutive surveys in 1990 and 2002. *Br Med J* 2004;328:500–501.

Neil HA, Huxley RR, Hawkins MM, et al. Comparison of the risk of fatal coronary heart disease in treated xanthomatous and nonxanthomatous heterozygous familial hypercholesterolaemia: a prospective registry study. *Atherosclerosis* 2003;170:73–78.

Pandhi D, Grover C, Reddy BSN. Type ha hyperlipoproteinemia manifesting with different types of cutaneous xanthomas. *Ind Pediatr* 2001;38:550–553.

Popescu I, Simionescu M, Tulbure D, et al. Homozygous familial hypercholesterolemia: specific indication for domino liver transplantation. *Transplantation* 2003;76:1345–1350.

Quaid KA. Psychological and ethical considerations in screening for disease. *Am J Cardiol* 1993;72:64D–67D.

Saito M, Tada Y, Harada-Shiba M, et al. Homozygous familial

hypercholesterolaemia: development of xanthogranuloma in a boy at puberty under long-term low-density lipoprotein apheresis and drug therapy. *Br J Dermatol* 2003;149:1302–1303.

Schuster H. Risk assessment and strategies to achieve lipid goals: lessons from real-world clinical practice. *Am J Med* 2004;116:26S–30S.

Soutar AK, Naoumova RP, Traub LM. Genetics, clinical phenotype, and molecular cell biology of autosomal recessive hypercholesterolemia. *Arterioscler Thromb Vasc Biol* 2003;23:1963–1970.

Sposito AC, Gonbert S, Bruckert E, et al. Magnitude of HDL cholesterol variation after high-dose atorvastatin is genetically determined at the LDL receptor locus in patients with homozygous familial hypercholesterolemia. *Arterioscler Thromb Vasc Biol* 2003;23:2078–2082.

Stein EA, Strutt K, Southworth H, et al. Comparison of rosuvastatin versus atorvastatin in patients with heterozygous familial hypercholesterolemia. *Am J Cardiol* 2003;92:1287–1293.

Tonstad S. Children and statins. *Acta Paediatr* 2003;92:1001–1002.

Vohnout B, Raslova K, Gasparovic J, et al. Lipid levels and their genetic regulation in patients with familial hypercholesterolemia and familial defective apolipoprotein B-100: the MEDPED Slovakia Project. *Atheroscler Suppl* 2003;4:3–5.

Zhao SP, Smelt AH, Leuven JA, et al. Changes of lipoprotein profile in familial dysbetalipoproteinemia with gemfibrozil. *Am J Med* 1994;96:49–56.

Chapter 12

Disorders with Chromosome Abnormalities

Kurt Hirschhorn, M.D. (KH) and Judith Willner, M.D. (JW)

Clinical
Pearls

Down Syndrome

Synonym	Trisomy 21 syndrome
Inheritance	Approximately 2% of cases secondary to an inherited translocation; otherwise not inherited
Prenatal Diagnosis	Amniocentesis/chorionic villus sampling (CVS): chromosome analysis reveals trisomy 21 Ultrasound: (second/third trimester)—constellation of abnormalities may suggest the diagnosis: hydrops fetalis, cystic hygroma, cardiac defects, nuchal edema, prune belly anomaly, duodenal obstruction Increased risk with low levels of alpha-fetoprotein in maternal serum—not specific or diagnostic for Down's syndrome
Incidence	Approximately 1:700, 45% of the affected with mothers >35 years old worldwide; 1:1,100, 20% of the affected with mothers >35 years old in the United States; approximately 1% recurrence risk for parents with affected trisomy 21 child because of nondisjunction; approximately 50% spontaneously abort in second trimester; M=F
Age at Presentation	Birth
Pathogenesis	Approximately 95% of cases secondary to nondisjunction at chromosome 21 during meiosis in one of the parents (maternally derived in 95%) resulting in trisomy 21; approximately 4% to 5% are secondary to a translocation (inherited and *de novo*); the remaining 1% to 2% are mosaics, occuring as a postzygotic event
Key Features	**Skin** Single palmar crease, flat nipples, increased nuchal skin folds in infancy, syringomas, elastosis perforans serpiginosa; xerosis and lichenification with age; increased infections **Hair** Alopecia areata **Craniofacial** Brachycephaly, flat face, flat nasal bridge with small nose, flat occiput; short, broad neck; small ears with dysplastic/absent earlobes **Eyes** Epicanthic folds, upslanting palpebral fissures, Brushfield spots, fine lens opacities, strabismus **Mouth** Small mouth with protruding scrotal tongue; fissured, thickened lips; dental anomalies, periodontal disease **Musculoskeletal** Short stature, hypotonia in infancy; small, broad hands with shortened metacarpals and phalanges; clinodactyly of fifth finger, wide gap between first and second toes, odontoid abnormalities, atlantoaxial instability; wide, flat iliac wings with narrow acetabular angle

Central Nervous System
   Mental retardation (IQ 30–50), seizures (10%)
Cardiovascular
   Congenital heart disease (atrioventricular communis and ventricular septal defects most common)
Gastrointestinal
   Duodenal atresia most common; other anomalies
Hematologic
   Acute myelogenous leukemia; transient leukemoid reaction and polycythemia (newborns); immunodeficiency
Endocrine
   Autoimmune hypothyroidism > hyperthyroidism
Genitourinary
   Micropenis, decreased male libido, increased impotency

Differential Diagnosis   None

Laboratory Data
Chromosomal analysis
X-ray pelvis
Thyroid function tests
Complete blood count
Echocardiogram

Management
Thorough physical examination and follow-up with primary care physician
Referral to symptom-specific specialist—cardiac surgeon/cardiologist, general surgeon, hematologist/oncologist, endocrinologist

Prognosis
While many are now living longer into their fifth and sixth decades of life, average life expectancy is still approximately 35 years; increased mortality in infancy secondary to congenital heart disease, neoplasms

Clinical Pearls

Fetal cells have been concentrated in maternal serum and fluorescent *in situ* hybridization has detected cells with 3 copies of 21. . . A more promising approach to noninvasive prenatal screening is first-trimester ultrasound looking for increased nuchal fold with abnormal maternal serum markers. . . Standard screening criteria include 35 and over, family history, previous child with Down's, translocation carrier. . . Many laboratories screen pregnant women who are 30 and over. . . Two clinical pearls I (*KH*) particularly like are the increased skin folds in the back of the neck and the "X" that is seen across the baby's crying face. . . When the baby's face squinches up, the upward slanted palpebral fissures appear to run in a line with the nasal-labial folds creating the "X". . . I (*JW*) look for an absence of breast tissue in a full-term baby. . . They all get an echo before they leave the hospital after birth. . . Congenital heart defects are the most common cause of early death. . . Our heart surgeons are moving in and repairing these kids within the first months of life. . . Later on they die of infection. . . Watch for Hirschsprung disease. . . The poorly formed odontoid process can shear their spine and leave them quadriplegic. . . Stimulation programs work best in Down's. . . Must remind parents to spend time with other children as well. . . Get other children involved in the care and stimulation of the baby. . . For reasons that are unclear, children with Down's love music. . . They calm down. . . They listen to it. . . Current recommendations are to mainstream high-functioning children with Down's as long as possible. . . They'll modify their behavior based on what they see around them. . . The Special Olympics has been great for their self-image. . . *Educating Peter*, a movie about mainstreaming a child with Down's, is beautifully done and should be seen.   *KH, JW*

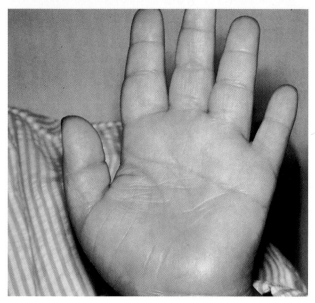

12.1. *Single horizontal palmar crease, single flexion crease on fifth finger, short fingers with broad hand. (1)*

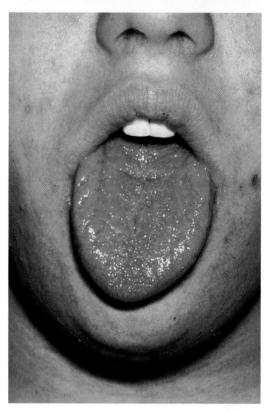

12.2. *Macroglossia with scrotal fissures. (133)*

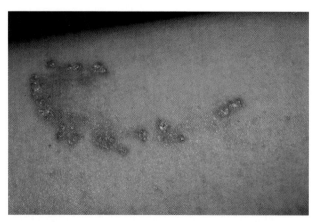

12.3. *Elastosis perforans serpiginosa in a patients with Down syndrome. (133)*

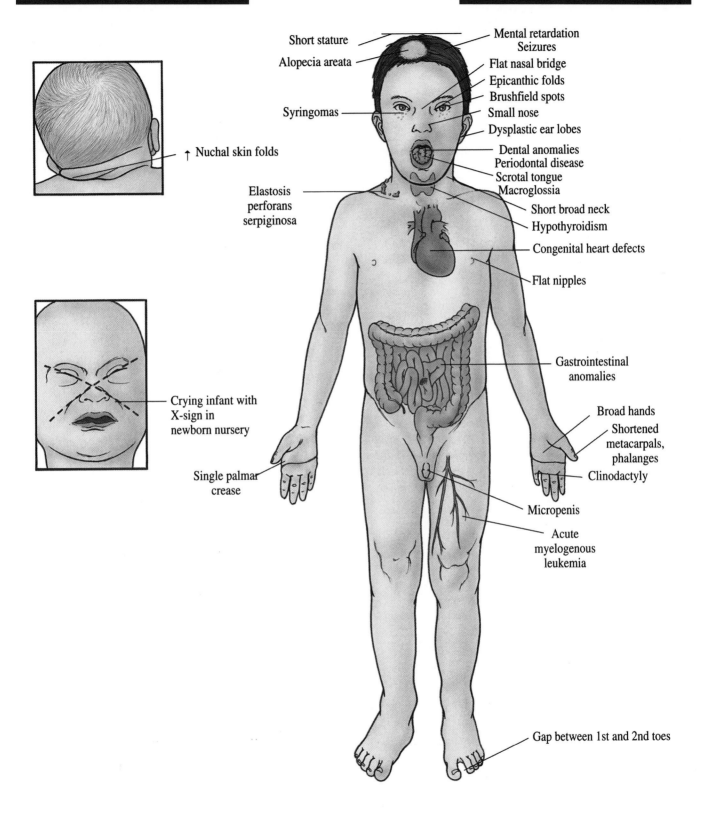

Short stature

Alopecia areata

Syringomas

Nuchal skin folds

Elastosis
perforans
serpiginosa

Crying infant with
X-sign in
newborn nursery

Single palmar
crease

Mental retardation
Seizures

Flat nasal bridge

Epicanthic folds

Brushfield spots

Small nose

Dysplastic ear lobes

Dental anomalies
Periodontal disease
Scrotal tongue
Macroglossia

Short broad neck

Hypothyroidism

Congenital heart defects

Flat nipples

Gastrointestinal
anomalies

Broad hands

Shortened
metacarpals,
phalanges

Clinodactyly

Micropenis

Acute
myelogenous
leukemia

Gap between 1st and 2nd toes

Turner Syndrome

Synonym

Gonadal dysgenesis
XO syndrome
Ullrich-Turner

Inheritance

Not inherited

Prenatal Diagnosis

Amniocentesis/CVS—chromosome analysis reveals XO karyotype
Ultrasound: (second trimester)—constellation of findings suggest diagnosis: cystic hygroma, hydrops fetalis, chylothorax, ascites

Incidence

1:2,500 to 5,000 female births; over 95% spontaneously abort in first trimester

Age at Presentation

Newborn: small for gestational age (SGA) baby with redundant neck skin, peripheral edema
Childhood: short stature, left-sided cardiac/aortic anomalies
Teenager: short stature, delayed puberty with primary amenorrhea

Pathogenesis

Partial or total loss of one X chromosome (XO monosomy) secondary to nondisjunction during gametogenesis in mother or father or a postfertilization mitotic error; 10% to 20% secondary to mosaicism

Key Features

Skin
    Redundant neck folds/webbed neck (remnant of fetal cystic hygroma), multiple pigmented nevi, increased keloid formation
Hair
    Low-set nuchal hairline
Nails
    Hypoplastic, hyperconvex, deep-set
Craniofacial
    Triangular facies with micrognathia, low-set ears, high-arched palate, ptosis
Musculoskeletal
    Short stature, shield chest with wide-set nipples, cubitus valgus, shortened fourth and fifth metacarpals

Lymphatic Vessels
Congenital hypoplasia of lymphatic channels with resultant transient peripheral lymphedema of hands and feet
Endocrine
Primary amenorrhea, gonadal dysgenesis/streak gonads, infertility
Cardiovascular
Multiple anomalies (coarctation of the aorta with secondary hypertension most common)
Kidney
Multiple anomalies (horseshoe kidneys most common)
Central Nervous System
Spatial relations deficit, hearing impairment

Differential Diagnosis

Noonan syndrome (p. 354)
Other short stature syndromes
Milroy disease

Laboratory Data

Chromosome analysis
Echocardiogram
Abdominal ultrasound

Management

Thorough physical examination by primary care physician
Referral to endocrinologist—cyclic estrogen replacement in second decade, growth hormone therapy
Referral to surgeon—repair of coarctation, webbed neck, renal anomalies

Prognosis

Normal life span with treatment of congenital anomalies; may have severe psychosocial impact given short stature, infertility, body habitus

Clinical Pearls

The clue in utero is an SGA fetus with a cystic hygroma on ultrasound. . . Some have picked up the cystic hygroma with a vaginal probe in the first trimester. . . The cardiologist seeing a girl with a coarctation of the aorta must check chromosomes. . . The girl who doesn't grow or stops growing needs to be evaluated for Turner's. . . Also, the girls with primary amenorrhea are worked up. . . Every kid gets an ultrasound of the heart and kidneys. . . Recently, a combination with low-dose estrogen-progesterone and growth hormone cycling in the first decade is being used so that they can develop secondary sexual characteristics and be brought onto the normal growth curve. . . Interestingly, the only thing wrong with their minds is that they have a poor sense of spatial relations. . . They have difficulty in mathematics, geometry. . . Poor sense of direction. . . Orientation is a problem. . . Plastics can tack down the webbed neck. . . Intelligence is perfectly normal. . . They may be high-functioning individuals. . . Although sterile, they can carry to term with donated ovum and hormonal supplementation. . . Must look for presence of 46 XY line (rule out mosaicism) because of risk for gonadal malignancy.   *KH, JW*

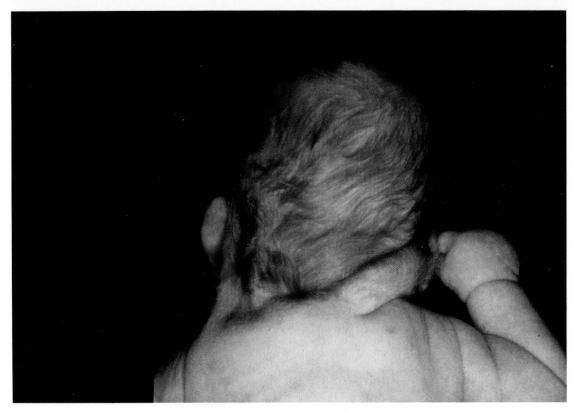

12.4. Redundant neck folds in infant. (48)

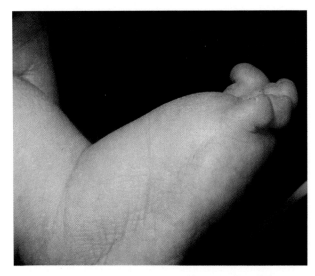

12.5. Transient lymphedema of foot in infant. (48)

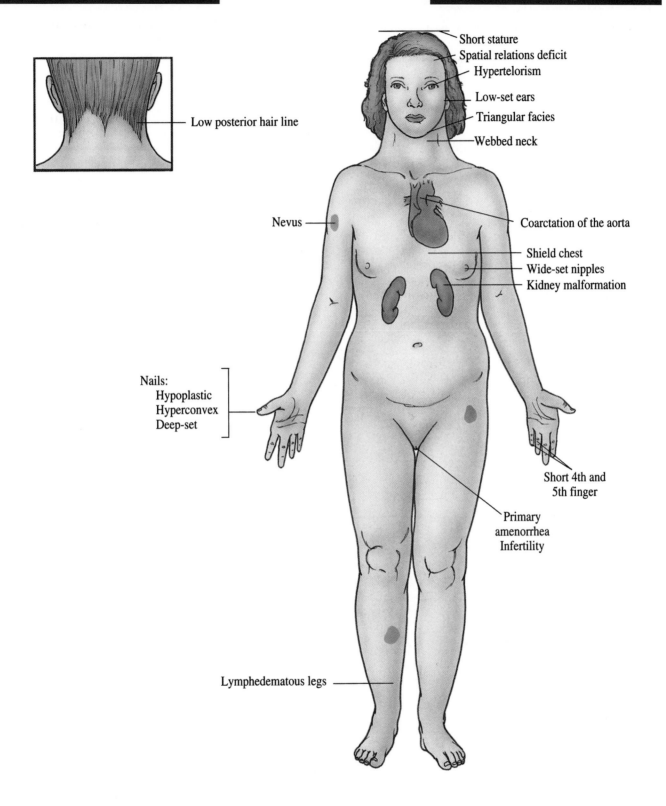

Low posterior hair line

Short stature
Spatial relations deficit
Hypertelorism
Low-set ears
Triangular facies
Webbed neck

Nevus

Coarctation of the aorta

Shield chest
Wide-set nipples
Kidney malformation

Nails:
Hypoplastic
Hyperconvex
Deep-set

Short 4th and
5th finger

Primary
amenorrhea
Infertility

Lymphedematous legs

Noonan Syndrome

Inheritance Autosomal dominant (30% to 75%); *PTPN11* gene on 12q24.1

Prenatal Diagnosis Ultrasound: cystic hygroma, polyhydramnios with normal karyotype
DNA analysis

Incidence Approximately 1:1,000 to 2,500 live births; M=F

Age at Presentation Birth

Pathogenesis A defect in *PTPN11*, a gene encoding the protein tyrosine phosphatase SHP2 and implicated in LEOPARD syndrome, has been linked to approximately 50% of cases; lymphedema thought to play a role in phenotype

Key Features

Skin
Lymphedema of lower extremities, pigmented nevi, café au lait macules
Hair
Coarse, light-colored, curly
Craniofacial
Hypertelorism, low-set ears with thickened helices, micrognathia, webbed neck with low posterior hairline, high-arched palate, ptosis
Musculoskeletal
Short stature, pectus excavatum/carinatum, cubitus valgus
Cardiovascular
Pulmonic valve stenosis (most common), atrial septal defects
Central Nervous System
Mental retardation (mild to severe)
Genitourinary
Cryptorchidism, hypogonadism

Differential Diagnosis Turner syndrome (p. 350)
Neurofibromatosis/Noonan's overlap

Laboratory Data Echocardiogram/electrocardiogram

Management Cardiac surgery
Referral to developmentalist/special school programs
Examine parents for subtle phenotypic changes

Prognosis Normal life span if cardiac defect treated and sequelae prevented

Clinical Pearls

If you look at the parents, you may pick up some of the signs of Noonan's. . . Interestingly, the pulmonic stenosis is thought to be secondary to a myxomatous degeneration of the valve leaflets. . . Possibly related to a congenital lymphatic channel defect. . . The babies need echoes. . . A developmentalist should follow the children and get them into special school programs so that they reach their fullest potential.
KH, JW

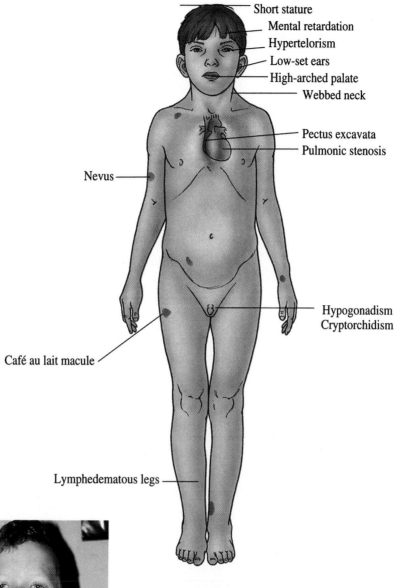

- Short stature
- Mental retardation
- Hypertelorism
- Low-set ears
- High-arched palate
- Webbed neck
- Pectus excavata
- Pulmonic stenosis
- Nevus
- Hypogonadism Cryptorchidism
- Café au lait macule
- Lymphedematous legs

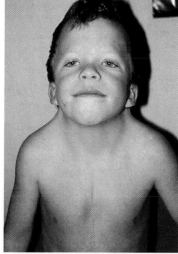

12.6. *Boy with short stature, webbed-neck, ptosis, low-set ears, pectus excavatum, and downward-sloping palpebral fissures. Note sternal scar after repair of atrial septal defect.* (134)

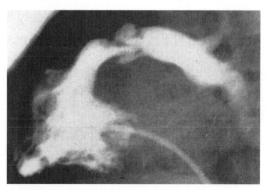

12.7. *Angiography demonstrating pulmonic valve stenosis.* (135)

Klinefelter Syndrome

Inheritance	Not inherited
Prenatal Diagnosis	Amniocentesis (second trimester): chromosome analysis
Incidence	Approximately 1:500 males; increased frequency with advanced maternal age
Age at Presentation	Childhood to puberty
Pathogenesis	Several X-aneuploidy variants (80%–47, XXY) secondary to nondisjunction in maternal or paternal meiosis producing phenotype

Key Features

Skin
Varicose veins, arterial and venous leg ulcers
Hair
Scant body and pubic hair
Musculoskeletal
Tall stature, low upper to lower body ratio with long legs, obesity, gynecomastia
Genitourinary
Small testes with/without small penis, hyalinization and fibrosis of seminiferous tubules, infertility with lack of spermatogenesis
Endocrine
Markedly decreased levels of testosterone
Central Nervous System
Delayed speech as child, dull mentality, antisocial behavioral disturbances

Differential Diagnosis	Homocystinuria (p. 332)
Laboratory Data	Chromosome analysis Decreased serum testosterone level; increased urinary gonadotropins
Management	Referral to endocrinologist—testosterone replacement at puberty Referral to psychologist/psychiatrist—therapy, behavioral modification Referral to vascular surgeon/dermatologist—leg ulcer care
Prognosis	Normal life span with improved secondary sexual characteristics with testosterone; infertile, many lead married lives

Clinical Pearls

If kids with learning difficulties and normal phenotypes had their chromosomes checked, we would pick up XXY's earlier. . . If these kids are picked up early enough and placed in learning disabled classes, perhaps this adult antisocial behavior can be prevented. . . Although generally infertile, rarely they can have kids with testicular aspiration and IVF. . . Like XYYs, they get in trouble with the police because of lower intelligence, poor judgement. . . They get caught. . . They are not aggressive. . . Starting testosterone therapy has made some of my (JW) patients feel uncomfortable because they're not used to the feelings they get. . . They're more labile. . . Prenatal counseling is very difficult if syndrome detected with amniocentesis. . . Parents frequently ask, "Will this child be homosexual?". . . And, of course, the answer is no, no more than anybody else. . . Many are diagnosed when they enter infertility clinics. . . Varicosities should be stripped to prevent stasis complications. . . Gynecomastia can be reduced surgically. . . "Normal" adolescents with excessive gynecomastia should be screened with chromosomes. . . Treat with testosterone as long as they want to maintain secondary sexual characteristics.   KH, JW

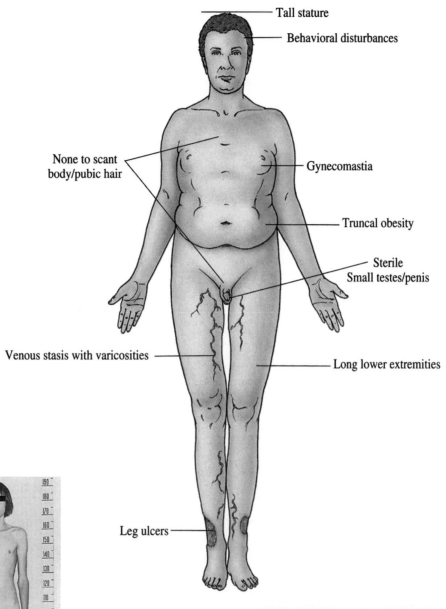

Tall stature

Behavioral disturbances

None to scant body/pubic hair

Gynecomastia

Truncal obesity

Sterile Small testes/penis

Venous stasis with varicosities

Long lower extremities

Leg ulcers

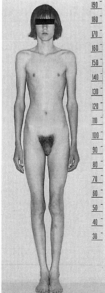

12.8. Eighteen-year-old male with long lower extremities, female distribution of pubic hair, and broad hips . (136)

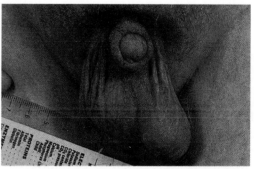

12.9. Micropenis with scant pubic hair in adult. (137)

Suggested Reading

Down Syndrome

Barlow GM, Chen XN, Shi ZY, et al. Down syndrome congenital heart disease: a narrowed region and a candidate gene. *Genet Med* 2001;3:91–101.

Bittles AH, Glasson EJ. Clinical, social, and ethical implications of changing life expectancy in Down syndrome. *Dev Med Child Neurol* 2004;46:282–286.

Burch JM, Weston WL, Rogers M, et al. Cutaneous pustular leukemoid reactions in trisomy 21. *Pediatr Dermatol* 2003;20:232–237.

Carey AB, Park HK, Burker WA. Multiple eruptive syringomas associated with Down's syndrome. *J Am Acad Dermatol* 1988;19:759–760.

Carter DM, Jegosothy BY. Alopecia areata and Down's syndrome. *Arch Dermatol* 1976;112:1397–1399.

Cheon MS, Shim KS, Kim SH, et al. Protein levels of genes encoded on chromosome 21 in fetal Down syndrome brain: challenging the gene dosage effect hypothesis (Part IV). *Amino Acids* 2003;25:41–47.

Cooley WC. Supporting the family of the newborn with Down syndrome. *Compr Ther* 1993;19:111–115.

De Pasquale R, Nasca MR, Musumeci ML, et al. Elastosis perforans serpiginosa in an adult with Down's syndrome: report of case with symmetrical localized involvement. *J Ear Acad Dermatol Venereol* 2002;16:387–389.

Durmowicz AG. Pulmonary edema in 6 children with Down syndrome during travel to moderate altitudes. *Pediatrics* 2001;108:443–447.

Gaulden ME. Maternal age effect: the enigma of Down syndrome and other trisomic conditions. *Mutat Res* 1992;296:69–88.

Goldberg MJ. Spine instability and the special olympics. *Clin Sports Med* 1993;12:507–515.

Harley EH, Collins MD. Neurologic sequelae secondary to atlantoaxial instability in Down syndrome. Implications in otolaryngologic surgery. *Arch Otolaryngol Head Neck Surg* 1994;120:159–165.

Hayes A, Batshaw ML. Down syndrome. *Pediatr Clin North Am* 1993;40:523–535.

Kabili G, Stricker R, Stricker R, et al. First trimester screening for trisomy 21: do the parameters used detect more pathologies than just Down syndrome? *Eur J Obstet Gynecol Reprod Biol* 2004;114:35–38.

Levy J. The gastrointestinal tract in Down syndrome. *Prog Clin Biol Res* 1991;373:245–256.

Lockwood CJ, Lynch L, Berkowitz RL. Ultrasonographic screening for the Down syndrome fetus. *Am J Obstet Gynecol* 1991;165:349–352.

Mathew P, Moodie D, Sterba R, et al. Long-term follow-up of children with Down syndrome with cardiac lesions. *Clin Pediatr* 1991;30:128.

Schepis C, Barone C, Siragusa M, et al. An updated survey on skin conditions in Down syndrome. *Dermatology* 2002;205:234–238.

Schepis C, Siragusa M, Palazzo R, et al. Perforating milia-like idiopathic calcinosis cutis and periorbital syringomas in a girl with Down syndrome. *Pediatr Dermatol* 1994;11:258–260.

Scherbenske JM, Benson PM, Rotchford JP, et al. Cutaneous and ocular manifestations of Down syndrome. *J Am Acad Dermatol* 1990;22:933–938.

Seashore MR. Chromosomal abnormalities in the newborn period. *Semin Perinatol* 1993;17:312–317.

Togawa Y, Nohira G, Shinkai H, et al. Collagenoma in Down syndrome. *Br J Dermatol* 2003;148:596–597.

van Trotsenburg AS, Vulsma T, van Santen HM, et al. Lower neonatal screening thyroxine concentrations in down syndrome newborns. *J Clin Endocrinol Metab* 2003;88:1512–1515.

Wind WM, Schwend RM, Larson J. Sports for the physically challenged child. *J Am Acad Orthop Surg* 2004;12:126–137.

Zipursky A, Peon A, Doyle J. Leukemia in Down syndrome: a review. *Pediatr Hematol Oncol* 1992;9:139–149.

Turner Syndrome

Becker B, Jospe N, Goldsmith LA. Melanocytic nevi in Turner syndrome. *Pediatr Dermatol* 1994;11:120–124.

Bronshtein M, Zimmer EZ, Blazer S. A characteristic cluster of fetal sonographic markers that are predictive of fetal Turner syndrome in early pregnancy. *Am J Obstet Gynecol* 2003;188:1016–1020.

Chipman JJ. Study design for final height determination in Turner syndrome: pros and cons. *Horm Res* 1993;39:18–22.

Edwards MJ, Graham JM Jr. Posterior nuchal cycstic hygroma. *Clin Perinatol* 1990;17:611–640.

Gibbs P, Brady, B, Gonzalez R, et al. Nevi and melanoma: lessons from Turner's Syndrome. *Dermatology* 2001;202:1–3.

Halac I, Zimmerman D. Coordinating care for children with Turner syndrome. *Pediatr Ann* 2004;33:189–196.

Hall JG, Gilchrist DM. Turner syndrome and its variants. *Pediatr Clin North Am* 1990;37:1421–1440.

Jobe S, Donohoue P, Di Paola J. Deep venous thrombosis and Turner syndrome. *J Pediatr Hematol Oncol* 2004;26:272.

Larralde M, Gardner SS, Torrado M, et al. Lymphedema as a postulated cause of cutis verticis gyrata in Turner syndrome. *Pediatr Dermatol* 1998;15:18–22.

Li CC, Chodirker BN, Dawson AJ, et al. Severe hemihypotrophy in a female infant with mosaic Turner syndrome: a variant of Russell-Silver syndrome? *Clin Dysmorphol* 2004;13:95–98.

Lippe B. Turner syndrome. *Endocrinol Metab Clin North Am* 1991;20:121–152.

Marinoni LP, Tangiguchi K, Giraldi S, et al. Cutis verticis gyrata in a child with Turner syndrome. *Pediatr Dermatol* 1999;16:242–243.

Naldi L. Turner's syndrome, melanocytic nevi and melanoma. *Dermatology* 2001;203:275.

Parvin M, Roche E, Costigan C, et al. Treatment outcome in Turner syndrome. *Ir Med J* 2004;97:12, 14–15.

von Kaisenberg CS, Nicolaides KH, Brand-Saberi B. Lymphatic vessel hypoplasia in fetuses with Turner syndrome. *Hum Reprod* 1999;4:823–826.

Wilson DM. Clinical actions of growth hormone. *Endocrinol Metab Clin North Am* 1992;21:519–537.

Zvulunov A, Wyatt DT, Laud PW, et al. Influence of genetic and environmental factors on melanocytic naevi: a lesson from Turner's syndrome. *Br J Dermatol* 1998;138:993–997.

Noonan Syndrome

Allanson J. The first Noonan syndrome gene: PTPN11, which encodes the protein tyrosine phosphatase SHP-2. *Pediatr Res* 2002;52:471.

Burch M, Sharland M, Shinebourne E, et al. Cardiologic abnormalities in Noonan syndrome: phenotypic diagnosis and echocardiographic assessment of 118 patients. *J Am Coll Cardiol* 1993;22:1189–1192.

Char F, Rodriguez-Fernandez HL, Scott CI Jr, et al. The Noonan syndrome—a clinical study of forty-five cases. *Birth Defects Orig Art Ser* 1972;VIII:110–118.

Duncan WJ, Fowler AS, Farkas LG, et al. A comprehensive scoring system for evaluating Noonan syndrome. *Am J Med Genet* 1981;10:37–50.

Gandhi SV, Howarth ES, Krarup KC, et al. Noonan syndrome presenting with transient cystic hygroma. *J Obstet Gynaecol* 2004;24:183–184.

George CD, Patton MA, el Sawi M, et al. Abdominal ultrasound in Noonan syndrome: a study of 44 patients. *Pediatr Radiol* 1993;23:316–318.

Lee NB, Kelly L, Sharland M. Ocular manifestations of Noonan syndrome. *Eye* 1992;6:328–334.

Loh ML, Vattikuti S, Schubbert S, et al. Mutations in PTPN11 implicate the SHP-2 phosphatase in leukemogenesis. *Blood* 2004;103:2325–2331.

Mendez HMM, Opitz JM. Noonan syndrome: a review. *Am J Med Genet* 1985;21:493–506.

Musante L, Kehl HG, Majewski F, et al. Spectrum of mutations in PTPN11 and genotype-phenotype correlation in 96 patients with Noonan syndrome and five patients with cardio-facio-cutaneou syndrome. *Eur J Hum Genet* 2003;11:201–206.

Ranke MB, Heidemann P, Knupfer C, et al. Noonan syndrome:growth and clinical manifestations in 144 cases. *Eur J Pediatr* 1988;148:220–227.

Sarkozy A, Conti E, Seripa D, et al. Correlation between PTPNl1 gene mutations and congenital heart defects in Noonan and LEOPARD syndromes. *J Med Genet* 2003;40:704–708.

Sharland M, Morgan M, Smith G, et al. Genetic counseling in Noonan syndrome. *Am J Med Genet* 1993;45:437–440.

Tartaglia M, Mehler EL, Goldberg R, et al. Mutations in PTPNII, encoding the protein tyrosine phosphatase SHP-2, cause Noonan syndrome. *Nat Genet* 2001;29:465–468.

Witt DR, Hoyme E, Zonana J, et al. Lymphedema in Noonan syndrome: clues to pathogenesis and prenatal diagnosis and review of the literature. *Am J Med Genet* 1987;27:841–856.

Wyre HW Jr. Cutaneous manifestations of Noonan's syndrome. *Arch Dermatol* 1978;114:929–930.

Zenker M, Buheitel G, Rauch R, et al. Genotype-phenotype correlations in Noonan syndrome. *J Pediatr* 2004;144:368–374.

Klinefelter Syndrome

Dissemond J, Schultewolter T, Brauns TC, et al. Venous leg ulcers in a patient with Klinefelter's syndrome and increased activity of plasminogen activator inhibitor-1. *Acta Derrn Venereal* 2003;83:149–150.

Eytan A, Paoloni-Giacobino A, Thorens G, et al. Fire-setting behavior associated with Klinefelter syndrome. *Int J Psychiatry Med* 2002;32:395–399.

Hecht F, Hecht BK. Behavior in Klinefelter syndrome, or where there is smoke there may not be a fire. *Pediatrics* 1990;86:1001–1002.

Hultborn R, Hanson C, Kopf I, et al. Prevalence of Klinefelter's syndrome in male breast cancer patients. *Anticancer Res* 1997;17:4293–4297.

Kenwriick S, Woffendin H, Jakins T, et al. Survival of male patients with incontinentia pigmenti carrying a lethal mutation can be explained by somatic mosaicism or Klinefelter syndrome. *Am J Hum Genet* 2001;69:1210–1217.

Mandoki MW, Sumner GS. Klinefelter syndrome: the need for early identification and treatment. *Clin Pediatr* 1991;30:161–164.

Nielsen J, Wohlert M. Sex chromosome abnormalities found among 34,910 newborn children: results from a 13-year incidence study in Arhus, Denmark. *Birth Defects* 1990;26:209–223.

Schwartz ID, Root AW. The Klinefelter syndrome of testicular dysgenesis. *Endocrinol Metab Clin North Am* 1991;20:153–163.

Simpson JL, de la Cruz F, Swerdloff RS, et al. Klinefelter syndrome: expanding the phenotype and identifying new research directions. *Genet Med* 2003;5:460–468.

Sorensen K. Physical and mental development of adolescent males with Klinefelter syndrome. *Horm Res* 1992;37:55–61.

Spier C, Shear NH, Lester RS. Recurrent leg ulcerations as the initial clinical manifestation of Klinefelter's syndrome. *Arch Dermatol* 1995;131:230.

Winter JS. Androgen therapy in Klinefelter syndrome during adolescence. *Birth Defects* 1990;26:235–245.

Chapter 13

Disorders with Short Stature

Clinical Pearls

Kurt Hirschhorn, M.D. (KH) and Judith Willner, M.D. (JW)

Cornelia de Lange Syndrome

Synonym	De Lange syndrome Brachmann-de Lange syndromse
Inheritance	Most cases are sporadic; autosomal dominant transmission favored in familial cases—variety of chromosomal abnormalities have been reported; recurrence risk estimated at 2% to 5% in families with affected child; nipped-β-like (*NIPBL*) gene on 5p13.1 has been identified in some cases
Prenatal Diagnosis	Fetal ultrasound—detection of intrauterine growth retardation and/or major structural abnormalities with positive family history
Incidence	Over 1:10,000 (estimate); M=F
Age at Presentation	Birth
Pathogenesis	Mutation in *NIPBL* gene may play a role in some cases

Key Features	**Skin**
	    Cutis marmorata, hirsutism, hypoplastic nipples and umbilicus
	Craniofacial
	    Synophrys, trichomegaly (long eyelashes), microcephaly, small nose, anteverted nostrils, long philtrum, downturned, thin lips, late erupting, widely spaced teeth, micrognathia, low-set ears, low hairline, short neck
	Central Nervous System
	    Severe mental retardation, psychomotor retardation, hypertonicity, low-pitched cry in infancy, behavioral problems
	Musculoskeletal
	    Short stature beginning prenatally, small hands and feet, malformed upper limbs/hands with fifth finger clinodactyly, proximally placed thumbs, simian crease; flexion contracture of elbows, syndactyly of second and third toes
	Genitourinary
	    Cryptorchidism, hypospadias, renal anomalies, bicornuate uterus
	Cardiovascular
	    Variety of congenital heart defects
	Ear-Nose-Throat
	    Hearing loss
	Lungs
	    Recurrent infection

Differential Diagnosis	Dup (3q) syndrome
Laboratory Data	Echocardiagram Abdominal ultrasound BEAR hearing evaluation Chest x-ray
Management	Close routine care with pediatrician—infection control; follow psychomotor, behavioral development Referral to symptom-specific specialist
Prognosis	Often premature death secondary to aspiration, recurrent pulmonary infection; usually severely retarded (IQ often < 35)

Clinical Pearls

Usually sporadic but there have been many familial reports. . . I (*KH*) have described a family with three affected children. . . May turn out to be a microdeletion syndrome. . . Newborns are very small for gestational age. . . Facies is striking, characteristic. . . Makes them look unhappy, almost like a Greek tragedy mask. . . Although usually severely retarded, some kids have borderline-normal IQs. . . Downturning, or carp-like mouth is typical. . . Probably a fairly common syndrome.   *KH, JW*

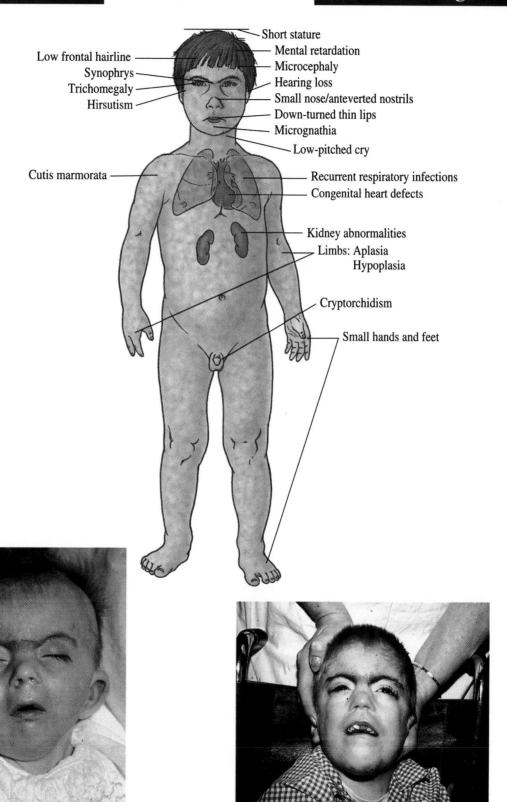

Short stature
Mental retardation
Microcephaly
Hearing loss
Small nose/anteverted nostrils
Down-turned thin lips
Micrognathia
Low-pitched cry

Low frontal hairline
Synophrys
Trichomegaly
Hirsutism

Cutis marmorata

Recurrent respiratory infections
Congenital heart defects

Kidney abnormalities
Limbs: Aplasia
        Hypoplasia

Cryptorchidism

Small hands and feet

13.1. *Infant with marked hirsutism on forehead, synophrys, trichomegaly, anteverted nostrils, long philtrum, and low-set ears.* (138)

13.2. *Similar features in a wheelchair-bound boy. Note late-erupting teeth.* (138)

363

Rubinstein-Taybi Syndrome

Inheritance

Sporadic; 1% recurrence rate within families of affected child; autosomal dominant transmission proposed; human CREB-binding protein (CREBBP) on 16p13.3

Prenatal Diagnosis

DNA analysis available in future

Incidence

Over 225 cases reported; 1:300 to 500 institutionalized, mentally retarded people over 5 years of age; M=F

Age at Presentation

Birth to neonatal period

Pathogenesis

Mutations in the *CREBBP* gene, a gene encoding a nuclear protein acting as a coactivator of cAMP regulated gene expression may be responsible for developmental abnormalities, neoplasms, and keloids

Key Features

Skin
　Capillary malformation (50%)
Musculoskeletal
　Broad thumbs and halluces (broad terminal phalanges with/without angulation deformity), short stature, stiff gait
Craniofacial
　Beaked nose with nasal septum below alae, broad nasal bridge, downslanting palpebral fissures, high-arched palate, epicanthal folds, "grimacing" smile, mild micrognathia, microcephaly
Central Nervous System
　Severe mental retardation with speech delay, motor retardation
Eyes
　Strabismus
Genitourinary
　Cryptorchidism (80%), variety of anomalies
Cardiovascular
　Congenital heart defects (35%)

Differential Diagnosis

None

Laboratory Data

X-ray of hands and feet

Management

Close routine care with primary care physician—follow psychomotor, language and speech development
Referral to symptom-specific specialist

Prognosis

May have increased mortality in infancy/early childhood secondary to respiratory distress/infections, feeding difficulties, cardiac failure; often normal life span with IQ ranging from 40 to 50

Clinical Pearls

Big thumbs, big toes, large beaked nose. . . Antimongolian eyes. . . Typical facies in nursery. . . Deletion in 16p has been described in a number of cases. . . Prenatally, best looking for the microdeletion. . . Severity of syndrome based on how much gene is clipped off. . . In our experience, fairly rare syndrome. . . Severely retarded. *KH, JW*

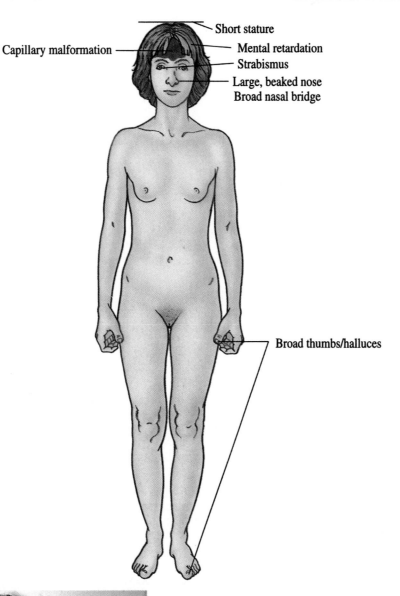

Short stature

Mental retardation

Capillary malformation

Strabismus

Large, beaked nose
Broad nasal bridge

Broad thumbs/halluces

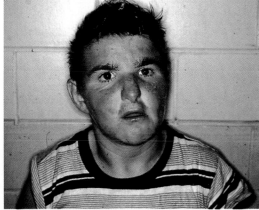

13.3. *Boy with beaked nose, nasal septum below alae, broad nasal bridge, and "grimacing smile." (139)*

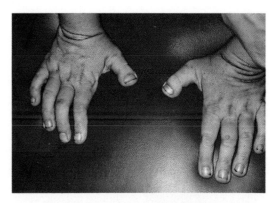

13.4. *Broad thumbs with angulation deformity. (139)*

Russell-Silver Syndrome

Synonym	Silver-Russell syndrome
Inheritance	Almost all cases are sporadic; rare reports of familial transmission
Prenatal Diagnosis	None
Incidence	Over 150 cases reported: M=F
Age at Presentation	Birth
Pathogenesis	Unknown

Key Features

Skin
Café au lait macules

Musculoskeletal
Short stature starting prenatally, motor milestones delayed, asymmetry of head, limbs or trunk, clinodactyly of fifth finger, syndactyly between second and third toes

Craniofacial
Thin lips with downturning at corners of mouth, triangular facies, delayed anterior fontanelle closure

Genitourinary
May have precocious sexual development, cryptorchidism/hypospadias, variety of anomalies noted

Gastrointestinal
Gastroesophageal reflux, esophagitis, food aversion, failure to thrive

Differential Diagnosis
Other small for gestational age (SGA) conditions
18p-syndrome
Trisomy 18 mosaicism
Proteus syndrome (p. 106)
McCune-Albright syndrome (p. 80)

Laboratory Data
Serum and urinary gonadotropin levels

Management
Supportive with routine care by primary care physician
Corrective shoes, braces if severe asymmetry
Referral to symptom-specific specialist
Psychosocial support given dwarfism, precocious puberty

Prognosis
Normal life span; functional impairment dependent on degree of asymmetry

Clinical Pearls

Approximately 10% have maternal uniparental disomy of chromosome 7 involving an imprinted region. . . We (geneticists) often don't see them in the nursery because they're not microcephalic. . . They show up later on with hypotonicity, characteristic facies. . . Features look delicate because of increased cranium:face ratio. . . Bony asymmetry anywhere. . . Probably heterogeneous group of causes. . . We follow one child who turned out to be a mitochondrial disorder. . . Important to make diagnosis to avoid a big pituitary work-up, growth hormone therapy. . . Motor milestones delayed but they catch up. . . Usually, normal intelligence.   *KH, JW*

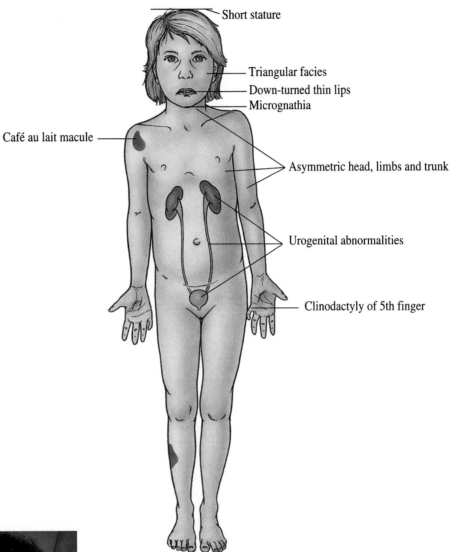

Short stature

Triangular facies

Down-turned thin lips

Micrognathia

Café au lait macule

Asymmetric head, limbs and trunk

Urogenital abnormalities

Clinodactyly of 5th finger

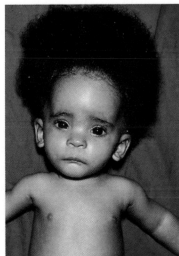

13.5. *West Indian infant with thin lips, downturning at corners of mouth, triangular facies. (140)*

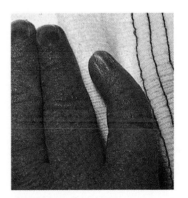

13.6. *Clinodactyly of fifth finger. (141)*

Familial Dysautonomia

Synonym	Riley-Day syndrome
Inheritance	Autosomal recessive; *IKBKAP* gene on 9q31–q33
Prenatal Diagnosis	DNA analysis
Incidence	1:3700 Ashkenazi Jews; M=F
Age at Presentation	Infancy to early childhood
Pathogenesis	Mutations on *IKBKAP* gene are responsible for phenotype; probable developmental arrest of unmyelinated sensory and sympathetic neurons with autonomic dysfunction

Key Features

Skin
Macular erythema increased on trunk, limbs with excitement, eating; hyperhidrosis; burns secondary to pain indifference; cold hands and feet

Craniofacial
Alert expression with decreased blink frequency, straight upper lip with smile

Gastrointestinal
Absence of fungiform papillae on tongue; excessive salivation; absent taste sensation; oromotor incoordination with poor suck at birth, tendency to misdirect and aspirate fluids, difficulty chewing, and drooling; gastroesophageal reflux; 40% exhibit vomiting crises associated with hypertension when stressed

Central Nervous System
Hypotonia in infancy, decreased deep tendon reflexes, insensitivity to pain, labile hypertension, orthostatic hypotension without compensatory tachycardia, dysarthria, prolonged nocturnal enuresis into the teens, breath-holding spells, normal intelligence

Eyes
Decreased corneal sensation/tear flow with corneal ulceration

Lungs
Excessive bronchial secretions, recurrent aspirations/infections; pulmonary failure

Musculoskeletal
Short stature, scoliosis, kyphosis, increased incidence of aseptic necrosis

Differential Diagnosis	Congenital sensory neuropathy; congenital universal indifference to pain; other chronic pulmonary diseases of childhood
Laboratory Data	Histamine skin test: 0.01 mL of 1:10,000 histamine injected intradermally—wheal without axon flare or pain; pilocarpine eyedrop test: 0.0625% pilocarpine eyedrops induce immediate pupillary constriction; increased urinary homovanillic acid to vanillylmandelic acid ratio
Management	Close follow-up with primary care physician—artificial tears, avoidance of aspiration, maintenance of proper nutrition with fundoplication, feeding gastrostomy; watch for musculoskeletal problems, orthostatic hypotension, vomiting "crises" Referral to orthopedist—scoliosis, fracture and joint repair
Prognosis	Fifty percent mortality before 30 years old resulting from pulmonary problems; adults at risk for cardiopulmonary arrests because of sympathetic and/or renal failure

Clinical Pearls

The gene has been found and 98% have the identical mutation on 9q. . . Prenatal diagnosis is being done here at Mt. Sinai. . . Felicia Axelrod is the world's expert at NYU's Dysautonomia Treatment and Evaluation Center. . . She takes phenomenal care of them, with kids surviving well beyond the reported life spans for this disease. . . One of her observations is that many are born breech. . . Apparently, the autonomic system may play a role in rotating into the vertex position. . . She has also noted that as they are surviving longer and getting older, they're developing an unusual nephropathy. . . Severe burns can be a big problem. . . Cover all radiators. . . Many come in with keratitis. . . Artificial tears are very important. . . Aspiration pneumonia is most common cause of death.   *KH, JW*

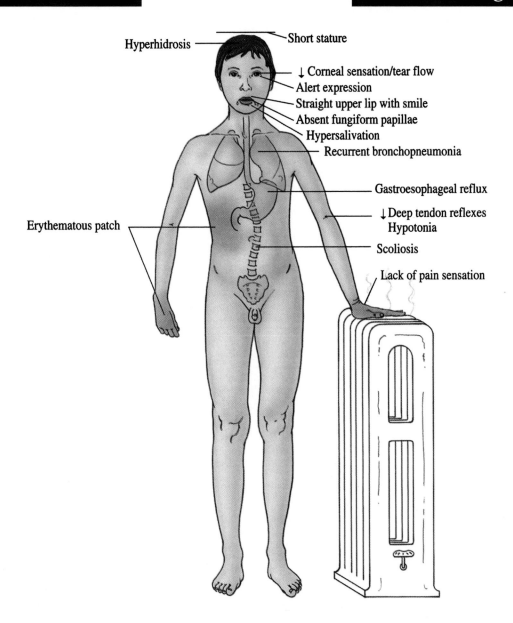

Hyperhidrosis

Short stature

↓ Corneal sensation/tear flow

Alert expression

Straight upper lip with smile

Absent fungiform papillae

Hypersalivation

Recurrent bronchopneumonia

Gastroesophageal reflux

↓ Deep tendon reflexes
Hypotonia

Erythematous patch

Scoliosis

Lack of pain sensation

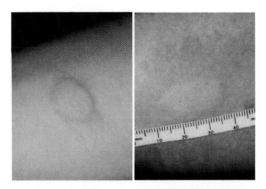

13.7. *Histamine skin test. Left. Abnormal test with wheal and absent axon flare; note erythema only at border of wheal. Right. Normal wheal with typical axon flare extending a few centimeters beyond wheal. (142)*

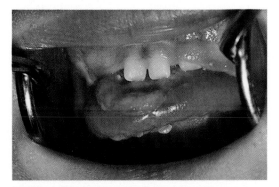

13.8. *Exophytic ulceration on tongue secondary to chronic trauma and indifference to pain. (143)*

Suggested Reading

Cornelia de Lange Syndrome

Arbuzova S, Nikolenko M, Krantz D, et al. Low first-trimester pregnancy-associated plasma protein-A and Cornelia de Lange syndrome. *Prenat Diagn* 2003;23:864.

Drolshagen LF, Durmon G, Berumen M, et al. Prenatal ultrasonographic appearance of "Cornelia de Lange" syndrome. *J Clin Ultrasound* 1992;20:470–474.

Goodban MT. Survey of speech and language skills with prognostic indicators in 116 patients with Cornelia de Lange syndrome. *Am J Med Genet* 1993;47:1059–1063.

Hawley PP, Jackson LG, Kurnit DM. Sixty-four patients with Brachmann-de Lange syndrome: a survey. *Am J Med Genet* 1985;20:453–459.

Hems TE, Godfrey A. Cosmetic surgery for Cornelia de Lange syndrome. *Br J Plast Surg* 1990;43:489–491.

Husain K, Fitzgerald P, Lau G. Cecal volvulus in the Cornelia de Lange syndrome. *J Pediatr Surg* 1994;29:1245–1247.

Ireland M, Burn J. Cornelia de Lange syndrome—photo essay. *Clin Dysmorphol* 1993;2:151–160.

Jackson L, Kline AD, Barr MA, et al. De Lange syndrome: a clinical review of 310 individuals. *Am J Med Genet* 1993;47:940–946.

Kline AD, Barr M, Jackson LG. Growth manifestations in the Brachmann-de Lange syndrome. *Am J Med Genet* 1993;47:1042–1049.

Levin AV, Seidman DJ, Nelson LB, et al. Ophthalmologic findings in the Cornelia de Lange syndrome. *J Pediatr Ophthalmol Strabismus* 1990;27:94–102.

Luzzani S, Macchini F, Valade A, et al. Gastroesophageal reflux and Cornelia de Lange syndrome: typical and atypical symptoms. *Am J Med Genet* 2003;119A:283–287.

McConnell V, Brown T, Morrison PJ. An Irish three-generation family of Cornelia de Lange syndrome displaying autosomal dominant inheritance. *Clin Dysmorphol* 2003;12:241–244.

Sataloff RT, Spiegel JR, Hawkshaw M, et al. Cornelia de Lange syndrome. Otolaryngologic manifestations. *Arch Otolaryngol Head Neck Surg* 1990;116:1044–1046.

Sekimoto H, Osada H, Kimura H, et al. Prenatal findings in Brachmann-de Lange syndrome. *Arch Gynecol Obstet* 2000;263:182–184.

Rubinstein-Taybi Syndrome

Bartsch O, Locher K, Meinecke P, et al. Molecular studies in 10 cases of Rubinstein-Taybi syndrome, including a mild variant showing a missense mutation in codon 1175 of CREBBP. *J Med Genet* 2002;39:496–501.

Cambiaghi S, Ermacora E, Brusesco A, et al. Multiple pilomatricomas in Rubinstein-Taybi syndrome. *Pediatr Dermatol* 1994;11:21–25.

Coupry I, Monnet L, Attia AA, et al. Analysis of CBP (CREBBP) gene deletions in Rubinstein-Taybi syndrome patients using real-time quantitative PCR. *Hum Mutat* 2004;23:278–284.

Coupry I, Roudaut C, Stef M, et al. Molecular analysis of the CBP gene in 60 patients with Rubinstein-Taybi syndrome. *J Med Genet* 2002;39:415–421.

De Silva B. What syndrome is this? Rubenstein-Taybi syndrome. *Pediatr Dermatol* 2002;19:177–179.

Hennekam RC. Rubinstein-Taybi syndrome: a history in pictures. *Clin Dysmorphol* 1993;2:87–92.

Hennekam RC, Tilanus M, Hamel BC, et al. Deletion at chromosome 16pl3. 3 as a cause of Rubinstein-Taybi syndrome: clinical aspects. *Am J Hum Genet* 1993;52:255–262.

Rubinstein JH. Broad thumb-hallux (Rubinstein-Taybi) syndrome 1957–1988. *Am J Med Genet Suppl* 1990;6:3–16.

Rubinstein-Taybi syndrome. Papers presented at the 9th annual David W. Smith Workshop on Malformations and Morphogenesis. Oakland, 1988 Proceedings. *Am J Med Genet Suppl* 1990;6:1–131.

Selmanowitz VJ, Stiller MJ. Rubinstein-Taybi syndrome. *Arch Dermatol* 1981;117:504–506.

Stevens CA, Hennekam RC, Blackburn BL. Growth in the Rubinstein-Taybi syndrome. *Am J Med Genet Suppl* 1990;6:51–55.

van Genderen MM, Kinds GF, Riemslag FC, et al. Ocular features in Rubinstein-Taybi syndrome: investigation of 24 patients and review of the literature. *Br J Ophthalmol* 2000;84:1177–1184.

Wiley S, Swayne S, Rubinstein JH, et al. Rubinstein-Taybi syndrome medical guidelines. *Am J Med Genet* 2003;119A:101–110.

Wood VE, Rubinstein JH. Surgical treatment of the thumb in the Rubinstein-Taybi syndrome. *J Hand Surg* 1987;12:166–172.

Russell-Silver Syndrome

Anderson J, Viskochil D, O'Gorman M, et al. Gastrointestinal complications of Russell-Silver syndrome: a pilot study. *Am J Med Genet* 2002;113:15–19.

Angehrn V, Zachmann M, Prader A. Silver-Russell syndrome: observations in 20 patients. *Helv Paediat Acta* 1979;34:297–308.

Beever CL, Penaherrera MS, Langlois S, et al. X chromosome inactivation patterns in Russell-Silver syndrome patients and their mothers. *Am J Med Genet* 2003;123A:231–235.

Hitchins MP, Stanier P, Preece MA, et al. Silver-Russell syndrome: a dissection of the genetic aetiology and candidate chromosomal regions. *J Med Genet* 2001;38:810–819.

Li CC, Chodirker BN, Dawson AJ, et al. Severe hemihypotrophy in a female infant with mosaic Turner syndrome: a variant of Russell-Silver syndrome? *Clin Dysmorphol* 2004;13:95–98.

Patton MA. Russell-Silver syndrome. *J Med Genet* 1988;25:557–560.

Perkins RM, Hoang-Xuan MT. The Russell-Silver syndrome: a case report and brief review of the literature. *Pediatr Dermatol* 2002;19:546–549.

Price SM, Stanhope R, Garrett C, et al. The spectrum of Silver-Russell syndrome: a clinical and molecular genetic study and new diagnostic criteria. *J Med Genet* 1999;36:837–842.

Silver HK. Asymmetry, short stature, and variations in sexual development: a syndrome of congenital malformations. *Am J Dis Child* 1964;107:495–515.

Tanner JM, Lejarraga H, Cameron N. The natural history of the Silver-Russell syndrome: a longitudinal study of thirty-nine cases. *Pediatr Res* 1975;9:611–623.

Wheeler PG, Bresnahan K, Shephard BA, et al. Short stature and functional impairment: a systematic review. *Arch Pediatr Adolesc Med* 2004;158:236–243.

Familial Dysautonomia Syndrome

Albanese SA, Bobechko WP. Spine deformity in familial dysautonomia (Riley-Day syndrome). *J Pediatr Orthop* 1987;7:179–183.

Axelrod FB. Familial dysautonomia. *Muscle Nerve* 2004;29:352–363.

Axelrod FB, Glickstein JS, Weider J, et al. The effects of postural change and exercise on renal haemodynamics in familial dysautonomia. *Clin Auton Res* 1993;3:195–200.

Axelrod FB, Goldberg JD, Ye XY, et al. Survival in familial dysautonomia: impact of early intervention. *J Pediatr* 2002;141:518–523.

Axelrod FB, Gouge TH, Ginsburg HB, et al. Fundoplication and gastrostomy in familial dysautonomia. *J Pediatr* 1991;118:388–334.

Axelrod FB, Iyer K, Fish I, et al. Progressive sensory loss in familial dysautonomia. *Pediatrics* 1981;67:517–522.

Axelrod FB, Pearson J. Congenital sensory neuropathies. Diagnostic distinction from familial dysautonomia. *Am J Dis Child* 1984;138:947–954.

Axelrod FB, Porges RF, Sein ME. Neonatal recognition of familial dysautonomia. *J Pediatr* 1987;110:946–948.

Blumenfeld A, Slaugenhaupt SA, Axelrod FB, et al. Localization of the gene for familial dysautonomia on chromosome 9 and definition of DNA markers for genetic diagnosis. *Nat Genet* 1993;4:160–164.

Dong J, Edelmann L, Bajwa AM, et al. Familial dysautonomia: detection of the IKBKAP IVS20(+6T—> C) and R696P mutations and frequencies among Ashkenazi Jews. *Am J Med Genet* 2002;110:253–257.

Glickstein JS, Schwartzman D, Friedman D, et al. Abnormalities of the corrected QT interval in familial dysautonomia: an indicator of autonomic dysfunction. *J Pediatr* 1993;122:925–928.

Huneycutt D, Folch E, Franco-Paredes C. Atypical manifestations of infections in patients with familial dysautonomia. *Am J Med* 2003;115:505–506.

Josaitis CA, Matisoff M. Familial dysautonomia in review: diagnosis and treatment of ocular manifestations. *Adv Exp Med Biol* 2002;506:71–80.

Kamboj MK, Axelrod FB, David R, et al. Growth hormone treatment in children with familial dysautonomia. *J Pediatr* 2004;144:63–67.

Lehavi O, Aizenstein O, Bercovich D, et al. Screening for familial dysautonomia in Israel: evidence for higher carrier rate among Polish Ashkenazi Jews. *Genet Test* 2003;7:139–142.

Mass E, Sarnat H, Ram D, et al. Dental and oral findings in patients with familial dysautonomia. *Oral Surg Oral Med Oral Pathol* 1992;74:305–311.

Pearson J, Gallo G, Gluck M, et al. Renal disease in familial dysautonomia. *Pediatrics* 1970;45:739–745.

Rechitsky S, Verlinsky O, Kuliev A, et al. Preimplantation genetic diagnosis for familial dysautonomia. *Reprod Biomed Online* 2003;6:488–493.

Tirosh I, Hoffer V, Finkelstein Y, et al. Heat stroke in familial dysautonomia. *Pediatr Neurol* 2003;29:164–166.

Support Groups

Clearinghouses

National Center for Education in Maternal and Child Health (NCEMH)
www.ncemch.org
2000 15th Street North
Suite 701
Arlington, VA 22201-2627
(703) 524-7802; Fax (703) 524-9335
Director of Information Services: Olivia Pickett

National Organization for Rare Disorders (NORD)
www.rarediseases.org
National Organization for Rare Disorders
55 Kenosia Avenue
P.O. Box 1968
Danbury, CT 06813-1968
(800) 999-6673; (203) 744-0100;
Fax (203) 798-2291
Executive Director: Abbey S. Meyers

Genetic Alliance
www.geneticalliance.org
4301 Connecticut Avenue
Washington, DC 20008
(202) 966-5557; Fax (202) 966-8553
Executive Director: Sharon F. Terry, M.A.

Center for Birth Defects Information Services
Dover Medical Building, Box 1776
30 Springdale Avenue
Dover, MA 02030
(508) 785-2525; Fax (508) 785-2526
Executive Director: Mary Louise Buyse, M.D.

March of Dimes Birth Defects Foundation
www.modimes.org
1275 Mamaroneck Avenue
White Plains, NY 10605
(888) 663-4637; (914) 428-7100;
Fax (914) 997-4763
Executive Director: Jennifer L. Howse, Ph.D.

Self-Help Clearinghouses

St. Clares Riverside Medical Center
25 Pocono Road
Denville, NJ 07834-2921
(201) 625-7101; Fax (201)625-8848
Director: Ed Madara

General

Alexander Graham Bell Association for the Deaf
www.agbell.org
3417 Volta Place, N.W.
Washington, DC 20007
(800) 432-7543; (866) 337-5220;
Fax (202)337-8314
Executive Director: K. Todd Houston, Ph.D.

American Association on Mental Retardation
www.aamr.org
444 North Capitol St., N.W., Suite 846
Washington, D.C. 20001-1512
(800) 424-3688; (202) 387-1968;
Fax (202)387-2193
Executive Director: Doreen M. Croser

American Association of University Centers on Disabilities
www.aucd.org
1010 Wayne Avenue, Suite 920
Silver Spring, MD 20910
(301) 588-8252; Fax (301) 588-2842
Executive Director: George Jesian, Ph.D.

American Foundation for the Blind
www.afb.org
11 Penn Plaza, Suite 300
New York, NY 10001
(800) 232- 5468; (212) 502-7600;
Fax: (212) 502-7777
Executive Director: Carl Augusto, CEO
Contact Person: Jacqueline Packer, Interim Director of Information

American Pseudo-Obstruction and Hirschsprung's Disease Society
158 Pleasant Street
North Andover, MA 01845
(800) 394-2747; (978) 684-4477;
Fax (978) 685-4488
Executive Director: Andrea M. Anastas, President

Children's Craniofacial Association
www.ccakids.com
13140 Coit Road
Suite 307
Dallas, TX 75240
(800) 535-3643; (214) 570-9099;
Fax (214) 570-8811
Executive Director: Charlene Smith

Coalition for Heritable Disorders of Connective Tissue
www.chdct.org
4301 Connecticut Avenue, N.W., Suite 404
Washington, DC 20008
(202) 362-9599; Fax (202) 966-8553
President: Sharon Terry

Immune Deficiency Foundatoin
www.primaryimmune.org
40 W. Chesapeake Avenue, Suite 308
Towson, MD 21204
(800) 296-4433; Fax (410) 321-9165
Executive Director: G. Richard Barr

International Skeletal Dysplasia Registry
www.csmc.edu/3805.html
Cedars-Sinai Medical Center
444 S. San Van Vicente Boulevard, Suite 604
Los Angeles, CA 90048

(800) CEDARS-1; (310) 423-9915;
Fax (310) 423-9946
Executive Director: David L. Rimoin, M.D., Ph.D.
Contact Person: MaryAnn Priore, Coordinator

The Leukemia and Lymphoma Society
www.leukemia.org
1311 Mamaroneck Avenue, 3rd Floor
White Plains, NY 10605
(914) 949-5213; Fax (914) 949-6691
Executive Director: Dwayne Howell, President, CEO

Major Aspects of Growth in Children Foundation
www.magicfoundation.org
6645 W. North Avenue
Oak Park, IL 60302
(800) 3MAGIC3; (708) 383-0808;
Fax (708) 383-0899
Executive Director: Mary Andrews

National Foundation for Facial Reconstruction
www.nffr.org
317 East 34th Street, Room 901
New York, NY 10016
(800) 422-FACE; (212) 263-6656;
Fax (212) 263-7534
Executive Director: Whitney Burnett
Contact Person: Michele Golombuski, Program Officer

National Scoliosis Foundation
www.scoliosis.org
5 Cabot Place
Stoughton, MA 02072
(800) 673-6922; (781) 341-6333;
Fax (781) 341-8333
Executive Director: Joseph P. O'Brien
Contact Person: Sandy Marcal, Office Manager

Organic Acidemia Association
www.oaanews.org
13210 35th Avenue North
Plymouth, MN 55441
(763) 559-1747; Fax (763) 694-0017
Executive Director: Kathy Stagni

Retinitis Pigmentosa International
www.rpinternational.org
P.O. Box 900
Woodland Hills, CA 91365
Fax: (818) 992-3265; (818) 992-0500;
Fax (818) 992-3265
Executive Director: Helen Harris, President

Syndromes

AEC (see Ectodermal Dysplasia)

Albinism

National Organization for Albinism and Hypopigmentation
www.albinism.org

P.O. Box 959
East Hampstead, NH 03826-0959
(800) 473-2310; (603) 887-2310;
    Fax (603) 887-6049
Executive Director: Michael McGowan,
President

Anhidrotic Ectodermal Dysplasia (see Ectodermal Dysplasia)

Ataxia-Telangiectasia

**National Ataxia Foundation
(Ataxia-Telangiectasi)**
www.ataxia.org
2600 Fernbrook Lane
Suite 119
Minneapolis, MN 5547
(763) 553-0020; Fax (763) 553-0167
Executive Director: Donna Gruetzmacher

Beckwith-Wiedemann Syndrome

Beckwith-Wiedemann Support Network
2711 Colony Road
Ann Arbor, MI 48104
(800) 837-2976; (734) 973-0263; Fax (734)
    973-9721
Executive Director: Susan Fettes

Bloom Syndrome

Bloom's Syndrome Registry
Laboratory of Human Genetics
New York Blood Center
310 East 67th Street
New York, NY 10021
(212) 570-3075; Fax (212) 570-3195
Contact Person: James L. German III,
M.D.

Chronic Granulomatous Disease

**Chronic Granulomatous Disease
Association**
2616 Monterey Road
San Marino, CA 91108-1646
(626) 441-4118
Contact Person: Mary A. Hurley

Cockayne Syndrome

Share and Care (Cockayne Syndrome)
P.O. Box 570618
Dallas, TX 75357
(972) 613-6273; Fax (972) 613-4590
Contact Person: Shirley Rodriguez,
Coordinator

Cornelia de Lange Syndrome

**Cornelia de Lange Syndrome
Foundation**
www.cdlsusa.org
302 West Main Street #100
Avon, CT 06001
(800) 223-8355; (860) 676-8166;
    Fax (860) 676-8337
Executive Director: Julie Mairano

Darier (see Ichthyosis)

Down Syndrome

**Association for Children with Down
Syndrome**
www.acds.org
4 Fern Place
Plainview, NY 11803
(415) 933-4700; Fax (516) 933-9524
Executive Director: Craig Lomma

National Down Syndrome Society
www.ndss.org
666 Broadway, Eighth Floor
New York, NY 10012
(800) 221-4602; Fax (212) 979-2873
Executive Director: Myra E. Madnick

Ectodermal Dysplasia

**National Foundation for Ectodermal
Dysplasias**
www.nfed.org
410 East Main Street, P.O. Box 114
Masoutah, IL 62258-0114
(618) 455-2020; Fax (618) 566-4718
Executive Director: Mary Kaye Richter

EEC (see Ectodermal Dysplasia)

Ehlers-Danlos Syndrome

Ehlers-Danlos National Foundation
www.ednf.org
6399 Wilshire Blvd., Suite 200
Los Angeles, CA 90048
(800) 956-2902; (323) 651-3038;
    Fax (323) 651-1366
Executive Director: Andrew McCluskey

Epidermolysis Bullosa

**Dystrophic Epidermolysis Bullosa
Research Association of America
(DEBRA)**
www.debra.org
5 West 36th Street, Suite 404
New York, NY 10018
(212) 868-1573; Fax (212) 868-9296
Executive Director: Dolores Cogliano,
Interim Executive Director

Familial Dysautonomia

Dysautonomia Foundation
www.familialdysautonomia.org
633 Third Avenue, 12th Floor
New York, NY 10017
(212) 949-6644
Executive Director: Lenore F. Roseman

Gardner Syndrome

Familial Polyposis Registry (U.S.)
Department of Colorectal Surgery
Cleveland Clinic Foundation
Cleveland, OH 44195-5001
(216) 444-6470; Fax (216) 445-8627
Executive Director: James Church, M.D.

Gaucher's Disease

National Gaucher Foundation
www.gaucherdisease.org
5410 Edison Lane, Suite 260
Rockville, MD 20852-3130
(800) 428-2437; (301) 816-1515;
    Fax (301) 816-1516
Executive Director: Rhonda Buyers

Harlequin Fetus (see Ichthyosis)

Hemochromatosis

Hemochromatosis Foundation
www.hemochromatosis.org
P.O. Box 8569
Albany, NY 12208
(518) 489-0972; Fax (518) 489-0227
Executive Director: Margit A. Krikker, M.D.

*Hereditary Hemorrhagic Telaniectasia
Syndrome*

**Hereditary Hemorrhagic Telangiectasia
Foundation Internationl**
www.hht.org
P.O. Box 8087
New Haven, CT 06530
(800) 448-6389; (410) 357-9932;
    Fax (410) 357-9931
Executive Director: Marianne Clancy

*Hidrotic Ectodermal Dysplasia (see
Ectodermal Dysplasia)*

Ichthyosis

**Foundation for Ichthyosis and Related
Skin Types (FIRST)**
www.scalyskin.org
650 N. Cannon Avenue, Suite 17
Lansdale, PA 19446
(800) 545-2386; (215) 631-1411; Fax (215)
    631-1413
Executive Director: Jean Pickford

X-linked ichthyosis: For steroid sulfatase
    assay, send 1 mL separated and frozen
    serum in EDTA test tube to:
Cedric H.L. Shackleton, PhD., DSc
Children's Hospital Oakland Research
    Institute
5700 Martin Luther King Jr Way
Oakland, CA 94609
(510) 450-7600; Fax (510) 450-7910

*Incontinentia Pigmenti (see
Ectodermal Dysplasia)*

Klinefelter Syndrome

Klinefelter Syndrome and Associates
www.genetic.org
P.O. Box 119
Roseville, CA 95678-0119
(888) 999-9428; (916) 773-2999; Fax (916)
    773-1449
Executive Director: Melissa Aylstock

Klippel-Trenaunay-Weber

Klippel-Trenaunay (K-T) Support Group
www.k-t.org
5404 Dundee Road
Edina, MN 55436
(952) 925-2596; Fax (952) 925-4708
Executive Director: Judy Vessey

Marfan Syndrome

National Marfan Foundation
www.marfan.org
22 Manhasset Avenue
Port Washington, NY 11050
(800) 8-MARFAN; (516) 883-8712;
    Fax (516) 883-8040
Executive Director: Caroline Levering

Menkes' Kinky Hair Syndrome (see Wilson's Disease)

Mucopolysaccharidoses

Zain Hansen MPS Foundation
23400 Henderson Rd
Covelo, CA 95420
(707) 983-0011
Executive Director: Tess Ives

Neurofibromatosis I

National Neurofibromatosis Foundation
www.nf.org
95 Pine Street, 16th Floor
New York, NY 10005
(800) 323-7938; (212) 344-NNFF;
    Fax (212) 747-0004
Executive Director: Peter Bellermann,
    President

Neurofibromatosis II

NF2 Sharing Network
10074 Cabachon Court
Ellicott City, MD 21042
(410) 461-2245 (voice); (410) 461-5213
Executive Director: Paul Mendelsohn

Acoustic Neuroma Association
www.anausa.org
600 Peachtree Parkway
Suite 108
Cumming, GA 30041-6899
(770) 205-8211; (770) 205-0239
Executive Director: Lois White

Niemann-Pick Disease

National Niemann Pick Disease Foundation
www.nnpdf.org
P.O. Box 49
415 Madison Avenue
Fort Atkinson, WI 53538
(877) CURE-NPC; (920) 563-0930;
    Fax (920) 563-0931
Executive Director: Nadine Hill

Noonan Syndrome

Noonan Syndrome Society
1278 Pine Avenue
San Jose, CA 95125
(408) 723-5188
Contact Person: Susan Espinoza, Parent
    Coordinator

Osteogenesis Imperfecta

Osteogenesis Imperfecta Foundation
www.oif.org
804 W. Diamond Avenue, Suite 210
Gaithersburg, MD 20878
(800) 981-2663; (301) 947-0083;
    Fax (301) 947-0456
Executive Director: Heller An Shapiro

Phenylketonuria

Children's PKU Network
www.pkunetwork.org
3790 Via de la Valle, Suite 120
Del Mar, CA 92014
(800) 377-6677; (858) 509-0767;
    Fax (858) 509-0768
Executive Director: Cindy Neptune

Porphyrias

American Porphyria Foundation
www.porphyriafoundation.com
P.O. Box 22712
Houston, TX 77227
(713) 266-9617; Fax (713) 266-9617 (phone
    first)
Executive Director: Desiree Lyon

Progeria

International Progeria Registry
New York State Institute for Basic
    Research
Department of Human Genetics
1050 Forest Hill Road
Staten Island, NY 10314
(718) 494-5333
Contact Person: W. Ted Brown, M.D.,
    Ph.D.

Pseudoxanthoma Elasticum

National Association for Pseudoxanthoma Elasticum
www.pxenape.org or www.napxe.org
8764 Manchester Road, Suite 200
St. Louis, MO 63114-2724
(314) 882-7273; Fax (314) 977-3587
Contact Person: Frances Benham

Rubinstein-Taybi Syndrome

Rubinstein-Taybi Parent Contact Group
www.rubinstein-taybi.org
P.O. Box 146
Smith Center, KS 66967
(888) 447-2989; (785) 697-2984;
    Fax (785) 697-2985
Contact Person: Lorrie Baxter

Russell-Silver Syndrome

Association for Children with Russell-Silver Syndrome
22 Hoyt Street
Madison, NJ 07940
(201) 377-4531; Fax (201) 822-2715
Executive Director: Jodi G. Zwain

Sturge-Weber Syndrome

Sturge-Weber Foundation
www.sturge-weber.com
P.O. Box 418
Mt. Freedom, NJ 07970
(800) 672-5482; (973) 895-4445;
    Fax (973) 895-4846
Contact Person: Karen Ball

Tuberous Sclerosis

National Tuberous Sclerosis Association
www.tsalliance.org
801 Roeder Road, Suite 750
Silver Spring, MD 20910
(800) 225-6872; (301) 562-9890;
    Fax (301) 562-9870
Executive Director: Michael Coburn

Turner Syndrome

Turner's Syndrome Society of the United States
www.turner-syndrome-us.org
14450 TC Jester, Suite 260
Houston, TX 77014
(800) 365-9944; (832) 249-9988;
    Fax (832) 249-9987
Executive Director: Merriott Terry

Von-Hippel-Lindau Syndrome

Von Hippel-Lindau Family Alliance
www.vhl.org
171 Clinton Road
Brookline, MA 02445-5815
(800) 767-4845; (617) 277-5667;
    Fax (617) 734-8233
Executive Director: Joyce Graff

Wilson's Disease

Wilson's Disease Association International
www.wilsonsdisease.org
1802 Brookside Drive
Wooster, OH 44691
(800) 399-0266; (330) 264-1450; (509) 757-6418
Executive Director: Kimberly Symonds

Xeroderma Pigmentosum

Xeroderma Pigmentosum Registry
University of Medicine and Dentistry of
    New Jersey
Department of Pathology
Med Sci Bldg Rm C-520
185 South Orange Avenue
Newark, NJ 07103-2714
(201) 982-4405
Executive Director: W. Clark Lambert,
    M.D, Ph.D.

Lab Testing Appendix

Acute Intermittent Porphyria (AIP)

Mayo Clinic
Biochemical Genetics Laboratory
200 First Street S.W.
Rochester, MN 55905
(800) 533-1710; (507) 266-1800;
Fax: (507) 284-1759
Directors: Sihoun Hahn, M.D., Ph.D.;
Dietrich Matern, M.D.; Joseph
McConnell, Ph.D.; John F. O'Brien,
Ph.D.; Piero Rinaldo, M.D., Ph.D.
E-mail: biochemicalgenetics@mayo.edu

Mount Sinai School of Medicine
Porphyria Laboratory
Center for Jewish Genetic Diseases
One Gustave L. Levy Place
Box 1498
New York, NY 10029
(212) 659-6783; Fax (212) 360-1809
Directors: Robert J. Desnick, M.D., Ph.D.;
Junaid Shabbeer, Ph.D.;
Kenneth H. Astrin, Ph.D.
Contact: Kenneth H. Astrin, Ph.D.
E-mail: kenneth.astrin@mssm.edu

Alkaptonuria

Duke University Medical Center
Pediatric Biochemical Genetics
Laboratory
P.O. Box 14991
99 Alexander Drive
Research Triangle Park, NC 27709
(919) 549-0445; Fax (919) 549-0709
Directors: David S. Millington, Ph.D.;
Dwight D. Koeberl, M.D., Ph.D.
E-mail: dmilli@acpub.duke.edu
Website: www.duke.edu/~M.D.feezor/
dukemedicalgenetics

Emory Biochemical Genetics Laboratory
2040 Ridgewood Drive, Lower Level
Atlanta, GA 30322
(404) 727-5782; Fax (404) 727-9398
Director: Chunli Yu, M.D.
Contact: Joyce Marshall
E-mail: jmarshall@genetics.emory.edu

OHSU Clinical Genetics Laboratories
Biochemical Genetics Laboratory
3181 S.W. Sam Jackson Park Road
Portland, OR 97239-3098
(503) 494-5400; Fax (503) 494-6922
Director: K. Michael Gibson, Ph.D.,
FACMG; Cary O. Harding, M.D.,
FACMG
Contact: Michelle R. Polinsky
E-mail: polinsky@ohsu.edu

Aplasia Cutis Congenita

Thomas Jefferson University
Department of Dermatology and
Cutaneous Biology
Bluemle Life Sciences Building
233 South 10th Street, Suite 450
Philadelphia, PA 19107
(215) 503-5785; Fax (215) 503-5788
Directors: Gabriele Richard and
Jouni Uitto

Contact: Elaine Pfendner, Ph.D. or
Gabriele Richard
E-mail: ellen.pfendner@mail.tju.edu,
gabriele.richard@mail.tju.edu

Argininosuccinic Aciduria

Baylor College of Medicine
Biochemical Genetics Laboratory
2450 Holcombe
Houston, TX 77021-2024
(800) 246-2436; Fax (713) 798-6584
Directors: V. Reid Sutton, M.D.,
William E. O'Brien, Ph.D.
Contact: Arthur W. Warman, MS
E-mail: genetictest@bcm.tmc.edu
Website: www.bcmgeneticlabs.org

Emory Biochemical Genetics Laboratory
2040 Ridgewood Drive, Lower Level
Atlanta, GA 30322
(404) 727-5782; Fax (404) 727-9398
Director: Chunli Yu, M.D.
Contact: Joyce Marshall
E-mail: jmarshall@genetics.emory.edu

Greenwood Genetic Center
Metabolic Laboratory
1 Gregor Mendel Circle
Greenwood, SC 29646
(800) 473-9411; (864) 941-8131;
Fax (864) 941-8133
Directors: Harold A. Taylor, Ph.D.;
Tim C. Wood, Ph.D.
Contact: Kim Stewart, M.T., ASCP
E-mail: kbstewart@ggc.org
Website: www.ggc.org

Massachusetts General Hospital
Amino Acid Disorder (Neurochemistry)
Lab
Charlestown Navy Yard
Building 149, 13th Street, 6th floor room
6310
Boston, MA 02129
(617) 726-3884; Fax (617) 726-5739
Director: Vivian E. Shih, M.D.
Contact: Roseann Mandell
E-mail: rmandell@partners.org

Mayo Clinic
Biochemical Genetics Laboratory
200 First Street S.W.
Rochester, MN 55905
(800) 533-1710; (507) 266-1800;
Fax (507) 284-1759
Directors: Sihoun Hahn, M.D., Ph.D.;
Dietrich Matern, M.D.; Joseph
McConnell, Ph.D.; John F. O'Brien,
Ph.D.; Piero Rinaldo, M.D., Ph.D.
E-mail: biochemicalgenetics@mayo.edu

Ataxia-Telangiectasia

UCLA Medical Center
Department of Pathology & Laboratory
Medicine
Division of Laboratory Medicine
10833 Le Conte Avenue
Los Angeles, CA 90095-1713
(310) 206-5294; Fax (310) 206-2757

Directors: Richard A Gatti, M.D.;
Wayne W Grody, M.D., Ph.D.
E-mail: rgatti@mednet.ucla.edu;
wgrody@mednet.ucla.edu

Johns Hopkins Hospital
DNA Diagnostic Laboratory
CMSC 10-106
600 N. Wolfe Street
Baltimore, MD 21287
(410) 955-0483; Fax (410) 955-0484
Director: Gary Cutting, M.D.
Contact: Barbara Karczeski
E-mail: bkarczes@jhmi.edu
Website: www.hopkinsmedicine.org/
dnadiagnostic

Basal Cell Nevus Syndrome

GeneDx, Inc.
207 Perry Parkway
Gaithersburg, MD 20877
(301) 519-2100; Fax (301) 519-2892
Directors: Sherri Bale, John Compton,
Anne Madalena
E-mail: genedx@genedx.com
Website: www.genedx.com

Yale University School of Medicine
DNA Diagnostics Laboratory
300 George Street
New Haven, CT 06511
(203) 785-2140; Fax (203) 785-6975
Director: Allen Bale, M.D.
E-mail: bale@biomed.med.yale.edu

Beckwith-Wiedemann Syndrome

Baylor College of Medicine
Kleborg Cytogenics Laboratory
2450 Holcombe
Houston, TX 77021-2024
1-800-411-GENE (4363); 713-798-6555;
Fax: 713-798-6584
Director: Sau W. Cheung
E-mail: genetictest@bcm.tmc.edu
Website: www.bcmgeneticlabs.org

Chapman Institute of Medical Genetics
DNA Laboratory
4502 E. 41st Street
Tulsa, OK 74135-2553
(918) 660-3838; (800) 299-7919;
Fax (918) 660-3840
Directors: Nancy Carpenter,
Frederick Schaefer
Contact: Jane Pritchard,
Frederick Schaefer
E-mail: janep@hillcrest.com;
fschaefer@hillcrest.com
Website: www.chapmangenetics.com

Comprehensive Genetic Services
Molecular Diagnostic Services
3720 North 124th Street
Milwaukee, WI 53222
(877)-COMPGENE; (414) 393-1000;
Fax (414) 393-1399
Directors: Anthony Garber, Ph.D.,
Christine Bryke, M.D., FABMG
E-mail: compgene@worldnet.att.net
Website: www.compgene.com

Lab Corp
Research Triangle Park
Center for Molecular Biology and
    Pathology
1912 Alexander Drive
P.O. Box 13973
Research Triangle Park, NC 27709
(919) 361-7700; (800) 533-0567;
    Fax 919-361-7798
Director: Kenneth Friedman, Ph.D.
E-mail: genetics@labcorp.com
Website: www.labcorp.com

Mayo Clinic
Molecular Genetics Laboratory
200 First Street S.W.
Rochester, MN 55905
(800) 533-1710; Fax (507) 284-0670
Directors: Stephen N Thibodeau, Ph.D.;
    D Brian Dawson, Ph.D.;
    W. Edward Highsmith, Ph.D.;
    Kevin Halling, M.D., Ph.D.
Contact: Kelle Steenblock, MS, CGC
Steenblock, MS, CGC
E-mail: gcmolgen@mayo.edu
Website: www.mayoclinic.org/
    laboratorygenetics-rst/molecular.html

Sacred Heart
Cytogenics Laboratory
P.O. Box 2555
Spokane, WA 99220-2555
(509) 474-4414; (509) 474-3328;
    Fax (509) 474-3490
Directors: Julie Hanna, M.S., Ph.D.,
    FACMG, Lisa Shaffer, Ph.D., FACMG
E-mail: hannaj@shmc.org;
    shaffer@shmc.org
Website: www.shmclab.org

Shodair Hospital
Genetics Laboratory
840 Helena Avenue
P.O. Box 5539
Helena, MT 59604
(800)-447-6614; (406) 444-7500;
    Fax (406) 444-1022
Directors: Mary M Haag, Ph.D.;
    John P Johnson, M.D.
Contact: Linda S Beischel, B.S., CLSp(MB)
E-mail: lbeischel@shodair.org

**Washington University School of
    Medicine**
Molecular Diagnostic Laboratory
Main Hematology, Barnes-Jewish
    Hospital
North Campus, Room 2320,
Mail Stop 90-28-372
216 South Kingshighway
St. Louis, MO 63110
(314) 454-7601; Fax (314) 454-8485
Director: Barbara Zehnbauer, Ph.D.,
    FACMG
Contact: Robert Timmerman, M.S.
E-mail: rjt9915@bjc.org

Bloom Syndrome

Baylor College of Medicine
Diagnostic Sequencing Laboratory
2450 Holcombe
Houston, TX 77021-2024

Phone: 713-798-6555
Fax: 713-798-6584
Director: Benjamin Roa
E-mail: genetictest@bcm.tmc.edu
Website: www.bcmgeneticlabs.org/

Boston University School of Medicine
Center for Human Genetics
715 Albany Street, W-4th Floor
Boston, MA 02118
(617) 638-7083; Fax (617) 638-7092
Director: Aubrey Milunsky
E-mail: amilunsk@bu.edu
Website: www.bumc.bu.edu/
    Departments/HomeMain.asp?
    DepartmentID=118

Genzyme Genetics
Molecular Diagnostic Laboratory
3400 Computer Drive
Westborough, MA 01581
800 848 4436; Fax 508 389 5577
Director: Elizabeth Rohlfs, Ph.D., FACMG
Website: www.genzymegenetics.com

Camey Complex

GeneDx, Inc.
207 Perry Parkway
Gaithersburg, M.D. 20877
(301) 519-2100; Fax (301) 519-2892
Directors: Sherri Bale, John Compton,
    Anne Madalena
E-mail: genedx@genedx.com
Website: www.genedx.com

CHILD Syndrome

Kennedy Krieger Institute
Clinical Mass Spectrometry Laboratory
707 North Broadway
Baltimore, MD 21205
(443) 923-2782; Fax (443) 923-2781
Director: Richard I. Kelley, M.D., Ph.D.
Contact: Lisa E. Kratz, Ph.D.
E-mail: kratz@kennedykrieger.org

Chronic Granulomatous Disease

GeneDx, Inc.
207 Perry Parkway
Gaithersburg, MD 20877
(301) 519-2100; Fax (301) 519-2892
Directors: Sherri Bale, John Compton,
    Anne Madalena
E-mail: genedx@genedx.com
Website: www.genedx.com

Congenital Erythropoietic Porphyria (CEP)

Mayo Clinic
Biochemical Genetics Laboratory
200 First Street S.W.
Rochester, MN 55905
(800) 533-1710; (507) 266-1800;
    Fax (507) 284-1759
Directors: Sihoun Hahn, M.D., Ph.D.;
    Dietrich Matern, M.D.; Joseph
    McConnell, Ph.D.; John F. O'Brien,
    Ph.D.; Piero Rinaldo, M.D., Ph.D.
E-mail: biochemicalgenetics@mayo.edu

Conradi-Hünermann Syndrome

Kennedy Krieger Institute
Clinical Mass Spectrometry Laboratory
707 North Broadway
Baltimore, MD 21205
(443) 923-2782; Fax (443) 923-2781
Director: Richard I. Kelley, M.D., Ph.D.
Contact: Lisa E. Kratz, Ph.D.
E-mail: kratz@kennedykrieger.org

Darier Disease

Thomas Jefferson University
Department of Dermatology and
    Cutaneous Biology
Bluemle Life Sciences Building
233 South 10th Street, Suite 450
Philadelphia, PA 19107
(215) 503-5785; Fax (215) 503-5788
Directors: Gabriele Richard and
    Jouni Uitto
Contact: Elaine Pfendner, Ph.D. or
    Gabriele Richard
E-mail: ellen.pfendner@mail.tju.edu,
    gabriele.richard@mail.tju.edu

Down Syndrome

All Children's Hospital
Cytogenetics and Molecular Cytogenetics
    Laboratory
801 6th Street South
St. Petersburg, FL 33701
(727) 767-8559; Fax (727) 767-8315
Director: Maxine J. Sutcliffe, Ph.D.,
    FACMG, FCCMG
E-mail: sutcliff@allkids.org
Contact: Doris P. Dumont, B.S., CLSp(Cg)
E-mail: dumontd@allkids.org

Mayo Clinic
Cytogenetics Laboratory
200 First Street S.W.
Rochester, MN 55905
(507) 538-2952; Fax (507) 284-0043
Directors: Gordon Dewald, Ph.D.;
    Syed Jalal, Ph.D.; Robert B. Jenkins,
    M.D., Ph.D.; Rhett P. Ketterling, M.D.;
    Daniel L. Van Dyke, Ph.D.
Website: www.mayoclinic.org/laboratory
    genetics-rst/cytogenetics.html

Dyskeratosis Congenita

GeneDx, Inc.
207 Perry Parkway
Gaithersburg, MD 20877
(301) 519-2100; Fax (301) 519-2892
Directors: Sherri Bale, John Compton,
    Anne Madalena
E-mail: genedx@genedx.com
Website: www.genedx.com

Ehlers Danlos Syndrome

**University of Washington Health
    Sciences Center**
Collagen Diagnostic Laboratory
Room D518 Health Sciences Building
1959 NE Pacific
Seattle, WA 98195
(206) 543-0459; Fax (206) 616-1899

Director: Peter H. Byers, M.D.
Contact: Barbara Kovacich
E-mail: kovacich@u.washington.edu

ARUP Laboratories
500 Chipeta Way
Salt Lake City, UT 84108-1221
(801) 583-2787; (800) 242-2787;
Fax: (801) 583-2712
Directors: Elaine Lyon, Ph.D.;
Edward R Ashwood, M.D.
Contact: Marzia Pasquali, Ph.D.
E-mail: pasquam@aruplab.com
Website: www.aruplab.com

Emory University
Biochemical Genetics Laboratory
2040 Ridgewood Dr., Lower Level
Atlanta, GA 30322
(404) 727-5782; Fax (404) 727-9398
Director: Chunli Yu, M.D.
Contact: Joyce Marshall
E-mail: jmarshall@genetics.emory.edu
Website: server2k.genetics.emory.edu/
lab/user

Epidermolysis Bullosa Simplex (EBS)
GeneDx, Inc.
207 Perry Parkway
Gaithersburg, MD 20877
(301) 519-2100; Fax (301) 519-2892
Directors: Sherri Bale, John Compton,
Anne Madalena
E-mail: genedx@genedx.com
Website: www.genedx.com

Thomas Jefferson University
Department of Dermatology and
Cutaneous Biology
Bluemle Life Sciences Building
233 South 10th Street, Suite 450
Philadelphia, PA 19107
(215) 503-5785; Fax (215) 503-5788
Directors: Gabriele Richard and
Jouni Uitto
Contact: Elaine Pfendner, Ph.D. or
Gabriele Richard
E-mail: ellen.pfendner@mail.tju.edu,
gabriele.richard@mail.tju.edu

Epidermolytic Hyperkeratosis
GeneDx, Inc.
207 Perry Parkway
Gaithersburg, MD 20877
(301) 519-2100; Fax (301) 519-2892
Directors: Sherri Bale, John Compton,
Anne Madalena
E-mail: genedx@genedx.com
Website: www.genedx.com

Erythrokeratoderma Variabilis

GeneDx, Inc.
207 Perry Parkway
Gaithersburg, MD 20877
(301) 519-2100; Fax (301) 519-2892
Directors: Sherri Bale, John Compton,
Anne Madalena
E-mail: genedx@genedx.com
Website: www.genedx.com

Thomas Jefferson University
Department of Dermatology and
Cutaneous Biology
Bluemle Life Sciences Building
233 South 10th Street, Suite 450
Philadelphia, PA 19107
(215) 503-5785; Fax (215) 503-5788
Directors: Gabriele Richard and
Jouni Uitto
Contact: Elaine Pfendner, Ph.D. or
Gabriele Richard
E-mail: ellen.pfendner@mail.tju.edu,
gabriele.richard@mail.tju.edu

Mount Sinai School of Medicine
Porphyria Laboratory
Center for Jewish Genetic Diseases
One Gustave L. Levy Place
Box 1498
New York, NY 10029
(212) 659-6783; Fax (212) 360-1809
Directors: Robert J. Desnick, M.D., Ph.D.;
Junaid Shabbeer, Ph.D.;
Kenneth H. Astrin, Ph.D.
Contact: Kenneth H. Astrin, Ph.D.
E-mail: kenneth.astrin@mssm.edu

Erythropoietic Protoporphyria (EPP)

Mayo Clinic
Biochemical Genetics Laboratory
200 First Street S.W.
Rochester, MN 55905
(800) 533-1710; (507) 266-1800;
Fax (507) 284-1759
Directors: Sihoun Hahn, M.D., Ph.D.;
Dietrich Matern, M.D.; Joseph
McConnell, Ph.D.; John F. O'Brien,
Ph.D.; Piero Rinaldo, M.D., Ph.D.
E-mail: biochemicalgenetics@mayo.edu

Fabry Disease

Baylor College of Medicine
Biochemical Genetics Laboratory
2450 Holcombe
Houston, TX 77021-2024
(800) 246-2436; Fax (713) 798-6584
Directors: V. Reid Sutton, M.D.,
William E. O'Brien, Ph.D.
Contact: Arthur W. Warman, MS
E-mail: genetictest@bcm.tmc.edu
Website: www.bcmgeneticlabs.org

Emory Biochemical Genetics Laboratory
2040 Ridgewood Drive, Lower Level
Atlanta, GA 30322
(404) 727-5782; Fax (404) 727-9398
Director: Chunli Yu, M.D.
Contact: Joyce Marshall
E-mail: jmarshall@genetics.emory.edu

GeneDx, Inc.
207 Perry Parkway
Gaithersburg, MD 20877
(301) 519-2100; Fax (301) 519-2892
Directors: Sherri Bale, John Compton,
Anne Madalena
E-mail: genedx@genedx.com
Website: www.genedx.com

Mount Sinai School of Medicine
International Center for Fabry Disease
Department of Human Genetics
Box 1498
Fifth Avenue at 100th Street
New York, NY 10029
(212) 659-6783; Fax: (212) 360-1809
Directors: Robert J. Desnick, M.D., Ph.D.;
Marie E. Grace, Ph.D.;
Junaid Shabbeer, Ph.D.
Contact: Kenneth H. Astrin, Ph.D.
E-mail: kenneth.astrin@mssm.edu
Website: www.mssm.edu/genetics/fabry

Familial Dysautonomia

Baylor College of Medicine
Diagnostic Sequencing Laboratory
2450 Holcombe
Houston, TX 77021-2024
(713) 798-6555; Fax (713) 798-6584
Director: Benjamin Roa
E-mail: genetictest@bcm.tmc.edu
Website: www.bcmgeneticlabs.org

Boston University School of Medicine
Center for Human Genetics
715 Albany Street, W-4th Floor
Boston, MA 02118
(617) 638-7083; Fax (617) 638-7092
Director: Aubrey Milunsky
E-mail: amilunsk@bu.edu
Website: www.bumc.bu.edu/
Departments/HomeMain.asp?
DepartmentID=118

Genzyme Genetics
Molecular Diagnostic Laboratory
3400 Computer Drive
Westborough, MA 01581
(800) 848 4436; Fax (508) 389 5577
Director: Elizabeth Rohlfs, Ph.D., FACMG
Website: www.genzymegenetics.com

Gardner Syndrome

Baylor College of Medicine
Diagnostic Sequencing Laboratory
2450 Holcombe
Houston, TX 77021-2024
1-800-411-GENE (4363); (713) 798-6555;
Fax (713) 798-6584
Director: Benjamin Roa
E-mail: genetictest@bcm.tmc.edu
Website: www.bcmgeneticlabs.org

Boston University School of Medicine
Center for Human Genetics
715 Albany Street, W-4th Floor
Boston, MA 02118
(617) 638-7083; Fax (617) 638-7092
Director: Aubrey Milunsky
E-mail: amilunsk@bu.edu
Website: www.bumc.bu.edu/
Departments/HomeMain.asp?
DepartmentID=118

Chapman Institute of Medical Genetics
DNA Laboratory
4502 E. 41st Street
Tulsa, OK 74135-2553
(918) 660-3838; (800) 299-7919;
  Fax (918) 660-3840
Directors: Nancy Carpenter,
  Frederick Schaefer
Contact: Jane Pritchard, Frederick Schaefer
E-mail: janep@hillcrest.com;
  fschaefer@hillcrest.com
Website: www.chapmangenetics.com

Huntington Medical Research Institutes
Molecular Oncology and Cancer Genetics
  Laboratory
99 North El Molino Avenue
Pasadena, CA 91101
(626) 795-4343; Fax (626) 795-5774
Director: Faye A. Eggerding, M.D., Ph.D.,
  FACMG
E-mail: eggerding@hmri.org
Website: home.pacbell.net/genedoc/
  Eggspage.html

Mayo Clinic
Molecular Genetics Laboratory
200 First Street S.W.
Rochester, MN 55905
(800) 533-1710; Fax (507) 284-0670
Directors: Stephen N. Thibodeau, Ph.D.;
  D. Brian Dawson, Ph.D.;
  W. Edward Highsmith, Ph.D.;
  Kevin Halling, M.D., Ph.D.
Contact: Kelle Steenblock, M.S., C.G.C.
E-mail: gcmolgen@mayo.edu
Website: www.mayoclinic.org/
  laboratorygenetics-rst/molecular.html

Memorial Sloan-Kettering Cancer Center
Diagnostic Molecular Genetics
1275 York Avenue
New York, NY 10021
(212) 639-5170; Fax: (212) 717-3571
Directors: Nathan A. Ellis, Ph.D.;
  Khedoudja Nafa, Ph.D.
Contact: Khedoudja Nafa, Ph.D.
E-mail: k-nafa@ski.mskcc.org

Myriad Genetics Laboratory
320 Wakara Way
Salt Lake City, UT 84108
(800) 469-7423 fax: (801) 584-3515
Director: Bryan Ward, Ph.D.
Contact: Client Services
E-mail: brca@myriad.com
Website: www.myriad.com/index.htm

**University of Pennsylvania School of
  Medicine**
The Genetic Diagnostic Laboratory
Department of Genetics
415 Curie Boulevard
Philadelphia, PA 19104-6145
(215) 573-9161; (215) 573-9166;
  Fax (215) 573-5940
Directors: Haig Kazazian, M.D.;
  Arupa Ganguly, Ph.D.
Contact: Lynn Godmilow, M.S.W., C.G.C.
E-mail: godmilow@mail.med.upenn.edu
Website: www.med.upenn.edu/genetics/
  core-facs/gdl

**Washington University School of
  Medicine**
Molecular Diagnostic Laboratory
Main Hematology
Barnes-Jewish Hospital
North Campus, Room 2320,
Mail Stop 90-28-372
216 South Kingshighway
St. Louis, MO 63110
(314) 454-7601; Fax (314) 454-8485
Director: Barbara Zehnbauer, Ph.D.,
  FACMG
Contact: Robert Timmerman, M.S.
E-mail: rjt9915@bjc.org

Gaucher Disease

**Children's Hospital and Regional
  Medical Center**
P.O. Box 5371
Seattle, WA 98105-0371
(206) 987-2216; Fax (206) 987-3840
Director: C. Ronald Scott, M.D.
Contact: Rhona Jack, Ph.D.
E-mail: rhona.jack@seattlechildrens.org

Mount Sinai School of Medicine
Lysosomal Enzymology
Fifth Avenue & 100th Street
New York, NY 10029
(212) 241-6947; Fax (212) 860-3316
Directors: Robert J. Desnick, M.D., Ph.D.;
  Marie E. Grace, Ph.D.
Contact: Administrative Staff

Hartnup Disease

Duke University Medical Center
Pediatric Biochemical Genetics
  Laboratory
P.O. Box 14991
99 Alexander Drive
Research Triangle Park, NC 27709
(919) 549-0445; Fax (919) 549-0709
Directors: David S. Millington, Ph.D.;
  Dwight D. Koeberl, M.D., Ph.D.
E-mail: dmilli@acpub.duke.edu
Website: www.duke.edu/~M.D.feezor/
  dukemedicalgenetics

Greenwood Genetic Center
Metabolic Laboratory
1 Gregor Mendel Circle
Greenwood, SC 29646
(800) 473-9411; (864) 941-8131;
  Fax (864) 941-8133
Directors: Harold A. Taylor, Ph.D.;
  Tim C. Wood, Ph.D.
Contact: Kim Stewart, MT, ASCP
E-mail: kbstewart@ggc.org
Website: www.ggc.org

OHSU Clinical Genetics Laboratory
3181 S.W. Sam Jackson Park Road
Portland, OR 97239-3098
(503) 494-2404; Fax (503) 494-6922
Directors: K. Michael Gibson, Ph.D.,
  FACMG; Cary O. Harding, M.D.,
  FACMG
Contact: Michelle R. Polinsky
E-mail: polinsky@ohsu.edu
Website: www.ohsu.edu/genetics

Yale University School of Medicine
Biochemical Disease Detection Lab
Department of Genetics
P.O. Box 20-8005
New Haven, CT 06520-8005
(203) 785-2662; Fax (203) 785-3535
Directors: Cheryl Lee Garganta, M.D.,
  Ph.D.; Margretta R Seashore, M.D.
Contact: Cheryl Lee Garganta, M.D., Ph.D.
E-mail: biochemical.lab@yale.edu

Hemochromatosis

Baylor College of Medicine
Diagnostic Sequencing Laboratory
2450 Holcombe
Houston, TX 77021-2024
(713) 798-6555; Fax (713) 798-6584
Director: Benjamin Roa
E-mail: genetictest@bcm.tmc.edu
Website: www.bcmgeneticlabs.org

Boston University School of Medicine
Center for Human Genetics
715 Albany Street, W-4th Floor
Boston, MA 02118
(617) 638-7083; Fax (617) 638-7092
Director: Aubrey Milunsky
E-mail: amilunsk@bu.edu
Website: www.bumc.bu.edu/
  Departments/HomeMain.asp?
  DepartmentID=118

Michigan State University
DNA Diagnostic Laboratory
Department of Pediatrics and Human
  Development
College of Human Medicine
B240 Life Science Building
East Lansing, MI 48824-1317
(517) 355-0733; Fax: (517) 353-8464
Director: Sarah H. Elsea, Ph.D., FACMG
Contact: Denise E. Olle
E-mail: denise.olle@ht.msu.edu
Website: www.Ph.D..msu.edu/DNA/
  home.html

*Hepatoerythropoietic Porphyria
(HEP)*

Mayo Clinic
Biochemical Genetics Laboratory
200 First Street S.W.
Rochester, MN 55905
(800) 533-1710; (507) 266-1800;
  Fax: (507) 284-1759
Directors: Sihoun Hahn, M.D., Ph.D.;
  Dietrich Matern, M.D.; Joseph
  McConnell, Ph.D.; John F. O'Brien,
  Ph.D.; Piero Rinaldo, M.D., Ph.D.
E-mail: biochemicalgenetics@mayo.edu

Mount Sinai School of Medicine
Porphyria Laboratory
Center for Jewish Genetic Diseases
One Gustave L. Levy Place
Box 1498
New York, NY 10029
(212) 659-6783; Fax (212) 360-1809

Directors: Robert J. Desnick, M.D., Ph.D.;
Junaid Shabbeer, Ph.D.;
Kenneth H. Astrin, Ph.D.
Contact: Kenneth H. Astrin, Ph.D.
E-mail: kenneth.astrin@mssm.edu

Hereditary Coproporphyria (HCP)

Mayo Clinic
Biochemical Genetics Laboratory
200 First Street S.W.
Rochester, MN 55905
(800) 533-1710; (507) 266-1800;
Fax: (507) 284-1759
Directors: Sihoun Hahn, M.D., Ph.D.;
Dietrich Matern, M.D.; Joseph
McConnell, Ph.D.; John F. O'Brien,
Ph.D.; Piero Rinaldo, M.D., Ph.D.
E-mail: biochemicalgenetics@mayo.edu

Hereditary Hemorrhagic Telangiectasia Syndrome

University of Pennsylvania School of Medicine
The Genetic Diagnostic Laboratory
Department of Genetics
415 Curie Boulevard
Philadelphia, PA 19104-6145
(215) 573-9161; (215) 573-9166
Fax (215) 573-5940
Directors: Haig Kazazian, M.D.;
Arupa Ganguly, Ph.D.
Contact: Lynn Godmilow, M.S.W., C.G.C.
E-mail: godmilow@mail.med.upenn.edu
Website: www.med.upenn.edu/genetics/
core-facs/gdl//

Hermansky-Pudlak Syndrome

GeneDx, Inc.
207 Perry Parkway
Gaithersburg, MD 20877
(301) 519-2100; Fax (301) 519-2892
Directors: Sherri Bale, John Compton,
Anne Madalena
E-mail: genedx@genedx.com
Website: www.genedx.com

University of Colorado School of Medicine
Department of Pediatrics,
Campus Box C-233
4200 East Ninth Avenue
Denver, CO 80262-0233
(303) 315-8415; Fax (303) 315-0349
Director: Elaine Spector, Ph.D.
E-mail: Elaine.spector@uchsc.edu
Website: www.uchsc.edu/sm/peds/
dnalab

Hidrotic Ectodermal Dysplasia

GeneDx, Inc.
207 Perry Parkway
Gaithersburg, MD 20877
(301) 519-2100; Fax (301) 519-2892
Directors: Sherri Bale, John Compton,
Anne Madalena
E-mail: genedx@genedx.com
Website: www.genedx.com

Pachyonychia Congenita

GeneDx, Inc.
207 Perry Parkway
Gaithersburg, MD 20877
(301) 519-2100; Fax (301) 519-2892
Directors: Sherri Bale, John Compton,
Anne Madalena
E-mail: genedx@genedx.com
Website: www.genedx.com

Homocystinuria

Emory Biochemical Genetics Laboratory
2040 Ridgewood Drive, Lower Level
Atlanta, GA 30322
(404) 727-5782; Fax (404) 727-9398
Director: Chunli Yu, M.D.
Contact: Joyce Marshall
E-mail: jmarshall@genetics.emory.edu

Mayo Clinic
Special Coagulation DNA Diagnostic
Laboratory
200 First Street S.W.
Rochester, MN 55905
(507) 266-1341; Fax (507) 284-8286
Directors: John Heit, M.D.;
Rajiv K. Pruthi, M.D.
Contact: Lisa Emiliusen, BA
E-mail: taylor.lisa2@mayo.edu

Quest Diagnostics, Inc.
Nichols Institute
14225 Newbrook Drive
Chantilly, VA 20153
(800) 336-3718; (703) 802-7100;
Fax (703) 802-7130
Director: V.M. Pratt, Ph.D.
Website: www.questdiagnostics.com

Hyperlipoproteinemias

ARUP Laboratories
500 Chipeta Way
Salt Lake City, UT 84108-1221
(801) 583-2787; (800) 242-2787;
Fax: (801) 583-2712
Directors: Elaine Lyon, Ph.D.;
Edward R. Ashwood, M.D.
Contact: Marzia Pasquali, Ph.D.
E-mail: pasquam@aruplab.com
Website: www.aruplab.com

Kimball Genetics
Molecular Genetics Laboratory
101 University Boulevard
Suite 350
Denver, CO 80206
(800) 320-1807; Fax (303) 388-9220
Director: Annette K. Taylor, Ph.D.,
FACMG
Contact: Juli A. Murphy, MS
E-mail: jamurphy@kimballgenetics.com
Website: www.kimballgenetics.com

University of Oklahoma Health Sciences Center
Molecular Pathology Laboratory
Department of Pathology
Biomedical Sciences Building
Rooms 411-417
940 Stanton L. Young Boulevard

Oklahoma City, Oklahoma 73104
(405) 271-5249; Fax (405) 271-2568.
Directors: Michael Talbert, M.D.;
S. Terence Dunn, Ph.D., DABCC
E-mail: michael-talbert@ouhsc.edu;
terry-dunn@ouhsc.edu

Incontinentia Pigmenti

Baylor College of Medicine
Diagnostic Sequencing Laboratory
2450 Holcombe
Houston, TX 77021-2024
(713) 798-6555; Fax (713) 798-6584
Director: Benjamin Roa
E-mail: genetictest@bcm.tmc.edu
Website: www.bcmgeneticlabs.org

Lamellar Ichthyosis

GeneDx, Inc.
207 Perry Parkway
Gaithersburg, MD 20877
(301) 519-2100; Fax (301) 519-2892
Directors: Sherri Bale, John Compton,
Anne Madalena
E-mail: genedx@genedx.com
Website: www.genedx.com

LEOPARD Syndrome

GeneDx, Inc.
207 Perry Parkway
Gaithersburg, MD 20877
(301) 519-2100; Fax (301) 519-2892
Directors: Sherri Bale, John Compton,
Anne Madalena
E-mail: genedx@genedx.com
Website: www.genedx.com

Harvard Partners Center for Genetics and Genomics
Laboratory for Molecular Medicine
65 Landsdowne Street 3rd floor,
Cambridge, MA, 02139-4232
(617) 768-8501; Fax (617) 768-8510
Directors: Raju Kucherlapati, Ph.D., Heidi
Rehm, Ph.D., Mei Peng, M.D., Ph.D.
E-mail: genome@rics.bwh.harvard.edu
Website: www.hpcgg.org/LMM/
index.html

Marfan Syndrome

Chapman Institute of Medical Genetics
DNA Laboratory
4502 E. 41st Street
Tulsa, OK 74135-2553
(918) 660-3838; (800) 299-7919;
Fax (918) 660-3840
Directors: Nancy Carpenter,
Frederick Schaefer
Contact: Jane Pritchard,
Frederick Schaefer
E-mail: janep@hillcrest.com;
fschaefer@hillcrest.com
Website: www.chapmangenetics.com

City of Hope National Medical Center
Clinical Molecular Diagnostic Laboratory
Fox South, Second Floor
1500 East Duarte Road
Duarte, CA 91010
(888) 826-4362; Fax (626) 301-8142

Director: Steve S. Sommer, M.D., Ph.D.
Contact: CM.D.L Client Services
E-mail: cM.D.l@coh.org
Website: www.cityofhope.org/cM.D.l

Comprehensive Genetic Services
Molecular Diagnostic Services
3720 North 124th Street
Milwaukee, WI 53222
(877)-COMPGENE; (414) 393-1000;
    Fax (414) 393-1399
Directors: Anthony Garber, Ph.D.,
    Christine Bryke, M.D., FABMG
E-mail: compgene@worldnet.att.net
Website: www.compgene.com

Johns Hopkins Hospital
DNA Diagnostic Laboratory
CMSC 10-106
600 N. Wolfe Street
Baltimore, M.D. 21287
(410) 955-0483; Fax (410) 955-0484
Director: Gary Cutting, M.D.
Contact: Barbara Karczeski
E-mail: bkarczes@jhmi.edu
Website: www.hopkinsmedicine.org/
    dnadiagnostic

Tulane University Health Sciences Center
Matrix DNA Diagnostic Laboratory
Center for Gene Therapy
J. Bennett Johnston Building
1324 Tulane Avenue, SL-99
New Orleans, LA 70112-2699
(504) 988-7706; Fax (504) 988-7704
Director: Darwin J. Prockop, M.D., Ph.D.
Contact: Charlene Crain, M.B.A., B.S.
E-mail: ccrain@tulane.edu

McCune-Albright Syndrome

Chapman Institute of Medical Genetics
DNA Laboratory
4502 E. 41st Street
Tulsa, OK 74135-2553
(918) 660-3838; (800) 299-7919;
    Fax (918) 660-3840
Directors: Nancy Carpenter, Frederick
    Schaefer
Contact: Jane Pritchard, Frederick
    Schaefer
E-mail: janep@hillcrest.com;
    fschaefer@hillcrest.com
Website: www.chapmangenetics.com

Menkes' Kinky Hair Syndrome

National Institute of Child Health and Human Development, NIH
Unit on Pediatric Genetics
Laboratory of Clinical Genomics
Building 10, Room 9S259
10 Center Drive MSC 1834
Bethesda, MD 20892-1834
(301)496-8368; Fax: (301)402-1073
Director: Stephen G Kaler, M.D., MPH
E-mail: kalers@mail.nih.gov

University of Chicago Genetic Services
5841 S. Maryland Avenue
Room L155, MC 0077
Chicago, IL 60637
(888) UC-GENES; (888) 834-3637;
    (773) 834-0555; Fax (773) 834-0556
Directors: Soma Das, Ph.D.;
    Christa Lese Martin, Ph.D.
E-mail: ucgslabs@genetics.uchicago.edu
Website: genes.uchicago.edu

Mucopolysaccharidoses

Emory Biochemical Genetics Laboratory
2040 Ridgewood Drive, Lower Level
Atlanta, GA 30322
(404) 727-5782; Fax (404) 727-9398
Director: Chunli Yu, M.D.
Contact: Joyce Marshall
E-mail: jmarshall@genetics.emory.edu

Greenwood Genetic Center
Metabolic Laboratory
1 Gregor Mendel Circle
Greenwood, SC 29646
(800) 473-9411; (864) 941-8131;
    Fax (864) 941-8133
Directors: Harold A. Taylor, Ph.D.;
    Tim C. Wood, Ph.D.
Contact: Kim Stewart, M.T., ASCP
E-mail: kbstewart@ggc.org
Website: www.ggc.org

Muir-Torre Syndrome

ARUP Laboratories
500 Chipeta Way
Salt Lake City, UT 84108-1221
(801) 583-2787; (800) 242-2787;
    Fax: (801) 583-2712
Directors: Elaine Lyon, Ph.D.;
    Edward R. Ashwood, M.D.
Contact: Marzia Pasquali, Ph.D.
E-mail: pasquam@aruplab.com
Website: www.aruplab.com

Baylor College of Medicine
Diagnostic Sequencing Laboratory
2450 Holcombe
Houston, TX 77021-2024
1-800-411-GENE (4363); 713-798-6555;
    Fax: 713-798-6584
Director: Benjamin Roa
E-mail: genetictest@bcm.tmc.edu
Website: www.bcmgeneticlabs.org

City of Hope National Medical Center
Clinical Molecular Diagnostic Laboratory
Fox South, Second Floor
1500 East Duarte Road
Duarte, CA 91010
(888) 826-4362; Fax (626) 301-8142
Director: Steve S. Sommer, M.D., Ph.D.
Contact: CM.D.L Client Services
E-mail: cM.D.l@coh.org
Website: www.cityofhope.org/cM.D.l

Huntington Medical Research Institutes
Molecular Oncology and Cancer Genetics
    Laboratory
99 North El Molino Avenue

Pasadena, CA 91101
(626) 795-4343; Fax (626) 795-5774
Director: Faye A. Eggerding, M.D., Ph.D.,
    FACMG
E-mail: eggerding@hmri.org
Website: home.pacbell.net/genedoc/
    Eggspage.html

Mayo Clinic
Molecular Genetics Laboratory
200 First Street S.W.
Rochester, MN 55905
(800) 533-1710; Fax (507) 284-0670
Directors: Stephen N. Thibodeau, Ph.D.;
    D. Brian Dawson, Ph.D.;
    W. Edward Highsmith, Ph.D.;
    Kevin Halling, M.D., Ph.D.
Contact: Kelle Steenblock, M.S., C.G.C.
E-mail: gcmolgen@mayo.edu
Website: www.mayoclinic.org/
    laboratorygenetics-rst/molecular.html

Memorial Sloan-Kettering Cancer Center
Diagnostic Molecular Genetics
1275 York Avenue
New York, NY 10021
(212) 639-5170; Fax: (212) 717-3571
Directors: Nathan A. Ellis, Ph.D.;
    Khedoudja Nafa, Ph.D.
Contact: Khedoudja Nafa, Ph.D.
E-mail: k-nafa@ski.mskcc.org

Myriad Genetics Laboratory
320 Wakara Way
Salt Lake City, UT 84108
(800) 469-7423 fax: (801) 584-3515
Director: Bryan Ward, Ph.D.
Contact: Client Services
E-mail: brca@myriad.com
Website: www.myriad.com/index.htm

Quest Diagnostics, Inc.
Nichols Institute
33608 Ortega Highway
San Juan Capistrano, CA 92690-6130
(800) 553-5445; (949) 728-4279;
    Fax (949) 728-4874
Director: Charles Strom, M.D., Ph.D.
Website: www.questdiagnostics.com

University of Pennsylvania School of Medicine
The Genetic Diagnostic Laboratory
Department of Genetics
415 Curie Boulevard
Philadelphia, PA 19104-6145
(215) 573-9161; (215) 573-9166
    Fax (215) 573-5940
Directors: Haig Kazazian, M.D.;
    Arupa Ganguly, Ph.D.
Contact: Lynn Godmilow, M.S.W., C.G.C.
E-mail: godmilow@mail.med.upenn.edu
Website: www.med.upenn.edu/genetics/
    core-facs/gdl

Multiple Carboxylase Deficiency

Duke University Medical Center
Pediatric Biochemical Genetics
    Laboratory
P.O. Box 14991

99 Alexander Drive
Research Triangle Park, NC 27709
(919) 549-0445; Fax (919) 549-0709
Directors: David S. Millington, Ph.D.;
Dwight D. Koeberl, M.D., Ph.D.
E-mail: dmilli@acpub.duke.edu
Website: www.duke.edu/~M.D.feezor/
dukemedicalgenetics

Pediatrix Screening
P.O. Box 219
Bridgeville, PA 15017
(866) 463-6436; (412) 220-2300;
Fax (412) 220-0784
Directors: Edwin W. Naylor, Ph.D., MPH;
Patricia D. Murphy, Ph.D.;
Donald Chace, Ph.D.
E-mail: pediatrixscreeninginformation
@pediatrix.com
Website: www.pediatrixscreening.com

OHSU Clinical Genetics Laboratories
Biochemical Genetics Laboratory
3181 S.W. Sam Jackson Park Road
Portland, OR 97239-3098
(503) 494-5400; Fax (503) 494-6922
Director: K. Michael Gibson, Ph.D.,
FACMG; Cary O. Harding, M.D.,
FACMG
Contact: Michelle R. Polinsky
E-mail: polinsky@ohsu.edu

Multiple Endocrine Neoplasia Type IIb

All Children's Hospital
Molecular Genetics Laboratory
801 6th Street South
St. Petersburg, FL 33701
(727) 767-8985; Fax: (727) 767-8516
Director: O Thomas Mueller, Ph.D.
E-mail: muellert@allkids.org

Comprehensive Genetic Services
Molecular Diagnostic Services
3720 North 124th Street
Milwaukee, WI 53222
(877)-COMPGENE; (414) 393-1000;
Fax (414) 393-1399
Directors: Anthony Garber, Ph.D.,
Christine Bryke, M.D., FABMG
E-mail: compgene@worldnet.att.net
Website: www.compgene.com

GeneDx, Inc.
207 Perry Parkway
Gaithersburg, MD 20877
(301) 519-2100; Fax (301) 519-2892
Directors: Sherri Bale, John Compton,
Anne Madalena
E-mail: genedx@genedx.com
Website: www.genedx.com

Henry Ford Hospital
DNA Diagnostic Laboratory
2799 W. Grand Boulevard
Detroit, MI 48202
(313) 916-7681; Fax: (313) 916-9476
Director: Kristin G Monaghan, Ph.D.,
FACMG
E-mail: kmonagh1@hfhs.org

Huntington Medical Research Institutes
Molecular Oncology and Cancer Genetics
Laboratory
99 North El Molino Avenue
Pasadena, CA 91101
(626) 795-4343; Fax: (626) 795-5774
Director: Faye A Eggerding, M.D., Ph.D.,
FACMG
E-mail: eggerding@hmri.org
Website: home.pacbell.net/genedoc/
Eggspage.html

Mayo Clinic
Molecular Genetics Laboratory
200 First Street S.W.
Rochester, MN 55905
(800) 533-1710; Fax (507) 284-0670
Directors: Stephen N. Thibodeau, Ph.D.;
D. Brian Dawson, Ph.D.;
W. Edward Highsmith, Ph.D.;
Kevin Halling, M.D., Ph.D.
Contact: Kelle Steenblock, M.S., C.G.C.
E-mail: gcmolgen@mayo.edu
Website: www.mayoclinic.org/
laboratorygenetics-rst/molecular.html

Ohio State University
Molecular Pathology Laboratory
121 Hamilton Hall
1645 Neil Avenue
Columbus, OH 43210
(614) 292-5484; Fax: (614) 292-7072
Director: Thomas W. Prior, Ph.D.,
FACMG
Contact: Thomas W. Prior, Ph.D.,
FACMG; Robert Pilarski, MS
E-mail: prior-1@medctr.osu.edu;
pilarski-1@medctr.osu.edu

Quest Diagnostics, Inc.
Nichols Institute
33608 Ortega Highway
San Juan Capistrano, CA 92690-6130
(800) 553-5445; (949) 728-4279;
Fax (949) 728-4874
Director: Charles Strom, M.D., Ph.D.
Website: www.questdiagnostics.com

All Children's Hospital
Molecular Genetics Laboratory
801 6th Street South
St. Petersburg, FL 33701
(727) 767-8985; Fax: (727) 767-8516
Director: O. Thomas Mueller, Ph.D.
E-mail: muellert@allkids.org

University of Pittsburgh Medical Center
Division of Molecular Genetics
3550 Terrace Street
7th Floor Scaife Hall
Pittsburgh, PA 15213-2500
(412) 383-8741 fax: (412) 383-9594
Director: Jeffrey A. Kant, M.D., Ph.D.
Contact: Laura Janocko, Ph.D.
E-mail: janockole@upmc.edu

**Washington University School of
Medicine**
Molecular Diagnostic Laboratory
Main Hematology
Barnes-Jewish Hospital

North Campus
Room 2320
Mail Stop 90-28-372
216 South Kingshighway
St. Louis, MO 63110
(314) 454-7601; Fax: (314) 454-8485
Director: Barbara Zehnbauer, Ph.D.,
FACMG
Contact: Robert Timmerman, M.S.
E-mail: rjt9915@bjc.org

Netherton Syndrome

Thomas Jefferson University
Department of Dermatology and
Cutaneous Biology
Bluemle Life Sciences Building
233 South 10th Street
Suite 450
Philadelphia, PA 19107
(215) 503-5785; Fax (215) 503-5788
Directors: Gabriele Richard and
Jouni Uitto
Contact: Elaine Pfendner, Ph.D. or
Gabriele Richard
E-mail: ellen.pfendner@mail.tju.edu,
gabriele.richard@mail.tju.edu

Neurofibromatosis I

Baylor College of Medicine
Kleborg Cytogenics Laboratory
2450 Holcombe
Houston, TX 77021-2024
1-800-411-GENE (4363); 713-798-6555;
Fax: 713-798-6584
Director: Sau W. Cheung
E-mail: genetictest@bcm.tmc.edu
Website: www.bcmgeneticlabs.org

Boston University School of Medicine
Center for Human Genetics
715 Albany Street, W-4th Floor
Boston, MA 02118
(617) 638-7083; Fax (617) 638-7092
Director: Aubrey Milunsky
E-mail: amilunsk@bu.edu
Website: www.bumc.bu.edu/

Brigham and Women's Hospital
BWH Cytogenics Laboratory
75 Francis Street
Amory Building
3rd Floor, Room #151
Boston, MA 02115
617-732-7981; Fax 617-975-0945
Director: Cynthia Morton, Ph.D.
E-mail: cytogenetics@partners.org
Website: www.brighamandwomens.org/
cytogenetics/default.asp

Comprehensive Genetic Services
Molecular Diagnostic Services
3720 North 124th Street
Milwaukee, WI 53222
(877)-COMPGENE; (414) 393-1000;
Fax (414) 393-1399
Directors: Anthony Garber, Ph.D.,
Christine Bryke, M.D., FABMG
E-mail: compgene@worldnet.att.net
Website: www.compgene.com

Johns Hopkins Hospital
DNA Diagnostic Laboratory
CMSC 10-106
600 N. Wolfe Street
Baltimore, MD 21287
(410) 955-0483; Fax (410) 955-0484
Director: Gary Cutting, M.D.
Contact: Barbara Karczeski
E-mail: bkarczes@jhmi.edu
Website: www.hopkinsmedicine.org/
dnadiagnostic

Lab Corp
Research Triangle Park
Center for Molecular Biology and
Pathology
1912 Alexander Drive
P.O. Box 13973
Research Triangle Park, NC 27709
919-361-7700; 800-533-0567;
Fax 919-361-7798
Director: Kenneth Friedman, Ph.D.
E-mail: genetics@labcorp.com
Website: www.labcorp.com

Sacred Heart
Cytogenics Laboratory
P.O. Box 2555
Spokane, WA 99220-2555
(509) 474-4414; (509) 474-3328;
Fax (509) 474-3490
Directors: Julie Hanna, M.S., Ph.D.,
FACMG, Lisa Shaffer, Ph.D., FACMG
E-mail: hannaj@shmc.org;
shaffer@shmc.org
Website: www.shmclab.org

University of Alabama at Birmingham
Medical Genomics Laboratory
Department of Genetics
Kaul 420
1530 3rd Avenue South
Birmingham, AL 35294-0024
(205) 996-2915; Fax (205) 996-2929
Director: Bruce Korf, M.D., Ph.D.
Contact: Ludwine Messiaen, Ph.D.
E-mail: lmessiaen@genetics.uab.edu

**University of Washington Medical
Center**
Genetics Lab
Clinical Lab, Room NW 220
University of Washington Medical Center
1959 NE Pacific Street
Seattle, WA 98195-7110
(206) 598-6429; Fax (206) 598-0304
Directors: Karen Stephens, Ph.D.,
Jonathan Tait, M.D., Ph.D.
Contact: Deborah Barden, Ph.D.
E-mail: barden@u.washington.edu
Website: depts.washington.edu/labweb

Neurofibromatosis II

Athena Diagnostics
Four Biotech Park
377 Plantation Street
Worcester, MA 01605
1-800-394-4493 or 1-508-756-2886;
Fax: 508-753-5601
Director: William Seltzer, Ph.D.,
FACMG

E-mail: genetics@athenadiagnostics.com
Website: www.athenadiagnostics.com/
site/content/index.asp

Massachusetts General Hospital
Neurogenetics DNA Diagnostic
Laboratory
149 13th Street, Room #6311
Charlestown, MA 02129
(617) 726-5721; Fax (617) 724-9620
Directors: Katherine Sims, M.D.,
Winnie Xin, Ph.D.
Contact: Jean Marie Danells
E-mail: jdanells@partners.org
Website: www.dnalab.org

Niemann-Pick Disease

Mayo Clinic
Biochemical Genetics Laboratory
200 First Street S.W.
Rochester, MN 55905
(800) 533-1710; (507) 266-1800;
Fax (507) 284-1759
Directors: Sihoun Hahn, M.D., Ph.D.;
Dietrich Matern, M.D.;
Joseph McConnell, Ph.D.;
John F. O'Brien, Ph.D.;
Piero Rinaldo, M.D., Ph.D.
E-mail: biochemicalgenetics@mayo.edu

Thomas Jefferson University
Lysosomal Diseases Testing Laboratory
Department of Neurology
1020 Locust Street
Room 394
Philadelphia, PA 19107
(215) 955-4923; Fax (215) 955-9554
Director: David Wenger, Ph.D.
E-mail: david.wenger@mail.tju.edu
Website: www.tju.edu/lysolab

Noonan Syndrome

Baylor College of Medicine
Diagnostic Sequencing Laboratory
2450 Holcombe
Houston, TX 77021-2024
(713) 798-6555; Fax (713) 798-6584
Director: Benjamin Roa
E-mail: genetictest@bcm.tmc.edu
Website: www.bcmgeneticlabs.org

GeneDx, Inc.
207 Perry Parkway
Gaithersburg, MD 20877
(301) 519-2100; Fax (301) 519-2892
Directors: Sherri Bale, John Compton,
Anne Madalena
E-mail: genedx@genedx.com
Website: www.genedx.com

Mount Sinai School of Medicine
Department of Human Genetics
New York, NY
(212) 241-6947; Fax (212) 860-3316
Director: Bruce D. Gelb, M.D.,
Ruth Kornreich, Ph.D.
Contact: Randi Zinberg, M.S., C.G.C.
E-mail: randi.zinberg@mssm.edu
Website: www.mssm.edu/genetics

Osteogenesis Imperfecta

**Tulane University Health Sciences
Center**
Matrix DNA Diagnostic Laboratory
Tulane Center for Gene Therapy
J. Bennett Johnston Building
1324 Tulane Avenue, SL-99
New Orleans, LA 70112-2699
(504) 988-7706; Fax: (504) 988-7704
Director: Darwin J. Prockop, M.D., Ph.D.
Contact: Charlene Crain, M.B.A., B.S.
E-mail: ccrain@tulane.edu

**University of Washington Health
Sciences Center**
Collagen Diagnostic Laboratory
Room D518 Health Sciences Building
1959 NE Pacific
Seattle, WA 98195
(206) 543-0459; Fax (206) 616-1899
Director: Peter H. Byers, M.D.
Contact: Barbara Kovacich
E-mail: kovacich@u.washington.edu

Peutz-Jeghers Syndrome

GeneDx, Inc.
207 Perry Parkway
Gaithersburg, MD 20877
(301) 519-2100; Fax (301) 519-2892
Directors: Sherri Bale, John Compton,
Anne Madalena
E-mail: genedx@genedx.com
Website: www.genedx.com

Ohio State University
Molecular Pathology Laboratory
121 Hamilton Hall
1645 Neil Avenue
Columbus, OH 43210
(614) 292-5484; Fax: (614) 292-7072
Director: Thomas W. Prior, Ph.D., FACMG
Contact: Thomas W. Prior, Ph.D.,
FACMG; Robert Pilarski, M.S.
E-mail: prior-1@medctr.osu.edu; pilarski-
1@medctr.osu.edu

Phenylketonuria

Boston University School of Medicine
Center for Human Genetics
715 Albany Street, W-4th Floor
Boston, MA 02118
(617) 638-7083; Fax (617) 638-7092
Director: Aubrey Milunsky
E-mail: amilunsk@bu.edu
Website: www.bumc.bu.edu/
Departments/HomeMain.asp?
DepartmentID=118

Clinic for Special Children
535 Bunker Hill Road
Strasburg, PA 17579
(717) 687-9407; Fax (717) 687-9237
Director: Erik G. Puffenberger, Ph.D.
Website: www.clinicforspecialchildren.org

ProGene, Inc.
University Children's Genetic Laboratory
4546 Sunset Boulevard
Mailstop 11

Los Angeles, CA 90027
(213) 381-2999; Fax (213) 381-6599
Director: Toni R. Prezant, Ph.D.
Contact: T. Tran, M.D., Ph.D.
E-mail: ucgl@progene.us

Porphyria Cutanea Tarda

Mayo Clinic
Biochemical Genetics Laboratory
200 First Street S.W.
Rochester, MN 55905
(800) 533-1710; (507) 266-1800;
Fax (507) 284-1759
Directors: Sihoun Hahn, M.D., Ph.D.;
Dietrich Matern, M.D.; Joseph
McConnell, Ph.D.; John F. O'Brien,
Ph.D.; Piero Rinaldo, M.D., Ph.D.
E-mail: biochemicalgenetics@mayo.edu

Mount Sinai School of Medicine
Porphyria Laboratory
Center for Jewish Genetic Diseases
One Gustave L. Levy Place
Box 1498
New York, NY 10029
(212) 659-6783; Fax (212) 360-1809
Directors: Robert J. Desnick, M.D., Ph.D.;
Junaid Shabbeer, Ph.D.;
Kenneth H. Astrin, Ph.D.
Contact: Kenneth H. Astrin, Ph.D.
E-mail: kenneth.astrin@mssm.edu

Progeria

The Progeria Research Foundation
P.O. Box 3453
Peabody, MA 01961-3453
(978) 535-2594; Fax: (508) 543-0377
Director: Leslie B. Gordon, M.D., Ph.D.
E-mail: lbgM.D.Ph.D.@aol.com
Website: www.progeriaresearch.org

**University of Colorado School of
Medicine**
Department of Pediatrics, Campus Box
C-233
4200 East Ninth Avenue
Denver, CO 80262-0233
(303) 315-8415; Fax (303) 315-0349
Director: Elaine Spector, Ph.D.
E-mail: Elaine.spector@uchsc.edu
Website: www.uchsc.edu/sm/peds/
dnalab

Richner-Hanhart Syndrome

Emory Biochemical Genetics Laboratory
2040 Ridgewood Dr., Lower Level
Atlanta, GA 30322
(404) 727-5782; Fax (404) 727-9398
Director: Chunli Yu, M.D.
Contact: Joyce Marshall
E-mail: jmarshall@genetics.emory.edu

Massachusetts General Hospital
Amino Acid Disorder (Neurochemistry)
Lab
Charlestown Navy Yard
Bldg 149, 13th Street, 6th floor room 6310
Boston, MA 02129
(617) 726-3884; Fax (617) 726-5739
Director: Vivian E. Shih, M.D.

Contact: Roseann Mandell
E-mail: rmandell@partners.org

Mayo Clinic
Biochemical Genetics Laboratory
200 First Street S.W.
Rochester, MN 55905
(800) 533-1710; (507) 266-1800;
Fax: (507) 284-1759
Directors: Sihoun Hahn, M.D., Ph.D.;
Dietrich Matern, M.D.;
Joseph McConnell, Ph.D.;
John F. O'Brien, Ph.D.;
Piero Rinaldo, M.D., Ph.D.
E-mail: biochemicalgenetics@mayo.edu

Pediatrix Screening
P.O. Box 219
Bridgeville, PA 15017
(866) 463-6436; (412) 220-2300;
Fax (412) 220-0784
Directors: Edwin W. Naylor, Ph.D.,
M.P.H.; Patricia D. Murphy, Ph.D.;
Donald Chace, Ph.D.
E-mail: pediatrixscreeninginformation@
pediatrix.com
Website: www.pediatrixscreening.com

OHSU Clinical Genetics Laboratories
Biochemical Genetics Laboratory/
3181 S.W. Sam Jackson Park Road
Portland, Oregon 97239-3098
Phone: (503) 494-5400; Fax (503) 494-6922
Director: K. Michael Gibson, Ph.D.,
FACMG; Cary O. Harding, M.D.,
FACMG
Contact: Michelle R. Polinsky
E-mail: polinsky@ohsu.edu

Stanford University Medical Center
Biochemical Genetics Laboratory
300 Pasteur Drive, H-315
Palo Alto, CA 94304
(650) 723-6858; Fax (650) 498-4555
Director: Tina M Cowan, Ph.D.
E-mail: tcowan@stanford.edu

Yale University School of Medicine
Biochemical Disease Detection Lab
Department of Genetics
P.O. Box 20-8005
New Haven, CT 06520-8005
(203) 785-2662; Fax (203) 785-3535
Directors: Cheryl Lee Garganta, M.D.,
Ph.D.; Margretta R Seashore, M.D.
E-mail: Biochemical.lab@yale.edu

Rubinstein-Taybi Syndrome

Baylor College of Medicine
Kleborg Cytogenics Laboratory
2450 Holcombe
Houston, TX 77021-2024
1-800-411-GENE (4363); (713) 798-6555;
Fax (713) 798-6584
Director: Sau W. Cheung
E-mail: genetictest@bcm.tmc.edu
Website: www.bcmgeneticlabs.org

Brigham and Women's Hospital
BWH Cytogenics Laboratory
75 Francis Street
Amory Building
3rd Floor, Room #151
Boston, MA 02115
(617) 732-7981; Fax (617) 975-0945
Director: Cynthia Morton, Ph.D.
E-mail: cytogenetics@partners.org
Website: www.brighamandwomens.org/
cytogenetics/default.asp

Case Western Reserve University
Center for Human Genetics Laboratory
11100 Euclid Avenue
Cleveland, OH 44106
(216) 983-1134; Fax (216) 983-1144
Director: Stuart Schwartz, Ph.D., FACMG
Contact: Tom Oravec
E-mail: tom.oravec@uhhs.com

Sacred Heart
Cytogenics Laboratory
P.O. Box 2555
Spokane, WA 99220-2555
(509) 474-4414; (509) 474-3328;
Fax (509) 474-3490
Directors: Julie Hanna, M.S., Ph.D.,
FACMG, Lisa Shaffer, Ph.D., FACMG
E-mail: hannaj@shmc.org;
shaffer@shmc.org
Website: www.shmclab.org

Russell-Silver Syndrome

LabCorp
Clinical Cytogenetics Laboratory
Research Triangle Park, NC
(800) 345-4363; Fax (919) 361-7755
Directors: Inder K. Gadi, Ph.D.;
Peter R. Papenhausen, Ph.D.;
Pal Singh-Kahlon, Ph.D.;
James Tepperberg, Ph.D.;
Eduardo S. Cantu, Ph.D.
Contact: Peter R. Papenhausen, Ph.D.;
James Tepperberg, Ph.D.
E-mail: papenhp@labcorp.com;
tepperj@labcorp.com

Mayo Clinic
Molecular Genetics Laboratory
200 First Street S.W.
Rochester, MN 55905
(800) 533-1710; Fax (507) 284-0670
Directors: Stephen N. Thibodeau, Ph.D.;
D. Brian Dawson, Ph.D.;
W. Edward Highsmith, Ph.D.;
Kevin Halling, M.D., Ph.D.
Contact: Kelle Steenblock, M.S., C.G.C.
E-mail: gcmolgen@mayo.edu
Website: www.mayoclinic.org/
laboratorygenetics-rst/molecular.html

University of Chicago
University of Chicago Genetic Services
5841 S. Maryland Avenue
Room L155, MC 0077
Chicago, IL 60637
(888) UC-GENES or (888) 834-3637;
(773) 834-0555; Fax (773) 834-0556
Directors: Soma Das, Ph.D.;
Christa Lese Martin, Ph.D.
E-mail: ucgslabs@genetics.uchicago.edu
Website: genes.uchicago.edu

Severe Combined Immunodeficiency

GeneDx, Inc.
207 Perry Parkway
Gaithersburg, M.D. 20877
(301) 519-2100; Fax (301) 519-2892
Directors: Sherri Bale, John Compton,
 Anne Madalena
E-mail: genedx@genedx.com
Website: www.genedx.com

Cincinnati Children's Hospital Medical Center
Molecular Genetics Laboratory
Children's Hospital Research Foundation
 building, Room 1040
3333 Burnet Avenue,
Cincinnati, OH 45229-3039
(513) 636-4474; Fax (513) 636-4373
Director: Richard Wenstrup, M.D.
Contact: Judith Johnson, M.S.;
 Thedia Watren
E-mail: moleculargenetics@cchmc.org

National Institutes of Health
Section of Immunological Genetics
Building 49, Room 4A14
49 Convent Drive, MSC 4442
Bethesda, MD 20892-4442
(301) 402-0911; Fax: (301) 402-2218
Director: Jennifer Puck, M.D.
Website: www.scid.net/nih.html

Sjögren-Larsson Syndrome

GeneDx, Inc.
207 Perry Parkway
Gaithersburg, MD 20877
(301) 519-2100; Fax (301) 519-2892
Directors: Sherri Bale, John Compton,
 Anne Madalena
E-mail: genedx@genedx.com
Website: www.genedx.com

Tuberous Sclerosis

Athena Diagnostics
Four Biotech Park
377 Plantation Street
Worcester, MA 01605
1-800-394-4493 or 1-508-756-2886;
 Fax: 508-753-5601
Director: William Seltzer, Ph.D., FACMG
E-mail: genetics@athenadiagnostics.com
Website: www.athenadiagnostics.com/
 site/content/index.asp

Massachusetts General Hospital
Neurogenetics DNA Diagnostic
 Laboratory
149 13th Street, Room #6311
Charlestown, MA 02129
(617) 726-5721; Fax (617) 724-9620
Directors: Katherine Sims, M.D.,
 Winnie Xin, Ph.D.
Contact: Jean Marie Danells
E-mail: jdanells@partners.org
Website: www.dnalab.org

University of Washington Medical Center

Genetics Lab
Clinical Lab, Room NW 220
University of Washington Medical Center
1959 NE Pacific Street
Seattle, WA 98195-7110
(206) 598-6429; Fax (206) 598-0304
Directors: Karen Stephens, Ph.D.,
 Jonathan Tait, M.D., Ph.D.
Contact: Deborah Barden, Ph.D.
E-mail: barden@u.washington.edu
Website: depts.washington.edu/labweb

Variegate Porphyria (VP)

Mayo Clinic
Biochemical Genetics Laboratory
200 First Street S.W.
Rochester, MN 55905
(800) 533-1710; (507) 266-1800;
 Fax: (507) 284-1759
Directors: Sihoun Hahn, M.D., Ph.D.;
 Dietrich Matern, M.D.; Joseph
 McConnell, Ph.D.; John F. O'Brien,
 Ph.D.; Piero Rinaldo, M.D., Ph.D.
E-mail: biochemicalgenetics@mayo.edu

Vohwinkel Syndrome

GeneDx, Inc.
207 Perry Parkway
Gaithersburg, MD 20877
(301) 519-2100; Fax (301) 519-2892
Directors: Sherri Bale, John Compton,
 Anne Madalena
E-mail: genedx@genedx.com
Website: www.genedx.com

University of Iowa
Molecular Otolaryngology Research
 Laboratories
Department of Otolaryngology
200 Hawkins Drive
21151 PFP
Iowa City, IA 52242
(319) 335-7997; Fax (319) 353-5869
Director: Richard Smith, M.D.
Contact: Carla Nishimura or
 Sai D. Prasad, B.S.
E-mail: carla-nishimura@uiowa.edu,
 sai-prasad@uiowa.edu

Von Hippel-Lindau Syndrome

Boston University School of Medicine
Center for Human Genetics
715 Albany Street, W-4th Floor
Boston, MA 02118
(617) 638-7083; Fax (617) 638-7092
Director: Aubrey Milunsky
E-mail: amilunsk@bu.edu
Website: www.bumc.bu.edu/
 Departments/HomeMain.asp?
 DepartmentID=118

Johns Hopkins Hospital

DNA Diagnostic Laboratory
CMSC 10-106
600 N. Wolfe Street
Baltimore, MD 21287
(410) 955-0483; Fax (410) 955-0484
Director: Gary Cutting, M.D.
Contact: Barbara Karczeski
E-mail: bkarczes@jhmi.edu
Website: www.hopkinsmedicine.org/
 dnadiagnostic

The Children's Hospital of Philadelphia

Molecular Genetics Laboratory
Abramson Research Center 1106F
34th & Civic Center Boulevard
Philadelphia, PA 19104
(215) 590-8736, (800) 669-2172;
 Fax: (215) 590-2156
Director: Catherine A. Stolle, Ph.D.
Contact: Raymond Colliton, M.S.
E-mail: colliton@email.chop.edu

Waardenburg Syndrome

Boston University School of Medicine
Center for Human Genetics
715 Albany Street, W-4th Floor
Boston, MA 02118
(617) 638-7083; Fax (617) 638-7092
Director: Aubrey Milunsky
E-mail: amilunsk@bu.edu
Website: www.bumc.bu.edu/

Wilson's Disease

Boston University School of Medicine
Center for Human Genetics
715 Albany Street, W-4th Floor
Boston, MA 02118
(617) 638-7083; Fax (617) 638-7092
Director: Aubrey Milunsky
E-mail: amilunsk@bu.edu
Website: www.bumc.bu.edu/
 Departments/HomeMain.asp?
 DepartmentID=118

Wiskott-Aldrich Syndrome

Cincinnati Children's Hospital Medical Center
Molecular Genetics Laboratory
Children's Hospital Research Foundation
 building, Room 1040
3333 Burnet Avenue,
Cincinnati, OH 45229-3039
(513) 636-4474; Fax (513) 636-4373
Director: Richard Wenstrup, M.D.
Contact: Judith Johnson, MS;
 Thedia Watren
E-mail: moleculargenetics@cchmc.org

Figure Credits

1. Marc E. Grossman MD, New York, New York
2. Heiko Traupe, MD, Munster, Germany
3. KP Steuhl, MD, Tubingen, Germany. Reproduced with permission from Steuhl KP, Anton-Lamprecht I, Arnold ML, et al. Recurrent bilateral corneal erosions due to an association of epidermolysis bullosa simplex Kobner and X-linked ichthyosis with steroid sulfatase deficiency: Graefe's. *Arch Clin Exp Ophthalmol* 1988;226:216–233, figures 3A and 4.
4. Lawrence A. Schachner, MD, Miami, Florida
5. Department of Dermatology, Columbia University, New York, New York
6. Tor Shwayder, MD, Detroit, Michigan. Reproduced with permission from Shwayder T, Ott F. All about ichthyosis. *Pediatr Clin North Am* 1991;38:835–857, figure 6.
7. Frances Lawlor, MD, London, England
8. Reproduced with permission from Levisohn D, Dintiman B, Rizzo WB. Sjogren-Larsson syndrome: case reports. *Pediatr Dermatol* 1991;8:217–220, figure 1.
9. Reproduced with permission from Ghadially R, Chong LP. Ichthyoses and hyperkeratotic disorders. *Dermatol Clin* 1992;10:597–607, figure 3.
10. Reproduced with permission from Ghadially R, Chong LP. Ichthyoses and hyperkeratotic disorders. *Dermatol Clin* 1992;10:597–607, figure 5.
11. DA Burns, MD, Leicester, England. Reproduced with permission from Shuttleworth D, Burns DA. Chondrodysplasia punctata-Conradi-Hunermann type. *Clin Exp Dermatol* 1986;11:73–78, figure 1.
12. Pr G. Lorette, Tours, France. Reproduced with permission from Lorette Pr. Chondrodysplasie ponctuee dominante liee a l'x: manifestations neonatales. *Ann Dermatol Venereol* 1991;118:773–775, figure 6h.
13. Adelaide A. Herbert, MD, Houston, Texas and Nancy Esterly, MD, Milwaukee, Wisconsin
13a. Shin-ich Ansai, MD, Akita, Japan
14. Vincenzo Navarro, MD, and Stefano Cambiaghi, MD, Center for Inherited Skin Diseases, University of Milan, Milan, Italy
15. Reproduced with permission from Griffiths WAD, Leigh IM, Judge MR. Disorders of Keratinization. In: Rook A, Wilkinson DS, Ebling FJG, eds. *Textbook of Dermatology*. Oxford: Blackwell Scientific, 1972:1325–1390, figure 30.39.
16. Reproduced with permission from Schnyder UW. Inherited keratodermas of palms and soles. In: Fitzpatrick TB, Arthur Z. Eisen, Klaus Wolff, et al, eds. *Dermatology in General Medicine*, 4th ed. New York: McGraw-Hill, 1993:557–564, figure 46–1b.
17. Julia P. Ellis, FRCP DCH, Swindon, England
18. Reproduced with permission from Peris K, Salvati EF, Torlone G, Chimenti S. Keratoderma hereditarium mutilans (Vohwinkel's Syndrome) associated with congenital deaf-mutism. *Br J Dermatol* 1995;132:617–620, figure 2.
19. Sharon Raimer, MD, Galveston, Texas
20. Gilles G. Lestringant, MD, Abu Dhabi, United Arab Emirates
21. Richard Gibbs, MD, New York, New York
22. Nicola Balato, MD, Napoli, Italy
23. Nicola Balato, MD, Napoli, Italy. Reproduced with permission from Balato N, Cusano F, Lembo G. Tyrosinemia type II in two cases previously reported as Richner-Hanhart syndrome. *Dermatologica* 1986;173:66–74, figure 3.
24. Reproduced with permission from Pehamberger H, Honigsmann H, Wolff K. Dysplastic nevus syndrome with multiple primary amelanotic melanomas in oculocutaneous albinism. *J Am Acad Dermatol* 1984;11:731–735, figures 1 and 2
25. Neal Gregory, MD, New York, New York
26. Reproduced with permission from Witkop CJ, Babcock, MN, Rao GHR, et al Albinism and Hermansky Pudlak syndrome in Puerto Rico. *Bol Asoc Med P R* 1990;82:333–339, figure 1.
27. Lawrence Anderson, MD, San Antonio, Texas
28. From Mancini AJ, Chan LW, Paller AS. Partial albinism with immunodeficiency: Griscelli syndrome: report of a case and review of the literature. *JAAD* 1998;38:295–300.
29. Ingrid Winship, MBchB, MD, Cape Town, South Africa
30. Reproduced with permission from Zitelli BJ, Davis HW, eds. *Atlas of Pediatric Physical Diagnosis*, 2nd ed. Gower Medical Publishing: New York, 1993; figure 10.26.
31. Maria Garzon, MD, New York, New York
32. J Aidan Carney, MD, Rochester, Minnesota. Reproduced with permission from Carney JA, Gordon H, Carpenter PC, et al. The complex of myxomas, spotty pigmentation, and endocrine overactivity. Medicine 1985;64:270, figures 1A and 4A.
33. Pediatric Radiology Department, Columbia-Presbyterian Medical Center, New York, New York
34. Lawrence Gordon, MD, New York, New York
35. Reproduced with permission from Resnick SD. Pediatric dermatology. In: Odom RB, ed. *Dermatology Board Review*. New York: Jarcom Inc., 1993.
36. Allen D. Elster, MD, Winston-Salem, North Carolina. Reproduced with permission from Pont MS, Elster AD. Lesions of skin and brain: modern imaging of the neurocutaneous syndromes. *AJR Am J Roentgenol* 1992;158:1193–1203, figures 1B, 7B, 12.
37. John Walczyk, MD, New York, New York
38. Allen D. Elster, MD, Winston-Salem, North Carolina
39. Jean L. Bologna, MD, New Haven, Connecticut. Reproduced with permission from Park S, Albert DM, Bolognia JL. Ocular manifestations of pigmentary disorders. *Dermatol Clin* 1992;10:609–622, figure 10h.
40. Reproduced with permission from Mulliken JB, Young AE. *Vascular Birthmarks*. Philadelphia: W.B. Saunders, 1988, figure 14.20A.
41. Tom Jessen, MD, Applegate, California. Reproduced with permission from Jessen RT, Thompson S, Smith EB. Cobb Syndrome. *Arch Dermatol* 1977;113:1587–1590, figure 1.
42. Reproduced with permission from Koos WT, Spetzler RF, Pendl G, et al. *Color Atlas of Microneurosurgery*. New York: Thieme Medical Pub, Inc.,1985, figure 395a.
43. Jacques Zeller, MD, and Pr J. Revuz, Creteil, France. Reproduced with permission from Zeller, J, Hovnanian A, Raulo Y, et al. Un cas de syndrome protee. *Ann Dermatol Venereol* 1991;118:786–787, figure 2.
44. Stephen J. Stricker, MD, Miami, Florida
45. M. Michael Cohen Jr, MD, Halifax, Nova Scotia, Canada. Reproduced with permission from Cohen MM Jr. A comprehensive and critical assessment of overgrowth and overgrowth syndromes. *Adv Hum Genet* 1989;18:181–303, 373–376, figure 7.
46. M. Michael Cohen Jr, MD, Hailfax, Nova Scotia, Canada
47. AT Moore, MA, FRCS, FRCOphth., Cambridge, England. Reproduced with permission from Moore AT, Maher ER, Rosen P, et al. Ophthalmological screening for von Hippel-Lindau Disease. *Eye* 1991;5:723–728, figure 3a.
48. Gregory Pastores, MD, New York, New York
48a. Pr. Jacques Remy, Lille, France.
49. Reproduced with permission from Tan OT. *Management and Treatment of Benign Cutaneous Vascular Lesions*. Philadelphia: Lea and Febiger, 1992, figure 1-17.
50. Paul Steven Collins, MD, St. Petersburg, Florida. Reproduced with permission from Collins PS, Han W, Williams LR, et al. Maffucci's syndrome (hemangiomatosis osteolytica): a report of four cases. *J Vasc Surg* 1992;16:364–371, figure 4.
51. Reproduced with permission from Tan OT. *Management and Treatment of Benign Cutaneous Vascular Lesions*. Philadelphia: Lea and Febiger, 1992, figure 12-12A.

52. Steven H. Gallo, MD, Louisville, Kentucky
53. Yoshihiko Nishimura M.D., Kyoto, Japan. Reproduced with permission from Seo W, Kishimoto M, Minato T, Nishimura Y. Submandibular hemangioma as the initial manifestation of Kasabach-Merritt Syndrome. *Int J Pediatr Otorhinolaryngol* 1993;25:269–276, figure 2.
54. Reproduced with permission from Metry DW, Dowd CF, Barkovich AJ, Frieden IJ. The many faces of PHACE Syndrome. *J Pediatr* 2001;139:117–123, figures 1 and 3.
55. Bernice R. Krafchik, MD, Toronto, Canada. Reproduced with permission from Mallory SB, Krafchik BR. What Syndrome is This? Ehlers-Danlos Syndrome. *Pediatr Dermatol* 1991;8:348–351, figures 1 and 2.
56. Pierre Soucy, MD, Ottawa, Canada. Reproduced with permission from Soucy P, Eidus L, Keeley F. Perforation of the colon in a 15-year-old-girl with Ehlers-Danlos Syndrome Type IV. *J Ped Surg* 1990;25:1180–1182, figure 1.
57. Toshiyuki Takahashi, MD, Tokyo, Japan. Reproduced with permission from Takahashi T, Koide T, Yamaguchi H, et al. Ehlers-Danlos with aortic regurgitation, dilation of the sinuses of Valsalva, and abnormal dermal collagen fibrils. *Am Heart J* 1992;123:1709, figure 1B.
58. Reproduced with permission from Rothe MJ, Grant-Kels JM, Kels BD. Ocular and cutaneous manifestations of heritable disorders of collagen and elastic tissue. *Dermatol Clin* 1992;10:591, figure 1.
59. Reproduced with permission from Nahas FX, Sterman S, Gemperli R, Ferreira MC. The role of plastic surgery in congenital cutis laxa-a 10 year follow-up. *Plast Reconstr Surg* 1999;104:1174–1178.
60. David A. Hanscom, MD, Seattle, Washington and Gillette Children's Hospital, St. Paul, Minnesota
61. Sarah Woodrow, MD, Suffolk, England. Reproduced with permission from Woodrow SL, Pope FM, Handfield-Jones SE. The Buschke-Ollendorff Syndrome presenting as familial elastic tissue naevi. *Br J Dermatol* 2001;144:890–893, figure 2.
62. Angela Christiano, PhD, New York, New York
63. J. Decroix, MD, Brussels, Belgium. Reproduced with permission from Malfait Y, Decroix J, Vandaele R, et al. Un nouveau cas de syndrome de Goltz. *Ann Dermatol Venereol* 1989;116:715–718, figure 3.
64. Konstantin N. Konstantinov, MD, PhD, La Jolla, California. Reproduced with permission from Konstantinov K, Kabakchiev P, Karchev T, et al., Lipoid proteinosis. *J Am Acad Dermatol* 1992;27:293–297, figure 2.

65. Reproduced with permission from Mallory SB, Krafchik BR. Hutchinson-Gilford Syndrome. *Pediatr Dermatol* 1990;7:317–319, figures 1 and 3.
66. David R. Bickers, MD, New York, New York
67. Gregory L. Skuta, MD, Oklahoma City, Oklahoma. Reproduced with permission from Johnson MW, Skuta GL, et al. Malignant melanoma of the iris in xeroderma pigmentosum. *Arch Ophthalmol* 1989;107:402–407, figure 4.
68. Philip R. Cohen, MD, Houston, Texas. Reproduced with permission from Cohen PR, Kohn SR, Kurzrock R. Association of sebaceous gland tumors and internal malignancy: the Muir-Torre syndrome. *Am J Med* 1991;90:606–613, figure 1.
69. Reproduced with permission from Yanoff M, Fine BS. *Ocular Pathology—A Color Atlas*. Philadelphia: J.B. Lippincott,1988, figure 633A.
70. Ezel Yavuzyilmaz, MD, Ankara, Turkey. Reproduced with permission from Yavuzyilmaz E, Yamalik N, Yetgin S, et al. Oral-dental findings in dyskeratosis congenital. *J Oral Pathol Med* 1992;21:280–284, figure 4.
71. Laszlo Torok, MD, Kecskemet, Hungary
72. Douglas M. Arendt, DDS, MS, San Diego, California. Reproduced with permission from Arendt DM, Frost R, Whitt JC, et al. Multiple radiopaque masses in the jaws. *JADA* 1989;118:349–351, figure 2.
73. W. Richard Green, MD, Baltimore, Maryland
74. Robert H. Sudduth, MD, Aurora, Colorado
75. Fausto Chilovi, MD, Werner Wallnoefer, MD, and Franco Perino, MD, Boizano, Italy
76. Pr. J. Sayag and MC Koeppel, MD, Marseille, France. Reproduced with permission from Koeppel MC, Lazzarini F, Lagrange B, Sayag J. Maladie de cowden. Polypes adenomateaux lentiginose peri-orificielle. *Ann Dermatol Venereol* 1990;117:455–458, figure 1.
77. Edwin Wortham V, MD, Richmond, Virginia
78. Melvin A. Block, MD, La Jolla, California
79. Reproduced with permission from Analisa Vincent A, Farley M, Chan E. Birt-Hogg-Dubé syndrome: a review of the literature and the differential diagnosis of firm facial papules. *JAAD* 2003;49:698–705.
80. Reproduced with permission from Choyke PL, Glenn GM, Walther MM, et al. Hereditary renal cancers. *Radiology* 2003; 226:33–46, figures 10a and 11b.
81. Mark A. Brenner, MD, New York, New York
82. Pr. Jean-Paul Denoeux, Amiens, France. Reproduced with permission from Labeille B, Turc Y, Lok C, et al.

Epidermolyse Bulleuse de Dowing-Meara. *Ann Dermatol Venereol* 1988;115:1117–1119, figures 1B and 4.
83. Eugene A. Bauer, MD, Stanford, California
84. Reproduced with permission from Lestringant GG, Akel SR, Qayed KI. The pyloric atresia-junctional epidermolysis bullosa syndrome. *Arch Dermatol* 1992;128:1083–1086, figure 1.
85. Melvin B. Heyman, MD, MPH, San Francisco, California
86. Professeur A.L. Claudy, Lyon, France
87. Peter D. Witt, MD, Madera, California
88. Shinichi Kiso, MD, Osaka, Japan. Reproduced with permission from Kiso S, Kashikhara T, Fujimori E, et al. Laparoscopic findings in hepatic coproporphyria. *Endoscopy* 1991;23:358–359, figure 1.
89. Reproduced with permission from Kiso S, Kashikhara T, Fujimori E, et al. Case of hepatic coproporphyria-laparoscopic findings and liver biopsy. *Gastroenterol Endosc* 1990;32:1685–1691, figure 5.
90. Reproduced with permission from Rector JT, Deloach-Banta L, Bartrett TL. Picture of the month—erythropoietic protoporphyria. Am J Dis Child 1993;147:73–74, figures 1 and 3.
91. D.G. Snels, Rotterdam, The Netherlands. Reproduced with permission from Snels DG, Bavinck JN, Muller H, Vermeer BJ. A female patient with the Rothmund-Thomson syndrome associated with anhidrosis and severe infection of the respiratory tract. *Dermatology* 1998; 196:260–263.
92. William D. James, MD, Washington, DC. Reproduced with permission from Vennos EM, Collins M, James WD. Rothmund-Thomson Syndrome: review of the world literature. *J Am Acad Dermatol* 1992;27:750–762, figure 5.
93. Elias I. Traboulsi, MD, Baltimore, Maryland
94. Mark R. Pittelkow, MD, Rochester, Minnesota
95. Ebrahim Galadari, MD, Al-Ain, United Arab Emirates. Reproduced with permission from Galadari E, Hadi S, Sabarinathan K. Hartnup disease. *Int J Derm* 1993;32:904, figures 1 and 2.
96. Eleanor E. Sahn, MD, Charleston, South Carolina. Reproduced with permission from Sahn EE, Migliardi RT. Crusted scalp nodule in an infant. *Arch Dermatol* 1994;130:105–110, figure 1.
97. Anthony R. Mattia, MD, Boston, Massachusetts
98. Reproduced with permission from Mallory SB, Krafchik BR. What syndrome is this? The hyper-immunoglobulin E syndrome. *Pediatr Dermatol* 1992;9:410–412, figure 1.

99. Robert C. Shamberger, MD, Boston, Massachusetts. Reproduced with permission from Shamberger RC, Wohl ME, Perez-Atayde A, et al. Pheumatocele complicating Hyperimmunoglobulin E Syndrome (Job's Syndrome). *Ann Thorac Surg* 1992;54:1206–1208, figure 2.

100. Reproduced with permission from Zitelli BJ, Davis HW, eds. *Atlas of Pediatric Physical Diagnosis*, 2nd ed. New York: Gower Medical Publishing, 1993, figure 4.48A.

101. Ricardo U. Sorensen, MD, New Orleans, Louisiana

102. Reproduced with permission from James WD. Cutaneous manifestations of internal diseases. In: Odom RB, ed. *Dermatology Board Preview*. New York: Jarcom Inc., 1993.

103. Leonard B. Weinstock, MD, St. Louis, Missouri

104. Prof. Emile Gautier, Colombier, Switzerland. Reproduced with permission from Gautier E, Frenk E, Uske A, et al. Maladie de Menkes. *Helv paediat Acta* 1989;43:333–344, figures 1, 2, and 4.

105. Rebekah M. Oyler, MD, Raleigh, North Carolina

106. Antoine Petit, MD, Argenteuil, France

107. Joseph C. Kvedar, MD, Charlestown, Massachusetts

108. Peter H. Itin, MD, Basel, Switzerland

109. Dr. Aryeh Metzker, Moshav Rishpon, Israel

110. Reproduced with permission from Landau M, Brenner S, Metzker A. Medical Pearl: an easy way to diagnose severe neonatal monilethrix. *J Am Acad Dermatol* 2002;46:111–112, figure 1.

111. Paulus T.V.M. de Jong, MD, Rotterdam, The Netherlands

112. Seval Olmez, MD, Ankara, Turkey

113. Bernice R. Krafchik, MD, Toronto, Canada

114. RM Trueb, MD, Zurich, Switzerland. Reproduced with permission from Trueb RM, Tsambaos D, Spycher MA, et al. Scarring Folliculitis in the ectrodactyly-ectodermal-dysplasia-clefting syndrome. Histologic, scanning electron-microscopic and biophysical studies of the hair. *Dermatology* 1997;194:191–194.

115. Reproduced with permission from Fosko SW, Stenn KS, et al. Ectodermal dysplasias associated with clefting: significance of scalp dermatitis. *JAAD* 1992;27:249–256.

116. Reproduced with permission from Mancini AJ, Paller AS. What syndrome is this? Ankyloblepharon-ectodermal defects—cleft lip and palate (Hay-Wells syndrome). *Pediatr Dermatol* 1997;14:403–405.

117. Reproduced with permission from Patil BB, Mohammed KK. Anklyoblepharon filiforme adnatum. *Eye* 2001;15:813–815, figure 1.

118. Kenneth J. Guidera, MD, Tampa, Florida

119. Kenneth J. Guidera, MD, Tampa, Florida. Reproduced with permission from Guidera KJ, Satterwhite Y, Ogden JA, et al. Nail Patella syndrome: a review of 44 orthopaedeic patients. *J Ped Orthop* 1991;11:737–742, figure 2.

120. Neil A. Fenske, MD, Tampa, Florida

121. Jose Abdenur, New York, New York

122. G. Trigonides, MD, Thessaloniki, Greece. Reproduced with permission from Trigonides G, Konstantinidis A, Markopoulos AK, et al. Angiokeratoma corporis diffusum (Anderson-Fabry Disease). *Ann Dent* 1988;47:13–15, figure 2.

123. Reproduced with permission from Zimran A, Kay A, Gelbart T, et al. Gaucher Disease. *Medicine* 1992;71: 337, figure 2.

124. Reproduced with permission from Zitelli BJ, Davis HW, eds. *Atlas of Pediatric Physical Diagnosis*, 2nd ed. New York: Gower Medical Publishing, 1993, figure 19.99.

125. Carl W. Demidovich, MD, Aurora, Colorado

126. Reproduced with permission from Ortonne JP, Mosher DB, Fitzpatrick TB. *Vitiligo and Other Hypomelanoses of Hair and Skin*. New York: Plenum Publishing Corp.,1983, figure 37.

127. Reproduced with permission from Jablonska Stefania, ed. *Scleroderma and Pseudoscleroderma*. Warsaw, Poland: Polish Medical Publishers, 1975, figure 16.12.

128. Alexander G. Bearn, MD, New York, New York. Reproduced with permission from Bearn AG, McKusick VA. Azure Lunulae. *JAMA* 1958;166:903–906, figure 1 (bottom).

129. I Bodokh, MD, Nice, France

130. Corwin Edwards, MD, Salt Lake City, Utah

131. Reproduced with permission from Yanoff M, Fine BS. *Ocular Pathology—A Color Atlas*. Philadlephia: J.B. Lippincott, 1988, figure 10.18A.

132. Kurt Hirschhorn, MD, New York, New York

133. William D. James, MD, Washington, DC. Reproduced with permission from Scherbenske JM, Benson PM, Rotchford JP, James WD. Cutaneous and ocular mainfestations of Down syndrome. *J Am Acd Dermatol* 1990;22:933–938, figures 1 and 3.

134. Mr. Nicholas Lee, FRCS, FRCOphth, London, England

135. Professeur C. Pernot and A.M. Worms, MD, Vandoeuvre, France. Reproduced with permission from Pernot C, Worms AM, Marcon F, et al. Le syndrome de Noonan et sa dysplasie cardio-vasculaire. Apropos de 64 observations. *Pediatrie* 1989;44: 437–447, figure 5.

136. Kurt Sorensen, MD, Risskov, Denmark. Reproduced with permission from Sorensen K. Physical and mental development of adolescent males with Klinefelter syndrome. *Horm Res* 1992;37:55–61, figure 3.

137. Reproduced with permission from Zitelli BJ, Davis HW, eds. *Atlas of Pediatric Physical Diagnosis*, 2nd ed. New York: Gower Medical Publishing, 1993, figure 1.23B.

138. M.M. Cohen, Jr, Halifax, Nova Scotia, Canada

139. M.M. Cohen, Jr, Halifax, Nova Scotia, Canada. Reproduced with permission from Cohen MM Jr. *The Child with Multiple Birth Defects*. New York: Raven Press, 1982, figures 3–7, 3–8.

140. Michael A. Patton, MD, London, England. Reproduced with permission from Patton MA. Russell-Silver syndrome. *J Med Gen* 1988;25: 557–560, figure 1.

141. Reproduced with permission from Zitelli BJ, Davis HW, eds. *Atlas of Pediatric Physical Diagnosis*, 2nd ed. New York: Gower Medical Publishing, 1993, figure 1.12B.

142. Felicia B. Axelrod, MD, New York, New York

143. Meir Rakocz, DMD, Tel-Hashomer, Israel

Index

Page numbers followed by italics indicate figures.

Index *(continued)*